Family in America

Family in America

Advisory Editors: David J. Rothman

Professor of History,
Columbia University

Sheila M. Rothman

SENESCENCE
THE LAST HALF OF LIFE

BY

G. STANLEY HALL, Ph.D., LL.D.

ARNO PRESS & THE NEW YORK TIMES

New York   1972

SENESCENCE
THE LAST HALF OF LIFE

SENESCENCE
THE LAST HALF OF LIFE

BY

G. STANLEY HALL, Ph.D., LL.D.

Author of "Adolescence," "Educational Problems," "Founders
of Modern Psychology," "Morale," "Recreations
of a Psychologist," etc.

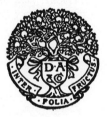

D. APPLETON AND COMPANY
NEW YORK :: MCMXXIII :: LONDON

FOREWORD

In this book I have tried to present the subjects of Old Age and Death from as many viewpoints as possible in order to show how the ignorant and the learned, the child, the adult, and the old, savage and civilized man, pagans and Christians, the ancient and the modern world, the representatives of various sciences, and different individuals have viewed these problems, letting each class, so far as I could, speak for itself. This part of the task has been long and arduous and my conspectus is not entirely encyclopedic, as it set out to be. I have also tried to develop an idea of death, and especially of old age, which I believe to be, if not essentially new, more true to the facts of life and mind than those now current, and which I think much needed by the world just now. Despite the great and growing interest that has impelled this study, its themes have proved increasingly depressing, so that its conclusion brings a unique relief that I may now turn to more cheerful occupations, although it would be craven to plead this as an extenuation of the shortcomings of which I am increasingly conscious. If I have at certain points drawn too frankly upon my own personal experiences with age I realize that this does not compensate for my limitations in some of the special fields I ventured to enter. I have had in mind throughout chiefly the nature and needs of intelligent people passing or past middle life quite as much as of those actually entering old age. It is hoped that the data here garnered and the views propounded may help to a better and more correct understanding of the nature and functions of old age, and also be a psychol-

v

FOREWORD

ogist's contribution to the long-desired but long-delayed science of gerontology.

It is a pleasant duty to express my personal obligations to the Library of Clark University and its staff, and particularly to my secretary, Miss Mary M. McLoughlin, who has not only typed and read the proof of all the book but has been of great assistance in finding references and made many helpful suggestions.

G. STANLEY HALL

INTRODUCTION

OUR life, bounded by birth and death, has five chief stages, each of which, while it may be divided into sub-stages, also passes into the next so gradually that we cannot date, save roughly and approximately, the transition from one period to that which succeeds it. These more marked nodes in the unity of man's individual existence are: (1) childhood, (2) adolescence from puberty to full nubility, (3) middle life or the prime, when we are at the apex of our aggregate of powers, ranging from twenty-five or thirty to forty or forty-five and comprising thus the fifteen or twenty years now commonly called our best, (4) senescence, which begins in the early forties, or before in woman, and (5) senectitude, the post-climacteric or old age proper. My own life work, such as it is, as a genetic psychologist was devoted for years to the study of infancy and childhood, then to the phenomena of youth, later to adulthood and the stage of sex maturity. To complete a long-cherished program I have now finally tried, aided by the first-hand knowledge that advancing years have brought, to understand better the two last and closing stages of human life.

In fact ever since I published my *Adolescence* in 1904 I have hoped to live to complement it by a study of senescence. The former could not have been written in the midst of the seething phenomena it describes, as this must be. We cannot outgrow and look back upon old age, for the course of time cannot be reversed, as Plato fancied life beginning in senility and ending in the mother's womb. The literature on this theme is limited and there are few specialists in gerontology even among physicians. Its physiological and pathological aspects have been treated not only for plants and animals but for man, and this has been done best by men in their prime. For its more subjective and psychological aspects, however, we shall always be dependent chiefly upon those who are undergoing its manifold metamorphoses and therefore lack the detachment that alone can give us a true and broad perspective.

Again, youth is an exhilarating, age a depressing theme. Both have their zest but they are as unlike as the mood of morning and evening, spring and autumn. Despite the interest that has impelled the preparation of these chapters there is, thus, a unique relief that they are done and that the mind can turn away from the contemplation of the terminal stage of life. An old man devoting himself for many months to the study of senectitude and death has a certain pathetic aspect, even to those nearest him, so that his very household brightens as his task draws toward its close. It was begun, not chiefly for others, even for other old people, but because the author felt impelled upon entering this new stage of life and upon retirement from active duties, to make a self-survey, to face reality, to understand more clearly what age was and meant for himself, and to be rightly oriented in the post-graduate course of life into which he had been entered. The decision to publish came later in the hope that his text might prove helpful, not only to fellow students in the same curriculum but to those just passing middle life, for the phenomena of age begin in the early forties, when all should think of preparing for old age.

Resent, resist, or ignore it as we will, the fact is that when we are once thought of as old, whether because of mental or physical signs or by withdrawal from our wonted sphere of activities, we enter a class more or less apart and by ourselves. We can claim, if we will, certain exemptions, privileges, immunities, and even demand allowances; but, on the other hand, we are liable to feel set aside by, or to make room for, younger people and find that even the new or old services we have a new urge to render may be declined. Many things meant or not meant to do so, remind us of our age. Friends and perhaps even critics show that they take it into consideration. Shortcomings that date from earlier years are now ascribed to age. We feel, often falsely, that we are observed or even spied upon for signs of its approach, and we are constantly tempted to do or say things to show that it is not yet upon us. Only later comes the stage of vaunting it, proclaiming openly our tale of years and perhaps posing as prodigies of senescence. Where the transition from leadership toward the chimney corner is sudden, this sense of aloofness and all its subjective experiences becomes acute, while only if it is very gradual may we pass into innocuous desuetude and hardly know it. Thus in all these and other ways isolation and the enhanced individuation characteristic of age separate us until in fact we feel more or less a caste apart. Despite all, however, there is a rapport between us oldsters, and we understand each other almost esoterically. We must accept and recognize this better knowledge of this stage of life as part of our present duty in the community.

Thus the chief thesis of this book is that we have a function in the world that we have not yet risen to and which is of the utmost importance—far greater, in fact, in the present stage of the world than ever before, and that this new and culminating service can only be seen and prepared for by first realizing what ripe and normal age really is, means, can, should, and now must do, if our race is ever to achieve its true goal. For both my purposes, the personal and later public one, it has seemed wisest to give much space to a conspectus of opinions by way of epitomes of the views of those who have considered the subject from the most diverse standpoints, and thus to let them speak for themselves. Both my own standpoint and my conclusions I believe to be justified by these data.

But, first, in a lighter and more personal vein and by way of further introduction, let me state that after six years of post-graduate study abroad, two of teaching at Harvard, and eight of professoring at the Johns Hopkins, I found myself at the head of a new university, from which latter post, after thirty-one years of service, I have just retired and become a pensioner. In this last left position I had to do creative educational work and shape new policies. I was given unusual freedom and threw my heart and soul into the work, making it more or less of a new departure. I nursed the infancy of the institution with almost maternal solicitude, saw it through various diseases incident to the early stages of its development, and steered it through several crises that taxed my physical and mental powers to their uttermost. In its service I had to do, as best I could, many things for which I was little adapted by training or talent and some of which were personally distasteful. But even to these I had given myself with loyalty and occasionally with abandon, as my "bit" in life, remembering that while men come and go, good institutions should, like Tennyson's brook, "go on forever."

There is always considerable publicity in such work and one has always to consider, in every measure, its effects upon the controlling board in whom the prime responsibility for its welfare is vested, the public, the faculty, and the students; and between the points of view of these four parties concerned there are often discrepancies so wide that if any of them knew how the others felt there might be serious trouble. Occasionally, too, my own opinion differed from all the others, and this involved a fifth factor to be reckoned with. Thus, much effort had to be directed toward compounding different interests and not infrequently the only way open seemed to be concealment, temporary at least, of the views of one of these elements, because untimely disclosure might have brought open rupture. However, I had muddled on as best I could, learning much tact and diplomacy and various mediatorial devices as the years rolled by.

And now I have resigned, and after months of delay and with gratifying expressions of regret, another younger captain, whom, happily, I can fully trust, is in my place. I had always planned that my retirement, when it came, should be complete. I would do my full duty up to the last moment and then sever every tie and entirely efface myself, so far as the institution I had served was concerned, and would distinctly avoid every worry, even as to the fate of my most cherished policies. This was only fair to my successor and all my interests must henceforth be vested elsewhere. But what a break after all these decades! It seemed almost like anticipatory death, and the press notices of my withdrawal read to me not unlike obituaries. The very kindness of all these and of the many private letters and messages that came to me suggested that their authors had been prompted by the old principle, *De mortuis nil nisi bonum.*

For more than forty years I have lectured at eleven o'clock and the cessation of this function leaves a curious void. My friends have already fancied that I tend to grow loquacious at that hour. If I speak or write now, it must be to a very different clientele. During all these years, too, I have held a seminary nearly every Monday night, and now when this evening comes around my faculties activate, even if *bombinantes in vacuo.* On those evenings I have been greatly stimulated by fa-

miliar contact with vigorous student minds, for on these
occasions they and I have inspired each other to some of
our best *aperçus*. But now this contact is gone forever.
My *Journal,* which for more than thirty years had taken
so much of my care and, at first in its nursling period,
of my surplus funds and had become for me an institution in itself, is also now transferred to better hands.

Thus, I am rather summarily divorced from my
world, and it might seem at first as if there was little
more to be said of me save to record the date of my
death—and we all know that men who retire often die
soon afterwards. So my prayer perhaps should be *Nunc
dimittis.* Ex-presidents, like founders of institutions,
have often lived to become meddling nuisances, so that
even those whom they have most profited, secretly and
perhaps unconsciously long to participate in an impressive funeral for them. What can remain but a trivial
postscript? And would not some of the suggested forms
of painless extinction be worthy of consideration? Of
course it is bitter to feign that I am suddenly dead to
these interests I have so long lived for, as all the proprieties demand I should do and as I inexorably will
to do for my very heart and soul went into them. But
I did not build a monument to myself in any sense but
strove only to fashion an instrument of service and
such I know it will remain—and, I hope, far more effectively than under my hand.

But I thank whatever gods there are that all this
painful renunciation has its very satisfying compensations and that there are other counsels than those of
despair, seeing which I can take heart again, and that
these are so satisfying that I do not need to have recourse to wood-sawing, like the Kaiser, though I have
a new sympathy even for him.

My very first and hardest duty of all is to realize
that I am really and truly old. Associated for so many

INTRODUCTION

years with young men and able to keep pace with them in my own line of work, carrying without scathe not a few extra burdens at times, and especially during the war, and having, varied as my duties were, fallen into a certain weekly and monthly routine that varied little from year to year, I had not realized that age was, all the while, creeping upon me. But now that I am out the full realization that I have reached and passed the scripturally allotted span of years comes upon me almost with a shock. Emerson says that a task is a life-pre-server, and now that mine is gone I must swim or go under. To be sure, I had been conscious during half a decade of certain slight incipient infirmities and had had moments of idealizing the leisure which retirement would bring. But when it came I was so overwhelmed and almost distracted by its completeness that I was at a loss, for a time, to know how to use it. I might travel, especially in the Orient, as I had long wanted to do, for I feel that I have a certain right to a "good time" for myself since my life has been a very indus-trious one and almost entirely in the service of others. I might live much out-of-doors on my small farm; read for pleasure, for I have literary tastes; move to a large city and take in its amusements, of which I am fond; devote myself more to my family, whom I now feel I have rather neglected; or give more time to certain avo-cations and interests in which I have dabbled but have never had time to cultivate save in the crudest way. Or, finally, I could do a little of all or several of these things in turn. But no program that I can construct out of such possibilities seems entirely satisfactory. I surely may indulge myself a little more in many ways but I really want and ought to do something useful and with a unitary purpose. Thus, I might have spent much time as *Senex quœrans institutum vitœ* but for the sav-ing fact that there are certain very specific things which

xiii

for years I have longed to do, and indeed have already well begun, and to which, with this new leisure, I can now devote myself as never before.

As preliminary to even this, it slowly came to me that I must, first of all, take careful stock of myself and now seek to attain more of the self-knowledge that Socrates taught the world was the highest, hardest, and last of all forms of knowledge. I must know, too, just how I stand in with my present stage of life. Hence I began with a physical inventory and visited doctors. The oculist found a slight but unsuspected defect in one eye and improved my sight, which was fairly good before, by better glasses. The aurist found even the less sensitive ear fairly good. Digestion was found to be above the average. I had for years been losing two or three pounds a year, but this rather than the opposite tendency to corpulence was pronounced good (*Corpora sicca durant*), and I was told that I might go on unloading myself of superfluous tissue for fifteen or twenty years before I became too emaciated to live, which humans, like starving animals, usually do on losing about one-third of their weight. My heart would probably last about the same length of time if I did not abuse it, and smoking in moderation, a great solace, was not forbidden. A little wine, "the milk of old age," was not taboo and I was given a prescription to enable me to get it if I desired, even in these prohibition days. One suggested that I insure my life heavily and another advised an annuity; but I thought neither of these quite fair in view of the above findings, for I did not wish to profiteer on my prospects of life.

This hygienic survey reinforced what I had realized before, namely, that physicians know very little of old age. Few have specialized in its distinctive needs, as they have in the diseases of women and children and the rest. Thus the older a man is, the more he must depend upon his own hygienic sagacity for health and long life. The lives of nearly all the centenarians I have been able to find show that they owe their longevity far more to their own insight than to medical care, and there seems to be a far greater individual difference of needs than medicine yet recognizes. Of the philosopher, Kant, it was said that he spent more mentality in keeping his congenitally feeble body alive and in good trim to the age of eighty than he expended in all the fourteen closely printed volumes of his epoch-making *Works*.

Thus, again, I realized that I was alone, indeed in a new kind of solitude, and must pursue the rest of my way in life by a more or less individual research as to how to keep well and at the top of my condition. In a word, I must henceforth, for the most part, be my own doctor. All of those I consulted agreed that I must eat moderately, slowly, oftener, less at a time, sleep regularly, cultivate the open air, exercise till fatigue came and then promptly stop, be cheerful, and avoid "nerves," worry, and all excesses. But with these commonplaces the agreement ceased. One said I needed change, as if, indeed, I was not getting it with a vengeance. One suggested Fletcherizing, while another thought this bad for the large intestine, which needed more coarse material to stimulate its action. One thought there was great virtue in cold, another in warm baths. Two prescribed a diet, while another said, "Eat what you like, with discretion." One suggested thyroid extract and perhaps Brown-Sequard's testicular juices, and there seemed to be a more general agreement that a man is as old, not as his heart and arteries as was once thought, but as his endocrine glands. One would give chief attention to the colon and recommended Metchnikoff's tablets. One prescribed Sanford Bennett's exercises which made him an athlete at seventy-two. Rubbing or self-massage on rising and retiring was commended. Battle Creek advises bowel movements not only daily but oftener, while others insist that constipation should and normally does increase with old age. Pavlovists, especially Sternberg in his writings, would have us trust appetite implicitly, believing that it always points true as the needle to the pole to the nutritive needs of both sick and well and that it gives the sole momentum to all the digestive processes, even down to the very end of the alimentary canal; while others prescribe everything chemically, calculating to a nicety the proportions of carbohydrates, fats, calories, and the rest, with no reference to gustatory inclination.

Perhaps I should try out all these suggestions in turn and seek to find by experiment which is really best for me. I almost have the will to do so because I certainly illustrate the old principle that as life advances we love it not less but more, for the habit of living grows so strong with years that it is ever harder to break it. All things considered, however, it would rather seem that the longer we live the harder it is to keep on doing so, and that with every year of life we must give more attention to regimen if we would put off the great life-queller, which all the world fears and hates as it does nothing else, beyond its normal term, which most generally agree is very largely heriditary. In fact, as Minot shows, all creatures begin to die at the very moment when they begin to live. All theories of euthanasia ignore the fact that death is essentially a negation of the will-to-live, so that a conscious and positive will-to-die is always only an artifact.

So much I gathered from the doctors I saw or read. Their books and counsels cost me a tidy sum but it was well worth it. I now know myself better than they, and it is much to realize that henceforth an ever-increasing attention must be given to body-keeping if one would stay "fit" or even alive. Now that the av-

INTRODUCTION

erage length of human life is increased and there are
more and more old people, a fact that marks the triumph
of science and civilization, there is more need of studying them, just as in recent decades children have been
studied, for medically, at least after the climacteric, they
constitute a class in the community that is somewhat
alien, its intrinsic nature but litle known, and the services it was meant to render but little utilized.[1]

As my horizon changed and I became more at home
with myself, and personal problems grew nearer and
clearer, I realized that I must make a new plan of life,
in which both tasks and also a program of renunciation
played a very prominent initial part. This began with a
literal house-cleaning. My home, from attic to cellar,
and even the large barn were more or less full of dis-
used articles of every kind—furniture and even wearing
apparel, still serviceable but displaced by better ones,
which it was now plain could never be of use to us but
might be so to others. About some of these so many
old associations clustered that it was a pang to part
with them, but it was selfish to keep them longer. And
so, by distribution to persons and institutions, then by
sales, and finally by dumpage, they were rigorously got-
ten rid of, room by room, and we all felt relieved physically, mentally, and morally, by this expropriation, even
though a few heirlooms were sacrificed. This process
has many analogies with those by which the body is rid
of waste material.

Next came books, of which my purchases, when I
was enthusiastic and had a passion for ownership and
completeness in my favorite topics, had been extravagant for my means and which, by many hundreds of
publisher's gifts for review in my journals, had over-

[1] In the preceding paragraphs I have incorporated, with minor changes,
parts of my anonymous article on "Old Age" in the *Atlantic Monthly* of
January, 1921, with the kind permission of the editor.

INTRODUCTION

flowed from both study and library into nearly every room. These, in open shelves for greater accessibility and laboriously and systematically arranged, could not be disturbed often or dusted and are a housekeeper's abomination. I had for years collected pamphlets and bound volumes on many topics in the vague hope of some future use, but which I now realize will never be warmed up again. So, section by section, shelf by shelf, I went over them, reserving all on topics I might yet study, and after inviting colleagues and the Library to take freely what they would I shipped the residue in boxes to antiquarian and second-hand dealers and accepted with equanimity the pittance they paid. This work done in leisure hours for months, was a wrenching process because every step in it involved the frustration of activities once thought possible but which now seemed to be no longer so. Little, thus, remained outside my own quite definitely narrowed field of work which I hope yet to do, and only a few gifts and sets, along with texts studied in younger and those taught in later days in which my descendants may sometime come to feel an interest, remain. This riddance of the residue of superfluous printed matter is not unlike anti-fat regimens, which are disagreeable but strengthening.

Next, I attacked a formidable pile of old lecture notes, beginning with a few small and faded records of college exercises in bound sheets, including the *Heften* of European courses, and finally the far more voluminous memoranda of my own lectures for nearly two-score years. How crude and impossible now were these earlier reminders of my professorial activity! What a prodigious amount of work, time, and even manual labor they involved! What hardihood of inference and conclusion! What immaturity and even foolhardiness of judgment on some of the greatest problems of life! If I wanted to dignify or even glorify my old age at the expense of my youth, here are abundant data for so doing. But I do not, and so I found peculiar pleasure in consigning, with my own hands, armfuls of such manuscript to the flames. How hard I rode my own hobbies! What liberties I took—and all with perfect innocence of intent—with the ideas of others, which insinuated themselves unconsciously into all of my mental complexes! And yet, at the same time, how voraciously I read, how copiously I quoted, and how radically I changed the form, substance, and scope of my favorite courses each year, slowly improving them in clarity and coherence! And how many special themes in my field, once central, have lapsed to secondary importance or become obsolete! Such breaks with the past, which psychology regards as analogues of a catharsis that relieves constipation, have a certain insurance value not only against ultra-conservatism but against the inveterate tendency of the old to hark back to past stages of life.

As a part of the process of reorientation I felt impelled, as I think natural enough for a psychologist, to write my autobiography and get myself in focus genetically. To this I devoted the first year after my retirement. It is now complete and laid safely away and may or may not be published sometime, although certainly not at present. Its preparation served me well in advancing my understanding of the one I know best of all, and I would earnestly prescribe such an occupation as one of the most pleasant and profitable services intelligent old people can render to themselves and perhaps their posterity and friends, if not to the world at large. The reading of "lives," too, is often one of the most absorbing and sometimes almost exclusive intellectual occupation of the old.

Incidental to this work I unearthed many written data of the past—my youthful diaries, school exercises, some two feet of letters from my parents, especially my mother, for more than a quarter of a century after I left home and before her death; and several hundred large envelopes of carefully filed correspondence with many friends and strangers on many topics. All these had to be at least cursorily glanced over. Part of this voluminous material no one, I am convinced, will ever care to reperuse. My own offspring have no interest in it, so why not consign it to oblivion now that it has served its final purpose? There is little of value to the living or of special credit to the dead in it all; so I conclude there is more of real piety, even to the memory of my mother, to select a number of the best of her missives which most clearly show her constant and affectionate solicitude and love, and burn all the rest. I am sure that both she and my father would heartily commend this course. So, as I watched them burn in the grate one solitary spring at evening twilight, I felt that I had completed a filial function of interment of her remains. No profane ear can now ever hear what she whispered into mine. She tried to convey everything good in her beautiful soul to me, her eldest, wanted me to do everything commendable that she could not and realize all her own thwarted ambitions. I hope that I may yet do something more worthy of her fondest hopes. If I seem to have cremated her very soul, or so much of it as she gave me, I feel that I have thus done the last and most sacred act of service which such a son can render such a mother.

By all this purgation I have, at any rate, saved my offspring from a task that could not be other than painful and embarrassing to them, and relieved them from inheriting a burden of impedimenta which they themselves would not have the hardihood to destroy, at least for years after my demise, and which could be of no earthly use to them or any one else.

And now it only remained for me to make my last

INTRODUCTION

will and testament and bequeath all that I have left
where I hope it may do most good. This should have
been done long ago but I have been withheld from this
duty, partly by preoccupation but far more by the instinctive reluctance all feel to thus anticipate their own
death. A dozen modes of disposing of my modest estate
had occurred to me and there were countless considerations to be weighed. Some provisions were obvious but
more were beset with a puzzling array of *pros* and *cons*.
But the time was over-ripe, and so I nerved myself for
this ordeal, feeling sure there would be regrets, revi-
sions, or perhaps codicils every year I lived. But when
it was duly signed and witnessed there was, on the
whole, great relief, as from having accomplished a long-
looming and difficult task.

For myself, I feel thrice fortunate in having really
found my *goru,* the one thing in which I am up to date
and seething with convictions, which I have never before had the courage to express, and that I can now
hope to devote myself to with all my spirit and understanding and with the abandon the subject really demands. I will not accept the subtle but persistently in-
trusive suggestion that it will do no good or that former
colleagues whom I esteem, and whose judgment I
greatly prize, will ignore it because other old men have
written fatuously. I can, at least, speak more honestly
than I have ever dared to do before, and if I am never
read or even venture into print, I shall have the satisfaction of having clarified and unified my own soul.

But before I can enter fully into the functions or the
service age ought to render and begin the one thing I
have always planned for this stage of life, I would know
more about what it really is, find out its status, estimate
its powers, its limitations, its physical and mental regimen; and especially, if I can, look death, which certainly
cannot be very far off, calmly in the face. It is in this

INTRODUCTION

final stage of preparation for what I yet hope to do later that I invite the reader to accompany me through the following pages in the fond hope that not only the old may be helped to better realize their estate and their responsibilities and duties in the world of today but that those just emerging from middle life and for whom the shadows have just begun to lengthen may be better fitted to meet old age when it overtakes them.

CONTENTS

CONTENTS

CONTENTS

CONTENTS

The early decades of age—The deadline of seventy —The patheticism of the old—The attitude of physicians toward them—Fluctuations of youth—Erotic decline—Alternations in the domain of sleep, food, mood, irritability, rational self-control, and sex— The dawn of old age in women—Dangers of the disparity when December weds May—Sexual hygiene for the old—Mental effects of the dulling of sensations—Lack of mental pabulum—The tedium vitæ—Changes in the emotional life—Age not second childhood—Women in the dangerous age— Need of a new and higher type of old age—Aristotle's golden mean and the magnanimous man—The age of disillusion—Increased power of synthesis— Nature's balance between old and young—Superior powers of the old in perspective and larger views— New love of nature and the country—Their preëminence in religion, politics, philosophy, morals, and as judges—Looking within and without—Merging with the cosmos.

The attitude of infancy and youth toward death as recapitulating that of the race—Suicide—The death-wish—Necrophilism—The Black Death—Depopulation by the next war—The evolutionary nisus and death as its queller—Death symbolism as pervasive as that of sex—Flirtations of youthful minds with the thought of death—Schopenhauer's view of death —The separation of ghosts from the living among primitive races—The thanatology of the Egyptians —The journey of the soul—Ancient cults of death and resurrection in the religions about the eastern Mediterranean, based on the death of vegetation in the fall and its revival in the spring, as a background of Pauline Christianity—The fading belief in immortality and Protestantism which now at funerals speaks only of peace and rest—Osler's five hundred deathbeds—Influential, plasmal, and personal im-

CONTENTS

SENESCENCE

CHAPTER I

THE YOUTH OF OLD AGE

The turn of the tide of life—Relative amount and importance of work accomplished before and after forty—The sexual life at the turn of the tide in man and woman—Osler's views and critics (E. G. Dexter, D. A. N. Dorland, E. S. P. Haynes)—Illustrations from Tolstoi, Fechner, Comte, Swedenborg—The typical cases of Segantini, Lenau, von Kleist, de Maupassant, Gogol, Scheffel, Ruskin and Nietzsche—Michaëlis's "dangerous age" in women—The difficulty in determining this age—The nature of the changes, conscious and unconscious, and the lessons that people in this stage of life should lay to heart—H. G. Wells and Ross.

THE easiest division of every whole is into two halves. Thus day and night are bisected by noon and midnight, the year by both the solstice and the equinox; the racer turns in the middle of his course; curricula, apprenticeships, and long tasks have, from immemorial time, celebrated the completion of their first moiety, and halfway houses divide established courses of travel. So, too, we speak of middle age and think vaguely of it as half way between birth and death or between adolescence and senescence. If we think of life as a binomial curve rising from a base line at birth and sinking into it at death, midway is the highest point with the longest ordinate; and as the crest of a wave has its spindrift, so life at this point often foams, or at least shows emulsive tendencies. We come in sight of the descent while the ascent behind is still visible. The man of thirty-five hopes to live the allotted span of seventy and at forty

I

he knows that in another two-score years his work will cease; and thus some comparison of the past and future is inevitable. Some begin taking stock of what has been and what remains to be done, reckoning only from the date of entering upon their careers and trying thus to judge its future by its past. Thus sooner or later there comes to all a realization that the tide that "drew us from out the boundless deep" begins to "turn again home."

These meridional perturbations usually come earlier in women than in men, and this has been called their "dangerous age." Both sexes realize that they face the bankruptcy of some of their youthful hopes, and certain temperaments make a desperate, now-or-never effort to realize their extravagant expectations and are thus led to excesses of many kinds; while others capitulate to fate, lose heart, and perhaps even lose the will-to-live. Osler was the evil genius, the croaking Poe raven of this period. If such pronouncements as his stimulate talent, which is longer lived, they depress genius, which blossoms earlier. On the height of life we ought to pause, circumspect, turn from the dead reckonings of the start, and ascend as into an outlook tower to see, before it is too late, if we need to reorient our course by the eternal stars. Here we begin the home stretch toward the finish. Change, or at least thoughts of change, arise even in those most successful, as biography so abundantly shows, while even partial failure impels many to seek new environments and perhaps callings and some are driven to mad new ventures. Most, however, despite a certain perturbation, go on perhaps a score of years, and instead of anticipating old age wait till it is upon them and they have to restrict their activities or retire; then only do they accept the burden of years. The modifications in the *vita sexualis* which middle life brings are only now beginning to be understood in their true sig-

THE YOUTH OF OLD AGE

nificance. Its first flush has come and gone and some settle to the tranquil fruition of a happy married life, while others stray into secret and forbidden ways or yield to the excitements of overindulgence just when Nature begins to suggest more moderation, so that love often grows gross just when its sublimation should begin to be most active. One close and experienced observer points out that the forties is the decade of the triangle, of the paramour, and of divorces for men, and that the preceding decade is so for women; but of course we have no confirmatory statistics for such a conclusion save only for divorce. The following epitomes represent the chief aspects and treatments of this period, although illustrations of its phenomena might be indefinitely multiplied.

The sensational press has so perverted the statements made by Dr. William Osler in his farewell address on leaving the Johns Hopkins University in 1905, and his remarks are so pithy, thinly and ineffectively as he tried to mask his earnestness with humor, that it seems worth while to quote his words, as follows: [1]

I have two fixed ideas well known to my friends, harmless obsessions with which I sometimes bore them, but which have a direct bearing on this important problem. The first is the comparative uselessness of men above forty years of age. This may seem shocking, and yet, read aright, the world's history bears out the statement. Take the sum of human achievement in action, in science, in art, in literature—subtract the work of the men above forty, and, while we should miss great treasures, even priceless treasures, we should practically be where we are to-day. It is difficult to name a great and far-reaching conquest of the mind which has not been given to the world by a man on whose back the sun was still shining. The effective, moving, vitalizing work of the world is done between the ages of twenty-five and forty years—these fifteen golden years of plenty, the anabolic or constructive period, in which there is always a balance in the mental bank and the credit is still good.

[1] *Scientific American*, March 25, 1905.

SENESCENCE

In the science and art of medicine there has not been an advance of the first rank which has not been initiated by young or comparatively young men. Vesalius, Harvey, Hunter, Bichat, Laennec, Virchow, Lister, Koch—the green years were yet on their heads when their epoch-making studies were made. To modify an old saying, a man is sane morally at thirty, rich mentally at forty, wise spiritually at fifty—or never. The young men should be encouraged and afforded every possible chance to show what is in them. If there is one thing more than another upon which the professors of the university are to be congratulated, it is this very sympathy and fellowship with their junior associates, upon whom really in many departments, in mine certainly, has fallen the brunt of the work. And herein lies the chief value of the teacher who has passed his climacteric and is no longer a productive factor; he can play the man midwife, as Socrates did to Theætetus, and determine whether the thoughts which the young men are bringing to the light are false idols or true and noble births.

My second fixed idea is the uselessness of men above sixty years of age, and the incalculable benefit it would be in commercial, political, and in professional life if, as a matter of course, men stopped work at this age. Donne tells us in his "Biathanatos" that by the laws of certain wise states sexagenarii were precipitated from a bridge, and in Rome men of that age were not admitted to the suffrage, and were called *depontani* because the way to the senate was *per pontem* and they from age were not permitted to come hither. In that charming novel, the "Fixed Period," Anthony Trollope discusses the practical advantages in modern life of a return to this ancient usage, and the plot hinges on the admirable scheme of a college into which at sixty men retired for a year of contemplation before a peaceful departure by chloroform. That incalculable benefits might follow such a scheme is apparent to any one who, like myself, is nearing the limit, and who has made a careful study of the calamities which may befall men during the seventh and eighth decades!

Still more when he contemplates the many evils which they perpetuate unconsciously and with impunity! As it can be maintained that all the great advances have come from men under forty, so the history of the world shows that a very large proportion of the evils may be traced to the sexagenarians—nearly all the great mistakes politically and socially, all of the worst poems, most of the bad pictures, a majority of the bad novels, and not a few of the bad sermons and speeches. It is not to be denied that

4

occasionally there is a sexagenarian whose mind, as Cicero remarks, stands out of reach of the body's decay. Such a one has
learned the secret of Hermippus, that ancient Roman, who, feeling that the silver cord was loosening, cut himself clear from all
companions of his own age, and betook himself to the company of
young men, mingling with their games and studies, and so lived
to the age of 153, *puerorum halitu refocillatus et educatus.* And
there is truth in the story, since it is only those who live with the
young who maintain a fresh outlook on the new problems of the
world.

The teacher's life should have three periods—study until
twenty-five, investigation until forty, professional until sixty, at
which age I would have him retired on a double allowance.
Whether Anthony Trollope's suggestion of a college and chloroform should be carried out or not, I have become a little dubious,
as my own time is getting so short.

E. G. Dexter [2] disputes Osler's conclusions by refer-
ring to such well-known cases as Gladstone, Bismarck,
von Moltke, Rockefeller, Morgan, etc., and finds that
according to the last census there are 4,871,861 persons
over sixty in the United States. He recognizes the fact,
however, that many corporations refuse to add new men
to their working force who are beyond forty years of
age. Dexter had previously tabulated the age of the
nearly 9,000 persons mentioned in the 1900 edition of
Who's Who and found that comparatively few who
were under forty attained the distinction of being included in this list. Of 6,983 men the median age was 54,
only one in six being below 40; that is, some 16 per cent
were within Osler's period of most effective work. But
he concludes that in *Who's Who* younger men did not
receive the recognition given to their older *confrères.*
This ratio he finds to be as follows:

20–29	30–39	40–49	50–59	60–69
3.9%	39.5%	36.4%	17.6%	2.4%

[2] See *Pop. Sci. Mo.,* July, 1902.

5

Thus the decade from 30 to 39 shows only very slightly greater productivity than the next one, and less than one-half made good, so far as public recognition is concerned, before the age of 40. This is irrespective of vocation.

In all the studies of genius[3] it would seem that musicians do their best work earliest and prodigies are most common in this field. In those callings that require a long preparation, science promises earliest recognition because this line of work is entered with better intellectual equipment. Here, too, belong professors, librarians, and teachers. Next come actors and authors, in whom ability is partly born and partly made. Compared with science, inventive genius gains a foothold on the ladder of fame late in life. The business man and financier, the lawyer, doctor, and minister, must often enter their profession from the bottom, and almost no great inventor is below forty. For woman, however, recognition comes earlier, and attractiveness of person has a greater premium here than with her brother. Having outlived her youth, however, progress is harder.

W. A. Newman Dorland[4] studied the histories of four hundred great men of modern times and concluded that they refute Osler's theory, the large majority of them being still active at sixty, although he distinguishes between workers and thinkers. He tells us that only that which is fittest survives and almost seems to imply that man became man when he was able to live and work productively after 40.[5] He considers old age one of the choicest products of evolution. His painstaking article is divided into three sections: (1) enumerating the great things done by men after 70; (2) by those between 60 and 70; (3) by those between 50 and 60. He thinks

---

[3] "Age and Eminence," *Pop. Sci. Mo.,* vol. 66, 1904–05, p. 538.
[4] *The Age of Mental Virility,* The Century Co., 1908.
[5] "What the World Might Have Missed," *Century,* 1908, p. 113, *et seq.*

that if Osler's dictum has any validity, it is found among manual laborers. It doubtless had its influence in the practice of so many industries that employ no new men above the age of 40.

E. S. P. Haynes [6] resents the idea that people should retire from public affairs at forty, although he recognizes that near this age in both men and women there is often an impatience with a future that promises to be just like the past and there is a peculiar liability to amorous, financial, or other adventures. If people do anything, they are labeled and so get into grooves, and their friends, if they break out in new lines, as for example, Ruskin did, are shocked. But the groove is liable to grow narrow, and when this is realized, abrupt changes may occur. Nature protests against decay and hence it is that we often see the spectacle of impatient old people who are in a hurry, due perhaps to a subconscious effort to feel young again. This is akin to the "dangerous age" in women. Life is not a bed of roses for those who have succeeded, for it is sometimes as difficult to retain as it is to achieve success. Very often our ideas, when we are young, are ahead of our age but the world may catch up with us in middle or later life. Very often, too, by ostentatiously turning their backs upon some new movement the old thereby compel the young to take it up in order to deploy themselves.

In this connection one may reflect, with Louise Creighton, that as older people caused the late war, while the younger fought it, when the latter came home the places that had to be found for them involved a great deal of displacement, so that the tension between old and young has been greatly increased since the close of the war. We also recall the view of George R. Sims,[7] that the effect of the war upon the old was depressing

[6] "The Age Limit," *Living Age,* 1914, p. 214.
[7] "The Old Folks and the War," *Living Age,* 1918.

because they felt they must die when the world was in darkness and without realizing the prayer of Simeon. The young anticipated the harvests of peace, but for the old the prospect of dying before this harvest was garnered was often pathetic.

Charles W. St. John [8] résumés the experimental studies of Ranschenburg and Balint which show that all activities of judgment, association, etc., are retarded, errors increased, and ideas impoverished in old age. De Fursac tabs the traits of normal senile dementia as (1) impaired attention and association; (2) inaccurate perception of the external world, with illusions and disorientation; (3) disordered memory, retrograde amnesia, and perhaps pseudo-reminiscence; (4) impoverishment of ideas; (5) loss of judgment; (6) loss of affectivity, along with morbid irritability; and (7) automatism. There may be ideas of persecution or delusions of greatness. Youthful items of experience hitherto only in the fringe of consciousness now press to the center, and youthful contents are revived. There is a tendency to depart from inductive procedure toward *a priori* methods, where feelings and beliefs are criteria, and especially, as Fechner showed, to introversion. There is less control and regression first shows itself in the intellect, which is last to develop.

St. John proceeds to characterize four eminent men who underwent more or less radical transformations in the early stages or youth of old age, as follows. Tolstoy [9] was a typical convert. He witnessed the horror of his grandmother's death, which profoundly affected all his later views. When he was about twelve, a schoolmate told him that there was no God and that all thought

[8] *The Psychology of Senescence,* Master's Thesis, Clark University, Worcester, Mass., 1912.
[9] P. Birukoff, *Leo Tolstoy, His Life and Work.* London, 1906; A. Maude, *The Life of Tolstoy,* London, 1908.

about Him was an invention; and he accepted this news and went on in a few years to Nihilism. In later life he asked himself if he should become "more famous than Gogol, Pushkin, Shakespeare, and Molière, what then?" and he could not answer. The ground crumbled under him. There was no reason to live. Every day was bringing him nearer to the precipice and yet he could not stop. He felt he could live no longer and the idea of suicide as a last resort was always with him and he had to practice self-deception to escape it. Yet he had a pagan love of life. He found his status summed up in an Eastern fable of a traveler who is attacked by a wild beast and attempts to escape by letting himself down into a dried-up well, at the bottom of which he finds a dragon, and so is forced to cling to a wild plant that grows on the wall. Suddenly he sees two mice (one black and one white—day and night) nibbling the plant from which he hangs and in despair he looks about, still with a faint hope of escape. On the leaves of this wild plant he sees a few drops of honey and even with fear at his heart he stretches out his tongue and licks them. Thus the dragon of death inevitably awaits him, while even the honey he tries to taste no longer rejoices him for it is not sweet. "I cannot turn my eyes from the mice or the dragon. Both are no fable."

Thus the fear of death which had long haunted him now excluded everything else and he was in despair. He turned to the working people, whom he had always liked, to study them and found that although they anticipated death they did not worry about it but had a simple faith that bridges the gulf between the finite and the infinite, although they held much he could not accept. Thus for a year while he was considering whether or not to kill himself, he was haunted by a feeling he describes as searching after God, not with his reason but with his feelings. Kant and Schopenhauer said that

9

man could not know Him. Tolstoy at first feared that these experiences presaged his own mental decline. He had joined the church and clung to orthodoxy for three years but in the end left and was later excommunicated. He became a peasant and finally left his pleasant home for a monastery, and as the church had failed he turned to the Gospels, the core of which he found in the Sermon on the Mount. Here was the solution of his problem. If everyone strives for self there is no happiness. Nor is there any love of family and friends alone, but love must extend to all mankind and even to being, and this must be all-embracing. No doubt of immortality can come to any man who renounces his individual happiness. Instead of God he now worships the world-soul and attains the goal of perfection he once sought in self-development.

Fechner,[10] born in 1801, made professor of physics in 1833, turned to more psychological studies in 1838. He had visual troubles and could not work without bandaging his eyes, lived in a blue room, had insomnia, and seemed about to die. But in 1843 he improved and felt he was called by God to do extraordinary things, prepared for by suffering. His philosophical inclinations now came into the foreground. He was on the way to the secret of the universe. He believed in insight rather than induction, and this was in the decades when German philosophy was at its lowest ebb. So his works fell dead. Not only Buchner and Moleschott but Kant belonged to what he called the "night side," for the latter's *Ding-an-Sich* was a plot to banish joy. Fechner knew no epistemology and thought we could come into direct contact with reality itself. Man lives three times: once before birth and in sleep; second alternating; and

---

[10] W. Wundt, *Gustav Theodor Fechner*, Leipzig, 1901; K. Lasswitz, *Gustav Theodor Fechner*, Stuttgart, 1896; G. S. Hall, *Founders of Modern Psychology*, New York, 1907.

finally in death comes to the eternal awakening. The spirit will then communicate with others without language and all the dead live in us as Christ did in His followers. The earth will return its soul to the sun. Visible phantoms may be degenerate souls. In his *Zendavesta* (Living Word) he gives us a philosophy that he deems Christian and that really sums up his final view of things. The childish view is nearest right and the philosopher only reverts to it. Fechner died November 18, 1887, at the age of eighty-six, and after his crisis was really more poet than scientist.

Auguste Comte, born 1798, married at the age of twenty-seven and was divorced at forty-four. He experienced losses by the failure of his publisher and had his first crisis when he was forty. He met Clotilde de Vaux when he was forty-seven but she died a year later. He then became the high priest of humanity, developing his *Politique Positive* and a new religion. His father, a government official, had given him an excellent scientific education, but during his early years his emotional life was entirely undeveloped and this now took the ascendency.[11]

Emanuel Swedenborg was born in 1688. He had his first vision in London in 1745 at the age of 57, became a seer and mystic, and changed from a subjective to an objective type of thought and developed his doctrine of correspondencies. The change was due to overwork and eye-strain, as was the case with Comte.[12]

Giovanni Segantini [13] affords us perhaps the very best

---

[11] See J. Croley, *The Love Life of Auguste Comte*, Modern Thinker, 2d ed., 1870; also J. Mill, *Auguste Comte and Positivism*, London, 1907, 5th ed.; also A. Poey, *The Three Mental Crises of Auguste Comte*, Modern Thinker, 2d ed., London, 1870.

[12] G. Trobridge, *Emanuel Swendenborg, His Life, Teachings, and Influence*, London, 1911; also B. White and B. Barrett, *Life and Writings of Emanuel Swedenborg*, 1876; also J. Wilkinson, *Emanuel Swedenborg, a Biography*, Boston, 1849. See also Emerson's essay.

[13] See Karl Abraham's work of this title (Leipzig, 1911), based on Seravia's biography.

picture of a man who died at the age of forty-three of what might be called meridional mental fever. His life was a struggle against an obsessive death thought and a compensatory will-to-live. His first painting, at the age of twelve, was of a child's corpse, which he tried to paint back into life. Haunted by the idealized image of his mother, who died when he was very young, and which he fancied he at length found in a peasant girl whom he made his model for years, this life-affirming motif was always in conflict with the thought of death, which in later years became an obsession. His struggle for sublimation was typified by his removal from the world and retirement to a high Alpine village where the mountains, in the ideal of which it was his final ambition to embody all the excelsior motives of life, so drew him that he had a passion for exploring their heights and once slept in the snow, to the permanent impairment of his health. He had several narrow escapes from death, which afterwards always provoked greater activity. He painted an upright corpse, the fall of which he thought (with the characteristic superstition of neurotics) was ominous. Death became, in the end, his muse as his mother had been in the earlier stages of his development. He seemed fascinated with the idea of anticipating death in every way, even though this was a more or less unconscious urge. It was as if he revolted against the ordinary fate of man to await its gradual approach with the soporific agencies that old age normally supplies, and was anxious to go forth and meet it face to face at the very summit of his powers. At times he let down all precautions and took great risks, so characteristic a result of acute disappointments or of general disenchantment with life.

He seemed to revel in the stimulus of the hurry-up motive that so often supervenes, but far more slowly, in those who realize that they have reached the zenith of their powers. Love of his mother made him an artist and he early married a wife who was the mother-image, which was never marred by any childish jealousy of his father, of whom he had known little, but was sublimated into love of mankind and even of animals. But his later greater love of death obscured the mother image and even overcame his passion for home, which he had idealized, and dominated his exquisite feeling for and worship of nature, which he always regarded as charged with symbolic meanings.

At a crisis in the early thirties a prevalent depressive mood gave way to the joy of creation, and his character and the method of his art seemed to undergo a transformation. His resentment at his own fate seemed to vent itself in the desire to banish if not, as Abraham thinks, to punish his mother by representing her in scenes of exquisite suffering; and when at the age of thirty-six his Alpinism made him at home only with the mountains the break with his past life became more and more marked. The ordinary vicissitudes of life were not sufficient and he wished to gamble not with the mere abatement or reinforcement of life but with life and death themselves. Even his dreams were haunted by a thanatic mood, and his superstitions were such that they almost made life itself a hateful dream. He tells us of fancying himself sitting in a retired nook that was at the same time like a church, when a strange figure stood before him, a creature of dreadful and repulsive form, with white gleaming eyes and yellow flesh tone, half cretin and half death. "I rose, and with impressive mien ordered it away after it had ogled me sideways. I followed it with my eye into the darkest corner until it had vanished." And this vision he thought ominous. When he turned around he shuddered, for the phantom was again before him. Then he arose like a fury, cursed and threatened it, and it vanished and did not return, for it was more obedient than Poe's Raven. His ambivalent reaction against this was not only to work harder but to affirm that there was no death and thus to revive much of the earlier religiosity of his childhood. One of his pictures was of a dying consumptive which he transformed into one of blooming life. More and more the death thought mastered his consciousness—almost as much as it did the soul of the insane painter, Wertz—and provoked him to greater enthusiasm and ever longer and more arduous programs for his future life. But from the subconscious he was always hearing more and more clearly the call of death, for which his deeper nature seems to have passionately longed, while the opposite will-to-live became more and more impotent. All his prodigious activity in later life seems to have been thus really due to a subdominant will to die. When he fell ill for the first time in his life, "the dark powers of his unconscious nature came in to help the disease and make the disintegrative process easier and to invite death," as if love of it were the consummation of his love of all things that lived, and the latter would not have been complete without the former.

Another case of a genius who hurried through the table d'hôte Nature provides and left the table sated to repletion when her regular guests were but half through the course was the German poet, Lenau.[14] Born in 1802, he studied philosophy, law, and medicine successively, sought contact with primeval nature in America at thirty, returned to find himself famous, and, after a period of prolonged chastity, became promptly infected with syphilis, falling a victim to insanity at forty-two and dying of progressive paralysis at forty-eight. Syphilis is perhaps the most psychalgic of all diseases that afflict man, for it not only poisons the arrows of love and

---

[14] J. Sadger, *Aus dem Liebeslebens Nicolaus Lenaus,* Leipzig, 1909, 96 p. See also his biography by B. E. Castle.

makes its ecstasy exquisite pain but weakens all the phyletic instincts, like the climacteric, and like it brings hyperindividuation in its train. He knew both the joys and the pains of life, the depths of misery and the heights of euphoria. Eros and Thanatos were inseparable in his soul, and both had their raptures and inspired him by turns. Amorousness brought acute religiosity, and between his erotic adventures he lapsed far toward the negation of all faiths and creeds. When not in love his violin was treated as a paramour, and he forgot it when the tender passion glowed again in his soul. I doubt if any poet ever had a truer and deeper feeling for nature or was a more eloquent interpreter of all her moods and aspects. He exhausted both homo- and heterosexual experiences, remaining through a series of love affairs, however, true to his Sophie, who was like his mother and with whom his relations were pure and whose influence was beneficent. Even before his infection megalomania alternated with misanthropy, and he had all the fluctuations of mood that are such characteristic stigmata of hysteria. Spells of lassitude alternated with Berserker energy; masochism with sadism; excesses, including those of drink, with spells of depression. In his aggressive moods he stormed up mountains, which to him were symbols of mental elevation, until he was completely exhausted. Sometimes he fancied himself a nobleman or even a monarch and always strove to reduce all about him to servile satellites. The Job-Faust-Manfred motive often took possession of him, and sometimes he played his violin half the night, dancing in rapt ecstasy and unable to keep time. In his periods of self-reproach after orgasms of ecstasy he became ascetic. His poetry and converse were, especially for such a man, singularly pure. He said he carried a corpse around within him. Most insanities are only an exaggeration or breaking out of previous traits, and this was exceptionally so in his case. At one time he seemed to want to break with all his old and to find a new set of friends.

In the high temperature at which he lived, with so many impulses that were either frustrated or crucified, always hot with love or its ambivalent hate, he died—not like Segantini, because he was hypnotized by death at the very acme of his power and willed it actively, though unconsciously, as surely as if he had committed suicide, but he rather turned to it from sheer repletion of life, most of the experiences of which he had exhausted. It was as if a congeries of souls took possession of him by turns, so that in middle life he had himself already played most of the parts in the drama and thus knew it far more exhaustively than those who lead more unitary lives, however prolonged they may be. He was by no means theoretically a miserabilist or even a pessimist but was simply burned out (*blasé, abgelebt*). As if to anticipate the *Weltschmerz* that his diathesis made it certain would later become acute, his passionate love for nature, deep and insightful as it was, did not prove an adequate compensation, and we cannot but wonder whether, if he had lived more normally and without infection to fourscore, his life would not inevitably have ended with the same, though less acute, general symptoms. Yet even he never cursed the fate that brought him into life or inveighed against his parentage. His life was like a candle in the wind blown every way by turns, now and then flaring up and emitting great light and heat, now almost put out, smoking, sputtering, and malodorous in a socket like a blue flame just before its final extinction.

The psychograph of the poet Heinrich von Kleist (d. 1811, *a.e.* 34) affords another example of a genius who died of premature old age near the period of its dawn or at the critical turn of the tide.[15] In the University his

[15] J. Sadger in *Grenzfragen des Nerven und Seelenlebens,* 1910, pp. 5-63.

passion for omniscience impelled him to enroll for so
many and diverse courses that his professors protested.
Later he actually tried eight and attempted to sample
other callings. "He would have liked to be everything."
In the space of fourteen years no less than nine women
had engaged his fancy, although none had made a deep
or lasting impression. He had also a veritable *Lust* for
traveling and after every important event in his life
resorted to this kind of fugue from reality to lose himself in new scenes. "There is nothing consistent in me
save inconsistency." His demands on his friends, and
also his ambitions, knew no bounds. He would "tear
the crown from Goethe's brow." He felt he must storm
all heights and do it now or never.

He, too, was bisexual in his instincts. He glorified
purity and sobriety as over-compensation for his shortcomings in both these respects. Much as he did, he never
could complete the great work he had long planned, and
despair at his impotence to achieve his ambitions made
him at last take flight to insanity as a refuge and finally
to joint suicide with a woman. Late in life he lost the
power to distinguish between fact and fancy, so fully
had his writing become a surrogate for life. Wagner
said that if life were as full as we wish it to be, there
would be no need of art, and von Kleist's biographer
seems to doubt whether to call his end a victory or a surrender. His wooing of death was not, like Segantini's,
a continuation and consummation of the thanatopsis
mood of adolescence but was rather due to a growing
endogenous lethargy and apathy. He lost his appetite
for life, from which he had expected more than it has
to give even to the most favored, and thus at the critical
age when men are prone to weigh themselves in the balance, he found incompleteness and inferiority both
within and without and so threw himself into the arms
of the Great Silencer. Everything conventional had

long since palled upon him. "His early fixation upon an unattainable goal was broken down and he pursued the unattainable until he fancied he found it in death." The outbreak of the Franco-Prussian War seemed, for a time, to afford him an outlet for his pent-up desires without compelling him to resort to illness.

In his ground *motif* De Maupassant [16] belongs to the same category as Lenau and von Kleist. He inherited neurotic trends from both parents and died in 1893 at the age of forty-three, having experienced most of the episodes of life and during his twelve productive years written fourteen volumes and climbed to the very summit of the French Parnassus. His morbidity was partly congenital and partly metasyphilitic. Had he lived his simple life in his Normandy home, instead of coming to Paris, he might have survived but he fell a victim to narcotics, ether, hashish, morphine, cocaine, Bacchus, and Venus. Like so many great men afflicted with the same disease, his symptoms showed many marked departures from its ordinary course, and before its active stage his divarications in the fields of various abnormal symptom-groups were many. His passion for the horrible is perhaps best illustrated in his shuddering "Horla."

Gogol's [17] life (d. 1852, *a.e.* 43) was full of contradictory completeness and incompleteness. He, too, desired not only to touch but to express life at every point, and his realism was in fact only self-expression. He lived through life as a fiction and tried to cast this fiction into the mold of actuality. He was a failure in nearly every department of life he tried and was a man whose character was made up of samples of every type of human nature. In him the creative impulse was not a

---

[16] G. Vorberg, *Guy de Maupassant's Krankheit*, 1908, 27 p.
[17] Otto Kaus, *Schriften des Vereins freie psychoanalytische Forschung*, No. 2, 1912, 81 p.

retreat from life but was an attempt to make a bridge between it and his soul. He was haunted by a feeling of inferiority which it was the passion of his life to overcome. When his aggressive feelings were strongest, he produced most, and failed as actor, teacher, clerk, and succeeded as poet and novelist because thus he could best wreak his inmost self upon expression. He was finally obsessed by a religious mania, became a mystic, and sought salvation by fasting and self-denial. Fear of death was a life-long obsession and he strove to conquer both love and death together by seeking and defying the latter. He decided to die by fasting and kneeling before the picture of the Mother of God. "Groaning and crying out with his last strength, he had dragged himself to the symbol of the highest feminine completeness, and when he found the 'Glorious Virgin' of his dreams his dissolution came." In his last moment he seems to have felt that he had overcome both death and woman, but only by yielding to them, and believed himself to be a martyr. It was the difficulty he found in bridging the chasm between his solitary, child-like self and the real world that made him a great creator of fiction, a practical failure, and a madman.

J. V. von Scheffel [18] exhibited a range of moods from humor and jollity to melancholia, and showed in his poems an entire absence of eroticism which was more or less compensatory. The bisexual instinct (he not only looked like a girl but sometimes disguised himself in woman's attire) was evoked by an earnest effort to see the world as woman did. He had an extraordinary variety of morbid attacks, hypochondria, delusions, headaches, morbid fear of death, anxiety, nightmares, weeping, etc. Schurmann even goes so far as to think that a cyclothymic diathesis or a tendency to periodic

---

[18] P. J. Moebius, *Ueber Scheffel's Krankheit,* 1907, p. 40.

attacks of various psychic morbidities is characteristic of genius, which finds occasional relief in attacks of insanity, like Cowper, Rousseau, Tasso, Hölderlin, and many others; and ascribes this in part to a hunger for a life larger and fuller than normality or sobriety can afford. This, however, is forbidden fruit, for nature punishes the enjoyment of it, if not by premature death at least by premature satiety with life.

John Ruskin's lifeline had marked nodes, the chief of which may be characterized as follows. Up to the early forties he had lived and written under the dominant influence of his father, who held very conservative views of religion; but the foundations of the son's faith were shaken and the tenet "which had held the hopes and beliefs of his youth and early manhood had proved too narrow. He was stretching forth to a wider and, as he felt, a nobler conception of life and destiny, but the transition was through much travail of soul." [19] He wrote, "It is a difficult thing to live without hope of another world when one has been used to it for forty years. But by how much the more difficult, by so much it makes one braver and stronger." And again, "It may be much nobler to hope for the advance of the human race only than for one's own immortality, much less selfish to look upon oneself merely as a leaf on a tree than as an independent spirit, but it is much less pleasant." Cook says that "he had been brought up as a Bible Christian in the strictest school of literal interpretation but he had also become deeply versed in some branches of natural science, and the truths of science seemed inconsistent with a literal belief in the Scriptures." He had been much influenced by Spurgeon, whom he knew well in private life, but made no secret of his adhesion to Colenso's heresies.

---

[19] E. T. Cook, *Life of John Ruskin*, London, 1911, vol. ii, p. 19.

No one understood the inmost causes of his muse as he grew melancholic. He was exhausted, dyspeptic, wanted to reconstruct society, had "the soul of a prophet consumed with wrath against a wayward and perverse generation," but also the heart of a lover of his fellow-men filled with pity for the miseries and follies of mankind. His mother recognized his tendency to misanthropy, and only at forty-two did he break away from parental discipline. "A new epoch of life began for me in this wise, that my father and mother could travel with me no more, but Rose [La Touche, the young girl with whom he was in love and who died when he was in the early fifties and left him forlorn] in heart was with me always, and all I did was for her sake." This was his first "exile." The clouds that had more than once lowered over his life settled in old age and he died in 1900 at the age of eighty-one. During most of the last ten years he presented one of the saddest of all the spectacles of old age, "dying from the top downward." He was apathetic, monosyllabic, could write little, and spoke less; and but for the kindly ministrations of Mrs. Severn and the thoughtfulness of Kate Greenaway almost nothing either in Brantwood or the great world without retained interest for him.

The middle-age crisis in Friedrich Nietzsche's life began when he left Bayreuth in August, 1876, after the performance of *The Ring of the Niebelung*. He was then thirty-two years of age. Now it was that his disenchantment with Wagner, whom he had regarded as a superman and often called Jupiter, "one who might bring the type of man to a higher degree of perfection," [20] began. He had thought Wagner "near to the divine," but he now found much of his music dull and recitative and thought that in *Parsifal* he had violated his own

---

[20] Frau Foerster-Nietzsche, *The Life of Nietzsche.*

atheism as a concession to the public; and so he "refused
to recognize a genius who was not honest with himself."
He abhorred Wagner's new "redemption philosophy" but
for months and years could not bring himself to an open
break with him and was for a long time plunged in the
depths of gloom. He now became truly lonely and went
through a complete inner revolution. He realized that
he must henceforth stand alone and work out the problem of life by himself. His anxiety as to how the venerable Wagner would receive his *Human, All Too
Human* was pathetic. When he found he could not publish it anonymously, he revised and toned down many of
his criticisms; and deep, indeed, was his grief when,
despite the almost fawning letter that accompanied a
copy of his book to Wagner, the latter lacked the greatness of soul to understand his sincerity and broke with
him forever. At the same time he was emancipating his
thought from Schopenhauer, who had hitherto been his
sovereign master in the philosophic field.

Now it was that he almost completely wrecked his life
by living according to the precepts of Cornaro, and his
letters show the intense struggle with which he finally
resolved to find his own way through life and to abandon
his soul to self-expression. He finally resigned his chair
of classic literature at Bâle and a little later sorted his
manuscripts and commissioned his sister to burn half of
them. This she refused to do, and it was just these that
were the basis of some of the best things he wrote later.
After trying residence in many places and various cures,
and experimenting with many regimens, he finally resolved to become his own doctor, and it was by his own
efforts that he succeeded in prolonging the efficient
period of his life. But he felt he had at last struck the
right road in *The Dawn of Day,* which marked the
opening of his campaign against popular morality.
From this time on, too, he had a deep, new, intense love

of nature and was inspired henceforth by the conviction that he must be the midwife of the superman in the world. This apostle of a "New Renaissance" was not unlike his Zarathustra, who retired to the mountains at thirty and at forty came down to the haunts of men with a new message for them.

The theme of Rostand's *Chanticleer* is the disillusion of that gorgeous barnyard fowl from the fond and at first secret conviction, which he later confessed to the pheasant hen, that it was his crowing that brought in the dawn and that if he failed in this function the world would lie in darkness. The tragedy of the play is the slow conviction that the sun could rise without him. In Nietzsche we see the exact reverse of this process. His delusions of greatness grew with years and eventually passed all bounds of sanity. He became jealous of Jesus and came to believe that he had brought the world a new dispensation and that his own work would some time be recognized as the dawn of a new era.

Robert Raymond [21] thinks it is pleasant to lie at anchor a while in port before setting sail for the last long voyage to the unknown. The passage from late youth to middle age has many of the same traits as growing old. We suddenly realize, perhaps in a flash, that life is no longer all before us. When youth begins to die it fights and struggles. The panic is not so much that we cannot do handsprings, but we have to compromise with our youthful hopes. We have been out of college perhaps twenty years. Napoleon lost Waterloo at 45, Dickens had written all his best at 40, and Pepys finished his diary at 37. We lose the sense of superfluous time and must hurry. We feel the futility of postponements and accept the philosophy of the second best as not so bad. We become more tolerant toward others and perhaps toward our-

[21] "On Growing Old," *Atlan.*, 1915, p. 803.

selves. We must not be too serious or yearn too much
for a lost youth. It is like the first anticipations of fall
in the summer.

F. von Mueller of Munich [22] says that we can never tell
when old age begins. Involution is closely connected
with evolution from the start. The lymphatics, tonsils,
and thymus begin to atrophy as soon as the development
of the sex organs comes. Among English button workers
it was found that young men did most; between the
ages of 40 and 45 they did 80 per cent of the work they
formerly did; 60 per cent in the fifty-fifth year, and 40
per cent after sixty-five. The power of observation is
so great in youth that seventy per cent of all our acquisitions are made at this stage. Originality comes later.
Age is more serious. There is less adaptation because
habit is growing rigid. The emotional life stiffens and
the intellectual narrows. There are more doubts. There
is a stronger-felt need of recognition from others that is
very deeply experienced in many ways. The capacity
for producing original ideas comes latest of all. It is
generally thought that the highest physical development
is before 30. Some investigators think that physical
deterioration begins with the brain but this is doubtful.

Bruce Birch [23] thinks the wreckage of youth spectac-
ular; that of old age less discernible because more subtle
and internal. The old should come to the fullest possible
maturity. Youth must be served. The church focuses
on young men. The old age here chiefly regarded is
from forty-five on. Most lack intelligent encouragement to go on. They are thought too old to need advice
and to only want comfort. Habits are supposed to be
formed. The old are not thought to be heart-searchers.
The fact is, senescence has very new and great

[22] "Concerning Age," *Sci. Amer. Sup.*, Nov. 15, 1919.
[23] "The Moral and Religious Psychology of Late Senescence," *Biblical World*, 1918, p. 75.

temptations, namely, to go on in the old way of habit and belief. The temptations of the old are largely of the spirit but sometimes also of the flesh and the devil. It is hard to keep up the struggle for personal righteousness and there are periods of storm and stress. The church has not done its duty here. Most think the most dangerous period is that of wild oats—between 16 and 26—but this writer says it is between 45 and 65 when there is the most wreckage.

1. There is a tendency to low ideals. Youth tends to lofty ideals and to realize them, but now hope often fails. With the abbreviation of life there is loss of initiative, perhaps sickness of hope deferred. Age thinks it has become all it can hope to be; so enthusiasm wanes and the *tedium vitae* makes us feel the game is not worth the candle and we are not willing to pay the price of sacrifice and struggle to maintain high ideals. So we aim lower. The *excelsior* motive is lost. So there is often a degeneration of moral character. Cheap pleasures satisfy—perhaps even those of the table, for this is the easiest way of reviving some of the tendencies of former life.

2. Hence lowering and liberalizing of conduct creeds. The frontal lobes shrink as the period of endeavor wanes. The edge of desire is dulled and so is the power to distinguish right and wrong, true and false. "Twice a child, once a man." The powers of imagination, aggression, and resistant effort flag, and we are content with the beaten path because the motor areas have decayed. There is ruttiness, the brain is set for habitual reactions, there are fixed points of view, the apperceptive mass is allowed to interpret all new ideas, and these cannot change it. Thus it is hard to adjust to progress. There is less resistance, self-control, courage for great deeds and high purposes, less tendency to ask advice of and be influenced by younger men. Politicians often

25

recognize this in putting forward respectable elderly, pliant candidates. One is often weak where he thinks himself strong because there is no fool like an old one. He may yield to selfishness, acquisitiveness, curiosity, secretiveness, envy, jealousy, avarice, and other primitive traits. There is too frequent moral collapse here.

3. There is a lessening of emotional intensity or stodginess. The imitative, religious, adventurous, belligerent, imaginative, initiative traits are developed early, and the younger man is the greater in the dominion of the emotions. But later poets turn to prose and others to more didactic activities. Scientists, philosophers, and statesmen are best when they are through this period. Disappointed men now become cynical, morose, petulant, or vicious as the intellect only rules. If the social and gregarious instinct fails, society may bore, friendships decline, and age may be lonely. Or, again, it may fall a prey to many dispositional, emotional, and obsessive feelings which may become insane. The patient may live in a logic-tight compartment. The obsession may be a hobby or a system of connected ideas with a strong emotional tone (complex). These are tendencies arising from instinct. When the social and sane instincts lose in the conflict, interest in the present may decline to indifference, and the obsessions may focus on real or fancied errors of the past—duty to a dead child, a business failure, etc. At any rate, there is a tendency to indulge temperament.

4. Failure in religious teaching. Versus "Be sure your sin will find you out" all the old realize that they have done much sin that is not found out and which, if it were exposed, would bring suffering, disgrace, public execration, and loss of vocation, property and friends. To fear only the consequences of evil is bad, and since they have escaped they feel a certain contempt of secular and moral law and take greater risks. The old man pre-

fers to be respectable and righteous, but he does not care if his unrighteousness is known or suspected if it is not made too public. Thus the old dread exposure more than they do sin.

5. The church offers too little to the old but wants to see old age tap new reservoirs of energy, vigor, joy, and enthusiasm. The best it can offer is faith in Jesus. Many would say it offers a larger intellectual view.

Karin Michaëlis [24] tells her story in the form of letters and a running journal. A poor girl, she early came to feel that with her beauty she could do anything and supremely longed for wealth. After just escaping marriage with a rich old man who educated her, she married a wealthy and most exemplary husband whom she divorced, after having lived tranquilly with him for a score of years, with no cause on either side but because she felt a growing passion for solitude. She retired to a desert island in a spacious new villa planned by an architect friend eight years younger than herself. After a year of isolation, slowly realizing that she is in love with the architect, as she had long been, she offers herself to him on any terms and is rejected. She then proposes to rejoin her husband but finds him engaged to a girl of nineteen.

The remarkable merit of this book that made it something of a sensation through all western Europe ten years ago is the masterly descriptions of the state of mind of women of a certain type, and perhaps to some extent of all, at the turn of life. While there is not a phrase in it that could shock the most fastidious, it is evident throughout that the author's soul is permeated with a sex consciousness that finds numberless indirect expressions and that she knows life and man chiefly from this standpoint, condones most of woman's errors,

---

[24] *The Dangerous Age*, London, 1912.

advises her friends to courses that convention forbids, etc. No one ever began to write such a book, not even Octave Feuillet in his *La Crise*. It all reads like a marvelous confession of things no woman ever said before or could say to a man. She says:

Somebody should found a vast and charitable sisterhood for women between forty and fifty, a kind of refuge for the victims of the years of transition, for during that time women would be happier in voluntary exile or at any rate entirely separated from the other sex. . . . We are all more or less mad, even though we struggle to make others think us sane.

There are moments when I envy every living creature who has the right to pair—either from hate or from habit. I am alone and shut out.

Women's doctors may be as clever and sly as they please but they will never learn any of the things women confide to each other. Between the sexes there lies not only a deep, eternal hostility but the involuntary abyss of a complete lack of reciprocal comprehension.

It would be better for woman if she walked barefoot over red-hot ploughshares for the pain she would suffer would be slight, indeed, compared to that which she must feel when, with a smile on her lips, she leaves her own youth behind and enters the region of despair we call growing old.

It may safely be said that on the whole surface of the earth not one man exists who really knows woman. If a woman took infinite pains to reveal herself to a husband or a lover just as she really is, he would think she was suffering from some incurable mental disease. A few of us indicate our true natures in hysterical outbreaks, fits of bitterness and suspicion, but this involuntary frankness is generally discounted by some subtle deceit.

If men suspected what took place in a woman's inner life after forty, they would avoid us like the plague or knock us in the head like mad dogs.

Are there honest women? At least we believe there are. It is a necessary part of our belief. Who does not think well of mother or sister, but who *believes entirely* in a mother or sister? Absolutely and unconditionally? Who has never caught mother or sister in a falsehood or a subterfuge? Who has not sometimes seen in the heart of mother or sister, as by a lightning flash, an abyss which the boundless love cannot bridge over? Who was ever really understood by mother or sister?

THE YOUTH OF OLD AGE

I envy every country wench or servant girl who goes off with her lover while I sit here waiting for old age.[25]

The author has been spoken of as a traitor to her sex, revealing all its freemasonry. Certainly no female writer ever emancipated herself more completely from man's point of view. There is no masculine note here. It would seem as if she aspired to be a specialist in feminine psychology. M. Prévost calls it a cinematograph of feminine thought set down without interposing between the author's mind and the paper the vision of a man. No extracts or epitome can do justice to the precision of style, the acuteness of self-observation, the range of social experience, and the depth of insight here shown in depicting the psychological processes that attend the beginnings of old age in women.

It is well at any stage of life, and particularly at its noonday, to pause and ask ourselves what kind of old people we would like, and also are likely, to be—two very different questions. In youth we have ideals of and fit for maturity. Why not do the same when we are mature for the next stage? Why should not forty plan for eighty (or at least for sixty) just as intently as twenty does for forty? At forty old age is in its infancy; the fifties are its boyhood, the sixties its youth, and at seventy it attains its majority. Woman passes through the same stages as man, only the first comes earlier and the last later for her. If and so far as Osler is right, it is because man up to the present has been abnormally precocious, a trait that he inherited from his shorter-lived precursors and has not yet outgrown, as is the case with sexual precocity, which brings premature age. Modern man was not meant to do his best work before forty but is by nature, and is becoming more and more so, an afternoon and evening worker. The coming superman will begin, not end, his real activity with the

---

[25] See W. L. Comfort's *Midstream* for the same crisis in men (1914).

29

advent of the fourth decade. Not only with many personal questions but with most of the harder and more complex problems that affect humanity we rarely come to anything like a masterly grip till the shadows begin to slant eastward, and for a season, which varies greatly with individuals, our powers increase as the shadows lengthen. Thus as the world grows intricate and the stage of apprenticeship necessarily lengthens it becomes increasingly necessary to conserve all those higher powers of man that culminate late, and it is just these that our civilization, that brings such excessive strains to middle life, now so tends to dwarf, making old age too often *blasé* and *abgelebt,* like the middle age of those roués who in youth have lived too fast.

There are many who now think more or less as does H. G. Wells [26] that the human race is just at its dangerous age and has, within the last few years, passed its prime; also that henceforth we must trust less to nature and place all our hope in and direct all our energy to nurture if the race is to escape premature decay. There is only too much to indicate that mankind, in Europe at least if not throughout the world, has reached the "dangerous age" that marks the dawn of senescence and that, unless we can develop what Renan calls "a new enthusiasm for humanity," a new social consciousness, and a new instinct for service and for posterity, our elaborate civilization with all its institutions will become a Frankenstein monster escaping the control of the being that devised and constructed it and will bring ruin to both him and to itself. Progressive eugenics, radical and world-wide reëducation, and the development of a richer, riper old age, are our only sources of hope for we can look to no others to arrest the degenerative processes of national and individual egoism. At any

---

[26] *The Salvaging of Civilization: The Probable Future of Mankind* New York, 1921. 199 p.

rate, we have to face a new problem, namely what is the old age of the world to be and how can we best prepare for it betimes?

As contrasted with Ireland, in which Ross [27] tells us "one-eighth of her people are more than sixty-five years old," we have considered ourselves as *par excellence* the land of young people and ideas. Our growth has been phenomenal and began and proceeded most opportunely, so that we profited to the full by steam, rapid transportation, invention, by our coal, oil, forests, and virgin soil, and especially by the ideals of liberty that were brought here by the first waves of immigrants to our shores. These were followed later, however, by those who had failed in the old world, by inferior and often Mediterranean stocks imported as tools or coming only in the hope of gain; but even this tide is now ceasing to flow. We are within measurable distance of the limits of our natural resources. Although the great war, the most stupendous, was also the most inconclusive ever fought, and although we reached our pinnacle in the idealism of Wilson's first visit to Europe, when the world came nearer than ever before since early Christianity, the Holy Roman Empire, and Comenius, to a merger of national sovereignty and a new world law backed by a new world power, this brief vision of a federated world has faded and we now realize that if we cannot make a break with history and leave much of it to the dead past, if we cannot transcend the boundaries that, especially in Europe, are now far too narrow for modern conditions, and if we cannot fearlessly enter upon the longer apprenticeship to life, which is now too short for mastery, we shall drift into far more disastrous wars that will leave even the victors exhausted, and mankind will either sink into an impotent senility or into a Tarzan bestialism, which from the standpoint of Clarence Day (*The Simian World*) would seem not impossible.

---

[27] *The Old World in the New*, 1914, p. 27.

CHAPTER II

THE HISTORY OF OLD AGE

The age of plants and animals—The Old Stone Age—Treatment of old age among existing savage tribes—The views of Frazer—The ancient Hebrews and the Old Testament—The Greeks (including Sparta, the Homeric Age, the status of the old in Athens, the views of Plato, Socrates' talks with boys, Aristotle)—The Romans—The Middle Ages—Witchcraft and old women—Attitude of children toward the old—Mantegazza's collection of favorable and unfavorable views of age—The division of life into stages—The relation of age groups to social strata—The religion of different ages of life—The Vedanta—The Freudian war between the old and the young—History of views from Cornaro to our own time—Bacon—Addison—Burton—Swift.

SOME plants live only a few hours; others, a few days; and very many only for a season. But trees are the oldest of all things that live. In the Canary Islands is an immense dragon tree, forty-five feet in circumference, which grows very slowly. This was vital enough to continue living fifty years after a third of it was destroyed. It must have been several thousand years old, but as its trunk was hollowed there was no way of ascertaining its age. In the Cape Verde Islands stood a tree thirty feet in diameter which Adanson estimated to be 5,150 years of age. Some of the old cypresses in Mexico are thought to be quite as old. The big trees of California are several thousand years old, the largest of which Sargent estimates to have lived 5,000 years. We have all seen cross-sections of the trunks of these monsters of the vegetable world with their concentric rings marked—"this growth was made during the year the Magna Charta was granted," "this when Christ was born," etc. Many botanists believe that trees of this sort do not die of old age as such, but of external accidents like lightning, tempests, etc.

As to animal longevity, no doubt there are real ephemerids. Life can also be prolonged by desiccation or by freezing. Certain it is that many species do not live to see their offspring. In many of the lower forms of life the larval is far longer than the adult stage. The seventeen-year locust, for example, lives out most of its time underground, the imago form continuing but little more than a month. Most butterflies are annual, although those that fail to copulate may hibernate and live through another season, while some are known to have lived several years. Worker bees do not survive the season but queens live from two to five years. J. H. Gurney[1] thinks the passerines are the shortest-lived birds, averaging from eight to nine years, that the lark, canary, bullfinch, gull, may live forty years, the goose fifty, and the parrot sixty. To the latter bird a mythical longevity is often assigned, one being said to have spoken a language that had become extinct. As to animals, domestication prolongs while captivity shortens their normal length of life. Longevity is often related to fertility. Beasts of prey breed slowly and live to be old, while the fecund rabbit is short-lived. But for increased fecundity species subject to high risk would die out. While there is a certain correlation between size and age, since large animals require more time to grow, it is extremely limited. Bunge thinks that in mammals the period the newborn take to double in size is an index of the normal duration of life; but this, too, has its limitations. Some stress diet as an essential factor and others think that length of life may be inversely as the reproductive tax levied upon the system. But of all these questions our knowledge is still very limited.

[1] *The Longevity of Birds.*

33

SENESCENCE

When Alexander conquered India, he took one of King Porus's largest elephants, Ajax, and labeled it, "Alexander, the son of Jupiter, dedicates this to the sun." This elephant is said to have been found 160 years later. This is the earliest record I find of animal longevity. We have many tables since Flourens attempted, with great pains, to construct one, and from the latest of these at hand I select the following of those animals popularly supposed to be able to attain one hundred years or more: carp, 100 to 150; crocodile, 100; crow, 100; eagle, 100; elephant, 150 to 200; parrot, 100; pike, 100; raven, 100; swan, 100; tortoise, over 100. In point of fact, as E. Ray Lankester [2] says, we know almost nothing definite of the length of life of larger animals. Flourens considered that in mammalia we could find a criterion of the end of the growth period in the union of the epiphyses of the bones throughout the skeleton, and laid down the law that for both mammals and man longevity is, on the average, about five times that of this period of growth. We know far more as to the span of the shorter- than of the longer-lived members of the brute creation. We also know far more of domestic animals than of their wild congeners. The former doubtless have lived longer because better protected. Darwin wrote that he had no information in regard to the longevity of the nearest wild representatives of our domestic animals or even of quadrupeds in general, and various experts whom Lankester addressed upon the subject informed him that almost nothing was known of reptiles or crustacea, while the ichthyologist, Gunther, said, "There is scarcely anything known about the age and causes of death of fishes," and Jeffreys, a molluscan expert, says the same of them. Insects, on the other hand, are a remarkable exception. Their life is so short that it can sometimes be observed almost con-

[2] *On the Comparative Longevity of Man and Animals*, 1870.

tinuously from ovum to ovum. There is in general, however, Lankester believes, a much closer relation between the life span of individuals of the same than between those of different species, specific longevity meaning the average length of life of the individual of the species. Of all this we know far more of man than of any other creature.

If age went with size, the extinct saurians would have attained the greatest age of all animals, and in fact they seem to have grown all their lives. However it may have been in past geologic ages, it may yet appear that man, on the average, lives longer than any brutes. This he should do if the civilization he has evolved really gives him a more favorable environment than nature and instinct have provided for him. Species, like individuals, very probably have a term of life and become extinct with age, as paleontology shows us not a few have done. But here, too, there is no sufficient basis of fact at present to warrant the generalizations so often met with concerning phyletic immortality or senescence. To some aspects of this theme I shall recur later in this volume.

Of the length of life of the predecessors of modern man we know almost nothing. In evolving as he did from anthropoid forms, he probably also considerably increased his span of life. It would seem, too, as if again in the transition from the unsocial, short, and still somewhat simian Neanderthal to that of the tall and more gregarious Crô-Magnon type he must have still further increased his longevity. But through all the paleolithic ages (lasting some 125,000 years as H. F. Osborn calculates [3]) there are no data either in the skeletal remains or in the implements he used that shed any clear light upon the subject; and the same is true of the neolithic cults that flowered in the lake- or pile-dwellings. Bones show different stages of development,

---

[3] *Men of the Old Stone Age*, New York, 1915, p. 40.

and teeth, always remarkably well preserved, often show the effects of use; a very few represent children but not one illustrates extreme old age according to the osseous or dental criteria of modern times. Hence we may conjecture that the attainment of great age under the conditions of life then prevailing was very rare. It would seem also that if life had been long and its experiences well ripened, preserved, and transmitted (so that each new generation would not merely repeat the life of that which had preceded it but profit by its lessons), progress would not have been so very slow, as it was. On the other hand, it might be urged perhaps with equal force that if, as with lower races now, most of the people who made prehistory not only matured but grew old early, and since age always tends to be conservative and unprogressive, it would make for retardation, even though it came in years that seem premature to us. Very probably even in these rude stages of life men who felt their physical powers beginning to abate—at least the more sagacious of them—had already hit upon some of the many devices by which the aging have very commonly contrived to maintain their position and even increase their importance in the community by developing wisdom in counsel, becoming repertories of tribal tradition and custom, and representatives of feared supernatural forces or persons, etc. But of all this paleo-anthropology has, up to date, almost nothing to tell us. Nor do we see much reason to believe it ever will. All these culture stages of the Old Stone Age have left us little but material vestiges of its industries—bones, a few carvings on cave walls or on bones and ivory, and very many chipped flints. Nothing of wood, skin, fiber or other material for binding, which must have been used, survives.[4] Much as these bones and stones tell us, they

---

[4] See my "What We Owe to the Tree-life of Our Ape-like Ancestors," *Ped. Sem.,* 23: 94-116, 1916.

have really done more to increase our curiosity than to satisfy it. We know almost nothing of how these thousands of generations of men viewed life or nature, or in what spirit and with what knowledge they met disease, age, and death.

What is called belief in another life is for primitives or children only inability to grasp completely the very difficult fact of death and to distinguish it from sleep. The disposition of some of the troglodyte skeletons suggests that these ancient forbears of our race were unable to realize that death ends all. Despite the close analogy and even kinship between human and animal life so deeply felt in early days, it was probably always somewhat harder for early man to conceive death for himself as complete cessation than to so conceive it for the higher forms of animal life with which his own was so intimately associated. Our ignorance of all these stages of human evolution becomes all the more pathetic as we are now coming to understand that it was then that all the deeper unconscious and dispositional strata of Mansoul, which still dominate us far more than we are even yet aware, were being laid down, and it is upon these traits that the later and conscious superstructure of our nature has been reared. Only hard things survive the ravages of time, and psychic traits and trends are the softest of all soft things, although they are no less persistent by way of biological and social inheritance than skeletons and flints.

Turning to the lower races of mankind that now survive and are accessible to study, we find only very few scattered, fragmentary, and often contradictory data as to old age. Yarrow has made a comprehensive study of mortuary customs, both of savages and man in the earlier stages of civilization. Mallory brought together what we know of sign language. Ploss has given us a compend on the child among primitives and, with Bartels, on woman. I have tried to compile the customs and ideas of pubescent initiation;[5] while animism, marriage rites, property and ownership, systems of kinship, mana concepts, hunting and trapping, war weapons, dances, ideas of disease and the function of the "medicine man," dwellings, dress, ornamentation, number systems, language, fire-making, industries, food, myths, and ceremonies galore, and many other themes have had comprehensive and comparative treatment. But I am able to find nothing of the kind (and Professor F. Boas, our most accomplished American scholar in this field, knows of nothing compendious) on old age in any language. Anthropology, therefore, has so far produced no gerontologists. I have looked over many volumes of travel and exploration among the so-called lower races of mankind, only to find nothing or brief and more or less incidental mentions of senescence. This neglect is itself significant of the inconspicuous rôle the old play in rude tribal life and also of the lack of vital interest in the theme by investigators.

From my own meager and inadequate gleanings in this field the unfavorable far outweigh the favorable mentions. The Encyclopedia Britannica tells us that from Herodotus, Strabo, and others we learn of people like the Scythian Massagetæ, a nomad race northeast of the Caspian Sea, who killed old people and ate them. For savages the practice of devouring dead kinsfolk is often regarded as the most respectful method of disposing of their remains. In a few cases this custom is combined with that of killing both the old and sick, but it is more often simply a form of burial. It prevails in many parts of Australia, Melanesia, Africa, South America, and elsewhere.

Reclus[6] tells us that among the various Siberian

---

[5] *Adolescence,* Ch. XIII, "Savage Pubic Initiations," etc.
[6] *Primitive Folk,* p. 42.

tribes aged and sickly people who are useless are asked if they have "had enough of it." It is a matter of duty and honor on their part to reply "yes." Thereupon an oval pit is roughly excavated in a burial ground and filled with moss. Heavy stones are rolled near, the extremities of the victim are bound to two horizontal poles, and on the headstone a reindeer is slaughtered, its blood flowing in torrents over the moss. The old man stretches himself upon this warm red couch. In the twinkling of an eye he finds that he is securely bound to the poles. Then he is asked "Art thou ready?" At this stage of the proceeding it would be folly to articulate a negative response. Moreover, his friends would pretend not to hear it. So his *moriturus saluto* is "Good night, friends." They then stop his nostrils with a stupefying substance and open his carotid and a large vein in his arm, so that he is bled to death in no time. Among most races, Reclus tells us, children are killed by being exposed; the old, by being deserted.

In Terra del Fuego, Darwin tells how Jimmy Buttons, a native, described the slaughter of the aged in winter and famine. Dogs, he said, catch otters; old women, not. He then proceeded to detail just how they were killed, imitated and ridiculed their cries and shrieks, told the parts of their bodies that were best to eat, and said they must generally be killed by friends and relatives.

Among the Hottentots, when their aged men and women can "no longer be of any manner of service in anything," they are conveyed by an ox, accompanied by most of the inhabitants of the kraal, to a solitary hut at a considerable distance and, with a small stock of provisions, laid in the middle of the hut, which is then securely closed. The company returns, deserting him forever. They think it the most humane thing they can do to thus hasten the conclusion of life when it has become a burden.

SENESCENCE

With at least one of the Papuan races in New Guinea, people when old and useless are put up a tree, around which the tribe sing "The fruit is ripe" and then shake the branches until the victim falls, tearing him to pieces and eating him raw. Among the Damaras the sick and aged are often cruelly treated, forsaken, or burned alive. In some of the East African tribes the aged and all supposed to be at the point of death are slain and eaten. One author tells us that among the Fijians the practice of burying alive is "so common that but few old and decrepit people are to be seen." In Herbert Spencer's anthropological charts we are told that among the Chippewas "old age is the greatest calamity that can befall a northern Indian for he is neglected and treated with disrespect."

C. Wissler [7] says, "As to the aged and sick, we have the formal practice of putting to death among some of the Esquimaux and other races." On the other hand, among all hunting people who shift from place to place the infirm are often of necessity left behind to their fate. Yet the reported examples of such cruelties can usually be matched by instances of the opposite tenor. He goes on to say that since the mythologies of various tribal groups contain rites showing retribution for such cruelties we must regard them as, on the whole, exceptional.

S. K. Hutton [8] says,

I found age a very deceptive thing. "Sixty-two" might be the answer from a bowed old figure crouching over the stove. I would have guessed twenty years more than that. The fact is, the Eskimo wears out fast. After fifty he begins to decline, and few live long after sixty. I have known a few over seventy, and the people told me with wonderment about an old woman who lived to be eighty-two and who worked to the last. But these

---

[7] *The American Indian*, p. 177.
[8] *Among the Eskimos of Labrador*, p. 111.

are great rarities. It must be a unique thing in one's lifetime to meet with an Eskimo great-grandmother. The very old people seem always to be active to the last. They have an unusual amount of vitality and die in the harness, dropping out like those too tired to go any further and passing away without illness or suffering. These are always those who have clung most closely to their own native foods and customs. Women who are too old and toothless to chew the boot-leather can still scrape the seal-skins, perhaps with a skill which the younger women lack; if they are too blind and feeble to scrape, they can sit behind a wall of snow upon the sea-ice and jig for the sleepy rock-cod through a hole.

C. A. Scott [9] tells us that in certain south Australian tribes it is taboo to catch or eat certain animals until a man has reached a prescribed advanced age, these animals being easiest to catch and the most wholesome and thus best adapted to old people's use. One of the chief maxims in Tonga is to reverence the gods, the chief, and old people. In Java, among the Iroquois, Dakotas, Comanches, the Hill tribes of India (Santals and Kukis), the Snakes and Zunis, much respect is shown to the aged.

K. Routledge [10] says, "part of the deference paid to advancing years, whether in men or women, is due to fear. Old age has something uncanny about it, and old persons could probably 'make medicine' or work havoc, were they so inclined." One chief said that in councils the old women would have their way because "it is a great work to have borne a child." A young warrior is taught to get out of the road for an old woman. She does not, however, take part in the sacrifices, although one called herself the wife of God and seemed to have established a sort of cult. This was because she was a woman of much character. Here the mothers take full

[9] "Old Age and Death," *Am. Jour. Psychol.*, October, 1896.
[10] *With a Prehistoric People: The Akikuyu of British East Africa*, p. 157.

41

part in initiations. The dignity and self-reliance of the older women is remarkable. When a woman is so old that she has no teeth she is said to be "filled with intelligence" and on her death receives the high honor of burial instead of being thrown out to the hyenas.

A. L. Cureau [11] tells us that the Negro is short-lived and that if some lucky star enables him to reach forty he becomes a man of importance, although death does not usually permit him to enjoy this distinction long. "During more than twenty years I never knew more than four or five who could have been considered sixty-five or seventy years of age, and even persons who were from fifty to sixty are very uncommon. At the age of thirty-five or forty they all exhibit signs of premature decrepitude." He thinks the death rate from forty to forty-five very high. Disease among the Africans is limited to only a few general troubles. Burial is usually by interment, although in some districts the dead are eaten, while elsewhere they are thrown into the river or left lying on the ground in some remote spot. Respect for the chief, however, continues to be observed even after his death. But customs are growing mild, and "if human sacrifice still takes place in locations that are most remote from our stations, the fact is kept a profound secret."

H. A. Junod [12] gives a melancholy picture of old age, especially for the leading man of the tribe. His wives die, his glory fades, his crown loses its luster and if it is scratched or broken he cannot repair it, he is forsaken, less respected, and often only a burden unwillingly supported. "The children laugh at him. If the cook sends them to their lonely grandfather with his share of food in the leaky old hut, the young rascals are capable of eating it on the way, pretending afterwards that they

[11] *Savage Man in Central Africa*, p. 176.
[12] *The Life of a South-African Tribe*, p. 131.

THE HISTORY OF OLD AGE

did what they were told." When, between two huts, under the shelter of the woods the old man warms his round-shouldered back in the rays of the sun, lost in some senile dream, his former friends point to him and say, "It is the bogie man, the ogre." Mature people show little more consideration for the old than do the young ones. Junod knew personally an old man and woman who, when their children moved to another part of the country, were left under a roof with no sides, without food, and were almost imbecile. "In times of war old people die in great numbers. During the movements of panic they are hidden in the woods, in the swamps or palm trees, while all the able-bodied population runs away. They are killed by the enemy, who spare no one, or they die in their hiding places of misery and hunger. Thus the evening of life is very sad for the poor Thonga." There are, however, children who to the end show devotion to their parents. Those old people are most to be pitied who fall to the charge of remote relatives.

A. Hrdlicka [13] says, "The proportion of nonagenarians, and especially centenarians, among the Indians is far in excess of that among native white Americans." As to the source of error, he thinks this is somewhat offset by the "marked general interest centering about the oldest of every tribe." He found twenty-four per million among the Indians as against three per million among native whites who had reached a hundred, and says, "The relative excess of aged persons (80 years and above) among the Indians would signify only that the infirmities and diseases known ordinarily as those of old age are less grave among them, a conclusion in harmony with general observation." Among the fifteen tribes embraced in this very careful and valuable investi-

[13] "Physiological and Medical Observations on the Indians of Southwest United States and Mexico," Bureau Amer. Ethnol., Bull. 34.

gation, Hrdlicka found in the old far less grayness and baldness and far better teeth than among the whites. They had more wrinkles but their muscular force was better preserved. Many debilitating effects among the whites are less so among the Indians. In general there is some bending and emaciation and the hair grows iron gray or yellowish-gray, but never white. Nor did he find among those of ninety a single one who was demented or helpless. The aged were generally more or less neglected, and had to care for themselves and help the younger. Owing to the diminution of the alveoli and adipose tissue, "the jaw looks more prominent, prognathism disappears, and the face looks shorter." There is an increase in the nasal index, the nose becomes broader and shorter, the malar bones more prominent. The eyes lose their luster and generally become narrowed, with adhesions at the canthi, particularly the external. The hardening of arteries is certainly not common. Of 716 well preserved males of 65, only 4 per cent showed baldness; and among 377 women there was but one slightly bald, the baldness being about equally common on vertex and forehead.

In W. I. Thomas's *Source Book for Social Origins* containing articles by various authors, we are told that among some of the Australian tribes old age is a very prominent factor in preëminence. After they have become feeble the old may have great authority, somewhat in proportion to what they know of ancient lore, magic, medicine, and especially if they are totem heads. Their authority is not patriarchal, and yet among the Yakuts, whether they are rich or poor, good or bad, the old are sometimes beaten by their children, especially if feebleminded. On the other hand, a weak man of seventy may beat his forty-year-old son who is strong and rich but in awe of his parent because he has so much to inherit from him. The transfer of authority and property to the son often comes very late. The greatest number of suicides is among the old people. A man who beat his mother said, "Let her cry and go hungry. She made me cry more than once and beat me for trifles," etc.

In this volume we are told, too, that even the Fuegians, who in times of scarcity kill and eat their old women for food, are generally affectionate, and until the whites interfered with their social order the old often had considerable authority. They sometimes prepare programs for ceremonials, which are very strictly observed by a hundred younger men. In some Australian tribes, too, a man's authority generally increases with age; and this is true, though less frequently, of women. The old enforce the strictest marriage rules and have much influence over the thoughts and feelings of the tribes. The old men often sit in a circle and speak on public matters, one after another, the young men standing outside in silence. A few old men may retire to discuss secret matters of importance. Offenders are often brought before them for trial and sentence. The old men of a tribe often band themselves together and by working on the superstitions of the tribe secure for themselves not only comfort but unbounded influence. In the famous Duk-Duk ceremonial they alone were in the secret, and all others were impressed with the supernatural character of the actors in these rites.

Ploss and Bartels [14] amplify the great changes senescence brings to women. Age not only obliterates race but sex. It often makes the most beautiful into the most ugly, for handsome old women among primitives are unknown. Children dread them. They often become careless of looks, the hand is claw-like, etc. A widespread German superstition is that if an old woman crosses the path of a hunter he will get nothing. They

---

[14] *Das Weib in der Natur- und Völkerkunde,* Chap. 74.

are ominous for marriages and some neurotics cannot look at them. They are sometimes said to have seven lives. Hans Sachs in poetry and Cranach in painting, in describing the fountains of youth, represent chiefly old women entering on the one side with every sign of decrepitude and coming out on the other beautiful, with wonderful toilets, and sometimes immediately engaging in orgies. Old women in early times sometimes had a guild, devised means of conjuration, made pacts or leagues with the devil, presided over the Walpurgis festivals, conjured with magic words, had evil eyes, knew strange brews, sometimes committed all kinds of lasciviousness with devils, might transform themselves into shapes as attractive as Circe for Ulysses or Medea for Jason, or take the more ominous forms of Hecate and Lamea. These maleficent creatures often allied themselves with black cats, serpents, owls, bats, had their salves and witch sabbaths, etc.

Frazer approaches this subject from a different angle. In the second chapter of his volume entitled *The Dying God* he tells us that in Fiji self-immolation is by no means rare, and the Fijians believe that as they leave this life they will remain ever after. This is a powerful motive to escape from decrepitude or from a crippled condition by voluntary death. "The custom of voluntary suicide on the part of the old men, which is among their most extraordinary usages, is connected with their superstitions regarding a future life." To this must be added the contempt that attaches to physical weakness among a nation of warriors, and the wrongs and insults that await those who are no longer able to protect themselves. So when a man feels age creeping on, so that he can no longer fully discharge the duties or enjoy the pleasures of life, he calls his relations, tells them he is worn out and useless, that they are ashamed of him, and he is determined to be buried. So on an appointed day they meet and bury him alive. In the New Hebrides the aged were buried alive at their own request. "It was considered a disgrace to a family of an old chief if he was not buried alive." A Jewish tribe of Abyssinia never let a person die a natural death, for if any of their relatives was near expiring the priest of the tribe was called to cut his throat. If this ceremony was omitted, they believed the departed soul had not entered the mansions of the blessed. Heraclitus thought that the souls of those who die in battle are purer than those who die of disease. In a South American tribe, when a man is at the point of death his nearest relatives break his spine with an axe, for to die a natural death is the greatest misfortune. In Paraguay, when a man grows weary of life, a feast is made, with revelry and dancing, and the man is gummed and feathered with the plumage of many birds and a huge jar is fixed in the ground, the mouth of which is closed over him with baked clay. Thus he goes to his doom "more joyful and gladsome than to his first nuptials."

With a tribe in northeastern Asia, when a man feels his last hour has come, he must either kill himself or be killed by a friend. In another tribe he requests his son or some near relative to dispose of him, choosing the manner of death he prefers. So his friends and neighbors assemble and he is stabbed, strangled, or otherwise slain. Elsewhere, if a man dies a natural death, his corpse must be wounded, so that he may seem to be received with the same honors in the next world as if he had died in battle, as Odin wanted for his disciples. The Wends once killed their aged parents and other kinsfolk and boiled and ate their bodies, and the old folk "preferred to die thus rather than drag out a weary life of poverty and decrepitude." Kings are killed when their strength fails. The people of Congo believed that if their pontiff died a natural death, the earth would perish,

since he sustained it by his power and merit, and that
everything would be annihilated. So his successor
entered his house and slew him with a rope or club. "The
king must not be allowed to become ill or senile lest with
his diminishing vigor the cattle should sicken and fail to
bear their increase, the crops should rot in the field, and
man, stricken with disease, should die." So the king
who showed signs of illness or failing strength was put
to death.

One of the fatal symptoms of decay was taken to be incapacity
to satisfy the sexual passion of his wives, of whom he has very
many distributed in a large number of huts at Fashoda. When
this ominous weakness manifested itself, the wives reported it
to the chiefs, who were popularly said to have intimated to the
king his doom by spreading a white cloth over his face and knees
as he lay slumbering in the heat of the sultry afternoon. Execution soon followed the sentence of death. A hut was especially
built for the occasion, the king was led to it and laid down with
his head resting on the lap of a nubile virgin, the door of the hut
was then walled up, and the couple were left without food, fire,
or water, to die of hunger and suffocation.

This custom persisted till five generations ago.
Seligmann shows that the Shilluk king was "liable
to be killed with due ceremony at the first symptoms of
incipient decay." But even while he was yet in the prime
of health and strength he might be attacked at any time
by a rival and have to defend his crown in a combat to
death. According to the common Shilluk tradition, any
son of a king had a right thus to fight the king in possession, and if he succeeded in killing him he reigned in his
stead. As every king had a large harem and many sons,
the number of possible candidates for the throne at any
time may well have been not inconsiderable, and the
reigning monarch must have carried his life in his hand.
But the attack on him could only take place by night
with any prospect of success. Then, according to cus-

tom, his guards had to be dismissed; so the hours of darkness were of special peril. It was a point of honor for the king not to call his herdsmen to his assistance. The age at which the king was killed would seem to have been commonly between forty and fifty. The Zulus put a king to death as soon as he began to have wrinkles and gray hair. Elsewhere kings were often killed at the end of a fixed term, perhaps because it was thought unsafe to wait for the slightest symptom of decay.

A unique and transformed survival of many such customs, according to Frazer, lingered in the vale of Nemi, idealized in Turner's picture. He tells us how in ancient times and long persisting there, like a primeval rock jutting out of a well shaven lawn, the priest-king watched all night with drawn sword. He was a murderer and would himself sooner or later be slain by his successor, for this was the rule of the sanctuary. The candidate for the priesthood could only succeed to office by slaying the priest, and having slain him he retained office until he himself was slain by one stronger or craftier. Although he held the title of king, no crowned head was ever uneasier. The least relaxation of vigilance put him in jeopardy. This rule had no parallel in historic antiquity but we must go farther back. Recent studies show the essential similarity with which, with many superficial differences, the human mind elaborated its first crude philosophy of life. Hence we must study outcrops of the same institution elsewhere, and Frazer tells us that the object of his book is, by meeting these conditions, to offer a fairly probable explanation of the priesthood of Nemi. Once, only a runaway slave could break off the mistletoe from the oak, and success in this enabled him to fight the priest in single combat; if he won he would become King of the Woods.

There are many unique features in the attitude of the Jewish mind toward old age. In Genesis 5: 3 *et seq.* the

ages of the antediluvian patriarchs are given. Adam
lived 930 years; Seth, 912; Enos, 905; Cainan, 970;
Mahalaleel, 895; Jared, 962; Enoch, 365; Methuselah,
969; Lamech, 777. All but four of them "begat" between 65 and 90—Adam at 130, Methuselah at 187,
Jared at 182, Noah at 500. By nearly all modern
scholars these great ages have been regarded as mythical, but so scientific and modern a student as T. E.
Young,[15] who is very skeptical about all later records of
great longevity, devotes a long chapter to these records,
which he is almost inclined to credit. He goes to
original sources, gives various hypotheses, epitomizes
diverse writers on the subject, and finally raises the
question whether or not in ancient days atmospheric
conditions, food, and a different and more uniform
climate might not have caused an unprecedented prolongation of human life. He does not, of course, credit
the ancient literature of India, where holy men are said
to have lived eighty thousand years and where in the
most flourishing period of Indian antiquity the term of
one hundred thousand was regarded as the average
length of the life of saints. He fully recognizes, too, the
influence of mystic numbers here, which persisted until
the age of the higher criticism, and is incredulous about
most of the modern records of centenarians. His point
of view is that man has now passed his acme and that a
slow decline of the human race, which will end in its
extinction, has already begun, masked as it is by modern
hygiene, which prolongs life beyond the average term
it would otherwise have reached. Thus human vitality
as measured by length of life is slowly but irresistibly
waning.[16]

---

[15] *On Centenarians and the Duration of the Human Race,* 1899.

[16] A few even recent writers have gone to the extreme of doubting the
authenticity of every record of human life beyond a century, although
Young seems to have demonstrated it in his twenty-two annuitants. All

THE HISTORY OF OLD AGE

The correspondence between organism and environment, which makes life perfect, was probably once better than now. Bacteriology is a factor never to be forgotten and there may be a new acidity of juices. Perhaps the energy of the sun is decreasing and also the productivity of the earth. Indeed, it is very probable that the solar system has attained its maturity or midway stage. From such data Young concludes, "The average intellectual condition of the present period, I should be inclined to surmise, exhibits no sign whatever of an ampler development." Knowledge has become mechanical and has lost its capacity as the instrument of self-cultivation. The highest faculties are decaying from cessation of activity and coherent function. Man has reached his limit. The utilities of civilization are

---

such contentions are only doctrinnaire. Lives exceptionally prolonged may be abnormal, like dwarfs and giants, and extreme skepticism here has hardly more justification than extreme credulity. In 1799 James Easton believed he had demonstrated that 712 persons between the years A.D. 66 and the above date had attained a century or upward. He found three whom he thought had lived between 170 and 175 years; two who had lived 160 to 170; three, 150–160; seven, 140–150; twenty-six, 130–140; eighty-four, 120–130; and thirteen hundred and ten, 100–110. Even Babbage assumed 150 as the limit of age in his abstract tables based upon seventeen hundred and fifty-one persons who had attained 100 or more. A. Haller (1766) accepted the age of Parr and Jenkins and is quite uncritical, saying that over one thousand men have lived to be 100–110, and twenty-five have lived to between 130–140. He even accepts Pliny's story of a man who lived to be 300, and another 340 years. Hufeland seems to approve the traditional 157 years of Epimenides, 108 of Gorgias, 139 of Democritus, 100 of Zeno, 105 of St. Anthony, and credited J. Effingham in Cornwall with 144 years. W. J. Thoms (*Human Longevity: Its Facts and Its Fictions,* 1873) is skeptical of great longevities and found no sure case of centenarians in any noble family. J. Pinney (1856) went to the limit of credulity, believing that there were three eras in which men lived to 900, 450, and 70 respectively. G. C. Lewis thinks there is no authentic record of a life exceeding 100 years. W. Farr in 1871 said that in 1821 there were 216 centenarians in England; in 1841, 249; 1851, 215; 1861, 201; 1871, 160, making a total of 1,041, of whom 716 were females. Walford (in his *Insurance Guide and Handbook*) compiled a list of 218 centenarians from what he deemed authentic sources, and J. B. Bailey in 1888 in his *Modern Methuselahs* discussed the question; while Humphry (1889) in his nine hundred returns, found 52 centenarians, 36 of whom were women.

51

also hindrances, so that the forces of evolution have spent their power.

The Hebrew conception of Yahveh generally made him old, the ancient of days without beginning or end; and the art of early Christendom where God the Father appears, usually represents Him as venerable with age, this trait being probably accentuated by contrast with His son, Jesus, who died in the prime of life. The ancient Hebrews had great respect for age, and many Biblical heroes from Abraham to Moses and some of the prophets were old in years and wisdom. The exhortation was to rise up before the hoary head and honor the face of the old man, and this has its nursery echo in the story of Elisha (II, Kings, 2: 23–24) whom little children came out of the city and mocked, saying "Go up, thou bald-head." He "turned back and cursed them in the name of the Lord, and there came forth two she-bears out of the wood and tare forty and two children of them." No passage in all the literature of the world has had such influence as Psalms 90: 10.[17] It is pathetic to see how incessantly this passage is quoted in the literature on old age and how not only among the Jews but perhaps quite as much, if not more, among the Christians, bibliolatry has made it accepted almost as a decree of fate.

Next most influential is the pessimistic view of senescence represented in Ecclesiastes, 12: 1–8. We quote Professor Paul Haupt's version,[18] with his explanations in parentheses:

Remember thy well (the wife and mother of thy children) in the days of thy vigor, ere there come the days of evil, and the years draw nigh in which thou wilt say I have no pleasure. Ere

---

[17] "The days of our years are three-score years and ten, and if by reason of strength they may be four-score years, yet is there strength, labor, and sorrow for it is cut off and we fly away."

[18] *Oriental Studies,* Boston, 1894.

is darkened the sun (sunshine of childhood), and the light of the day, and the moon (more tempered light of boyhood and early manhood), and the stars (the sporadic moments of happiness in mature age), and the clouds return after the rain (for the old, clouds and rainy days increase) ; when the keepers of the house (hands) tremble, and the men of power (the bones, especially the backbone) bend themselves; the grinding maids (teeth) cease and the ladies that look out through the lattices (eyes) are darkened; the doors are shut toward the street (secretion and excretion cease) ; he riseth at the voice of the birds (awakens too early), and all the daughters of song are brought low (grows deaf), he is afraid of that which is high, and fears are in the way (avoids climbing and high places) ; the almond tree blossometh (he grows gray), the locust crawleth along with difficulty, the caper-berry breaketh up (the soul is freed), the silver (spinal) cord is snapped asunder, the golden bowl (brain) crushed in, the bucket at the well smashed (heart grows weak), and the wheel breaketh down at the pit (machinery runs down). Man is going to his eternal house (the grave), and the mourners go about in the street. Vanity of vanities (all is transitory), saith Ecclesiastes, all is vanity, and all that is coming is vanity.

L. Löw [19] collects from the Scripture and post-Biblical Talmud, German and other literature, instances of rejuvenescence in the old which ancient Hebrew writers seem to have stressed. We all know that sight sometimes comes back, perhaps to a marked degree, but Löw quotes cases where wrinkles vanished, the hair was restored to its youthful shade and increased in quantity, while teeth, after years of decay, have sometimes grown from new roots—occasionally more than once. In many cases sex potency has been restored as well as muscular strength, freshness of complexion, and, more rarely, hearing. Myths, of course, of many races detail cases where magic sleep lasting many, perhaps a hundred, years has converted age into youth, and in Semitic folklore this is often connected with the passage, "The righteous shall renew their strength like the eagle." The

*Das Lebensalter in der Jüdischen Literatur, 1875.

Hebrews were perhaps even more fond than other people of dividing life into periods, usually in conformity to the magic numbers 3, 4, 7, etc. The comparison of age with the four seasons was very common, and here we may perhaps mention Lotze's effort to harmonize the life span with the four temperaments. For him, childhood is sanguine on account of the ease of excitation, the keenness of response to sensation, the ready passage of impulse to action, and the fluctuations of mood. Youth he calls melancholic and emotionally characterized by *Stimmungen.* It judges the items of experience by their effect upon feeling and upon self, and oscillates readily and widely from pleasure to pain. Mature manhood is choleric, practical, executive, with definiteness of aim and fulfillment of ideas and even phantasies but with less excitability of emotion; while old age is phlegmatic, seeks repose, and has been taught by experience to abate the life of affectivity and take the attitude of *laissez faire.*

In the modern Jewish family the authority of and respect for the father is great, more among the orthodox and conservative than the liberal and reformed wing of Judaism. The grandfather and -mother are always provided for, although their authority and influence are generally greatly diminished.

Perhaps mention should here be made of the very interesting medieval legend of Ahasuerus, the Wandering Jew, although it is of Christian origin. This cobbler, past whose shop Jesus bore the Cross on the way to Calvary, reproached Him, and Jesus, turning, sentenced him to "tarry till I come," which meant that his punishment was to remain alive on earth until the second coming of the Messiah. In some of the many forms of this tradition he is represented at the time as being of about Jesus' age and every time he reached a hundred as being set back again to this stage of life; while in others he is described with ever increasing symptoms of age, and in Doré's illustrations he is depicted as wandering the earth, appearing here and there and, when recognized, generally mysteriously vanishing, ever seeking death, visiting graveyards and regions smitten with plague and famine, rushing into the mêlée of battles, etc.—but all in vain. He longs with an ever increasing passion to pay the debt of nature but is unable to do so and must rove the earth until the Judgment Day, when he hopes his penalty may be remitted and that he may keep some "rendezvous with Death." [20]

In ancient Greece we may begin with Sparta and its very unique *gerousia,* the council of twenty-eight old men who must be over sixty, when the duty to bear arms ceased and when by the original law of Sparta men were put to death. This council of old men at the height of its power is sometimes compared with that of the boulé in Athens but was even greater, for although it held its mandate from the people and its members were annually elected, they could depose the five ephors and the kings and even cause them to be put to death. J. P. Mahaffy [21] condemns the parochial politics of Sparta, where ignorant old men watched over and secured the closest adhesion of the state to the system of a semifabulous legislator, and compares the rigidity of the Spartan system, not based on written laws, with the effects of excessive reverence of ancestors in China in retarding progress. [22] He thinks that here we have "one of the

---

[20] M. D. Conway, *The Wandering Jew,* 1881, and T. Kappstein, *Ahesver in der Weltpoesie,* 1906.

[21] *Greek Life and Thought,* London, 1896.

[22] E. Bard, in *Chinese Life in Town and Country,* p. 39, says, "In the worship of ancestors we have the keystone to the arch of the social structure of this strange country [China]. Hundreds of millions of living Chinese are bound to thousands of millions of dead ones. The cult induces parents to marry off their children almost before maturity so that they should have offspring to make their lives after death pleasant by means of worship and oblations. No matter how great the squalor,

most signal instances in history of the vast mischief done by the government of old men. All the leading patriots, nay all the leading politicians, were past their prime. There was not a single young man of ability taking part in public affairs." This, he thinks, was more or less true of Athens in the early days, and he goes on to say that if any young orator tried to advance new ideas, the old masters, who had the ear of the assembly, were out upon him as a hireling and traitor so that he had to retire from the agora into private life, and some were thus driven into exile. He even holds that the sudden growth of the philosophic schools a little later was due to the activities that but for this diversion would have been directed to politics.

But in Greece at its best opposite influences were at work and generally predominated. In the Homeric age "the king or chief, as soon as his bodily vigor passed away, was apparently pushed aside by younger and stronger men. He might either maintain himself by extraordinary usefulness, like Nestor, or be supported by his children, if they chanced to be affectionate and dutiful; but except in these cases his lot was sad indeed." [23] Achilles laments that nearby chiefs are ill-treating the aged Peleus, and we see Laertes, the father of Ulysses, exiled to a barren farm in the country and spending the later years of his life in poverty and hardship. Hence when we see princes who had sons that might return any day to avenge them treated in such a way, we must infer that unprotected old age commanded

there must be many children in the family," etc. "Funeral expenses for parents are the most sacred of all obligations, and it is not uncommon for the living to sell their estates to the very last foot and often their houses to be able to render proper homage to the deceased." Presents of coffins, elaborate ones, are often very common. The sons of a deceased parent must at least wear mourning for three years, though this has been lately reduced to twenty-seven months. The expenses of elaborate funerals are enormous.

[23] Mahaffy, *Social Life in Greece from Homer to Menander,* p. 34.

very little veneration among the Homeric Greeks, so that worn-out men received scant consideration.   Among friends and neighbors in peace and in good humor they were treated with consideration, but with the first clash of interests all this vanished.   Interference of the gods to protect their weakness was no longer believed in. Thus the exact prescription of the conduct of the young toward the elders in Sparta was an exception, and their treatment of old age as illustrated by the well-worn story of an old man coming into the theater at Athens and looking in vain for a seat until he came near the Spartan embassy, which at once rose and made room for him, was suggestive.   It was well added that while the Athenians applauded this act it is doubtful if they imitated it.   Probably the disparagement of old age prompted Athenian gentlemen to resort to every means to prolong their youth.   Zeus came to rule the turbulent and self-willed lesser gods on Olympus, who were perpetually trying to evade and thwart him, by occasionally terrifying them, and he seemed to be able to count on no higher principle of loyalty.

The Greeks loved wealth because it gave pleasure, and perhaps in this fact we have one key to another horror that old age had for them.   Mimnermus tells us to enjoy the delights of love, for "when old age with its pains comes upon us it mars even the fair, wretched cares besiege the mind; nor do we delight in beholding the rays of the sun but are hateful to boys and despised among women, so sore a burden have the gods made old age." "When youth has fled, short-lived as a dream, forthwith this burdensome and hideous old age looms over us hateful and dishonored, which changes the fashion of man's countenance, marring his sight and his mind with its mist."   Pindar asks why those who must of necessity meet the fate of death should desire "to sit in obscurity vainly brooding through a forgotten old age without sharing a single blessing." He and Aeschylus take a somewhat less unfavorable view of age, although even Pindar calls it "detested." Sophocles is the only dramatist who, at least in one passage, welcomes its approach, although there are nowhere bitterer words concerning it than those of the chorus of Œdipus at Coloneus, "That is the final lot of man, even old age, hateful, impotent, unsociable, friendless, wherein all evil of evil dwells." Thus, in general, Greek writers take a very gloomy view of it, never calling it beautiful, peaceful, or mellow, but rather dismal and oppressive. The best they say of it is that it brings wisdom.

R. W. Livingstone[24] says:

> When youth wore away, he [the Greek] felt that what made life most worth living was gone. In part perhaps it was that old age had terrors for the Greeks which we do not feel. They were without eyeglasses, ear-trumpets, bath-chairs, and an elaborate system of *apéritifs,* which modern science has devised to assist our declining years. Yet even with these consolations it may be doubted whether the Greek would have faced old age with pleasure. At least to judge from Greek literature, he lamented its minor discomforts less than the loss of youth's intense capacity for action and enjoyment. People who prize beauty and health so highly can hardly think otherwise when age comes.

Again, old men in Greece had to contend with the younger generation upon even terms and without the large allowance conceded them by modern sentiment and good manners. At Athens legal proceedings of children to secure the property of their parents were very common—and that, too, without medical evidence of incapacity. Aristophanes complains of the treatment of older men by the newer generation and in his *Wasps* makes an old man say that his only chance of respect or even safety is to retain the power of acting as a juryman,

---

[24] *The Greek Genius and Its Meaning to Us,* 1912.

so exacting homage from the accused and supporting himself by his pay without depending on his children. When he comes home with his fee they are glad to see him. Indeed, thus he might support a second wife and younger children and not be dependent for his daily bread upon his son's steward. In the tragedies the old kings are represented as acquiescing, though not without complaint, in the weakness of their position and submitting to insults from foes and rivals. There seems no such thing as patient submission for an aged sovereign. Nor did his own excellence nor the score of former battles secure for him the allegiance of his people when his vigor had passed. This was all because in spite of the modicum of respect that all must yield to old age at its best, the violent nature of the Periclean politics and the warlike temper of early days made vigor in their leaders a necessity. The nation was strong, always seeking to advance and enlarge, and its maxim seemed to be that of Hesiod, "Work for youth; counsel for maturity; prayers for old age." The Greeks, realizing the danger of relying too much upon experience as the source of wisdom, saw that when the maturity of age is passed and the power of decision begins to wane, trusting to the leadership of the old may be dangerous. By a law often relied on, old men could be brought into court by their children and be found incapable of managing their property, which was then transferred to their heirs; and this helps to explain why sometimes old people, beginning to feel their uselessness, committed suicide rather than become an encumbrance.

Plato [25] makes one of his characters say:

I and a few other people of my own age are in the habit of frequently meeting together. On these occasions most of us give way to lamentations and regret the pleasures of youth, and call

---

[25] *Republic,* 329.

up the memory of love affairs, drinking parties, and similar proceedings. They are grievously discontented at the loss of what they consider great privileges and describe themselves as having lived well in those days whereas now they can hardly be said to live at all. Some also complain of the manner in which their relations insult their infirmities or make this a ground for reproaching old age with the many miseries it occasions them.

Plato did not himself agree with this view but thought the cause of this discontent lay not in age itself but in character. Still the humanist view of life does tend to some such position, and the Greeks really felt that it was better to be the humblest citizen of Athens than to rule in Hades.

Two unique characters stand out with great clearness and significance. The first is that of the Homeric Nestor, who had lived through three generations of men and in whom Anthon says Homer intended to exemplify the greatest perfection of which human nature is capable. His wisdom was great, as was his age, and both grew together. In his earlier years he had been as great in war as he became in counsel later. Very different is the figure of Tithonus, whom Tennyson has made the theme of one of his oft-quoted poems. He was a mortal, the son of a king, but Aurora became so enamored of him that she besought Zeus to confer upon him the gift of immortality. The ruler of Olympus granted her prayer and Tithonus became exempt from death. But the goddess had forgotten to crave youth along with immortality and accordingly, after his children had been born, old age slowly began to mar the visage and form of her lover and spouse. When she saw him thus declining she still remained true to him, kept him "in her palace, on the eastern margin of the Ocean stream, 'giving him ambrosial food and fair garments.' But when he was no longer able to move his limbs she deemed it the wisest course to shut him up in his chamber, whence his feeble voice was incessantly heard. Later poets say that out of compassion she turned him into a cicada."

It is gratifying to turn from the depressing attitude toward old age that was characteristic of the Hellenic mind as a whole, because it came nearer than any other to being the embodiment of eternal youth, and to glance at the unique and, we must believe on the whole, very wholesome and suggestive relation that so often subsisted between men, not to be sure very old (unless in the case of Socrates) but aging and young men and even boys.

It was assumed that every well-born and -bred young male must have an older man as his mentor and to be without one was, to some degree, regarded as discreditable. Thus juniors sometimes came to vie with each other in their efforts to win the regard of their seniors, especially if they were prominent; while the latter, in turn, felt that it was a part of their duty to the community and to the state to respond to such advances, even to make them. These friendships between ephebics and sages were, at their best, highly advantageous to both. The man embodied the boy's ideal at that stage of life when he realized that all excellencies were not embodied in his father and when home relations were merging into those of citizenship. To win the personal attention and interest of a great man who would occasionally exercise the function of teacher, foster parent, guardian, godfather, adviser, or patron, brought not only advantage but distinction if the youth was noble and beautiful. On the other hand, Plato thought no man would wish to do or say a discreditable thing in the presence of a youth who admired him but would wish to be a pattern or inspirer of virtue. He seems to have been the first to realize that there is really nothing in the world quite so worthy of love, reverence, and service, as ingenuous youth fired with the right ambitions and smitten with a passion to both know and be the best possible. The period between the dawn of sex and complete nubility has always been the chief opportunity of the true teacher or initiator of its apprentice into life.

Here we must recall the very pregnant sense in which, as I have tried in my *Adolescence* to set forth at greater length, education in its various implications began in the initiations of youth by their elders into the pubertal stage of life and slowly extended upward toward the university, and downward toward the kindergarten, as civilization advanced. The world has always felt that these pre-marital years, when the young have such peculiar needs and are subjected to so many dangers, are the great opportunity for the transmission of knowledge and influence from the older to the younger generation.

Thus while Socrates loved to mingle with men of all classes and ages, his most congenial companions were those of a younger generation. With the gracious boy, Charmides, "beautiful in mind and body, a charming combination of moral dignity and artless sprightliness," he discussed temperance in the presence of his guardian, Critias. With Theætetus, "the younger Socrates," like his master more beautiful in mind than in body, he conversed about the nature of knowledge, in the presence of his tutor. With the fair and noble young Lysis, invoked to do so by his lover, Hypothales, he discourses on the right words or acts best calculated to ingratiate himself with his ward, and the theme is friendship. In the presence and with the coöperation of four youths he discusses courage with General Laches, and to young Clineas and his adviser he narrates his amusing encounter with Euthydemus and his brother, the bumptious young Sophists, the "eristic sluggers." He explains the true nature of his own art to Ion, the Homeric rhapsodist. In the Meno he brings out the essential points of the forty-seventh proposition of Euclid from the mind of an ignorant slave boy.[26]

This relation of old and younger men was thought to keep youth plastic, docile, and receptive, if not a trifle feminine. Plato would have these pairs of friends fight side by side to inspire each other with courage. But this relation, as we all know, had its dangers and often lapsed to homosexuality and inversion. In the Symposium, Alcibiades, that most beautiful and alluring of male coquettes, describes Socrates as a paragon of chastity because he remained cold and unmoved by all the seductive blandishments he could bring to bear upon him. This vice, now so fully explored by Krafft-Ebing, Tarnowski, Moll, Ellis, and Freud and his disciples, is favored by war, the seclusion of women as in Turkey, and even by female virtue; but the Platonic view was that true love was a wisdom or philosophy, although possibly they did not realize that even the custom of the Sophists, who first took pay for teaching—a practice they thought profanation—was nevertheless a step toward the reform of degraded boy love.

The chief function of wise and older men toward their juniors, they thought, was to prevent the premature hardening of opinions into convictions and to keep their minds open and growing. As we now often say that the chief function of religion and sex is to keep each other pure, so they thought that wisdom culminated in eros, which in turn found its highest deployment in the love of knowledge, which Aristotle later described as the theoretic life, the attainment of which he deemed the supreme felicity of man. From all this it follows that those who achieve complete ideal senescence are those who have entirely sublimated eroticism into the passion for truth and pursue it with the same ardor that in their

---

[26] *Talks with Athenian Youth*, tr. anon., New York, 1893, 178 p.

prime attracted them to the most beautiful of the other sex; and that their chief function to the next generation is to lay in it the foundations for the same gradual transfer and transformation of it as old age advances.

Aristotle's [27] physical theory of old age is that heat is lost by gradual dissipation, very little remaining in old age—a flickering flame that a slight disturbance could put out. The lung hardens by gradual evaporation of the fluid and so is unable to perform its office of heat regulation. He assumes that heat is gradually developed in the heart. The amount produced is always somewhat less than that which is given off and the deficiency has to be made good out of the stock with which the organism started originally, that is, from the innate heat in which the soul was incorporate. This eventually is so reduced by constant draughts made upon it that it is insufficient to support the soul. The natural span of life, he says, differs greatly in length in different species, due to material constitution and the degree of harmony with the environment. But still, as a general rule, big plants and animals live longer than smaller ones; sanguineous or vertebrates longer than invertebrates; the more perfect longer than the less perfect; and long gestation generally goes with long duration. Thus bulk, degree of organization, period of gestation, are correlated. Great size goes with high organization.

In his *Rhetoric*,[28] as is well known, Aristotle gives old age an unfavorable aspect. He says in substance that the old have lived many years and been often the victims of deception, and since vice is the rule rather than the exception in human affairs, they are never positive about anything. They "suppose" and add "perhaps" or "possibly," always expressing themselves in doubt and never

---

[27] *Aristotle on Youth and Old Age, Life and Death and Respiration*, tr. by Ogle, London, 1897, 135 p.
[28] Book II, Chap. 13.

64

positively. They are uncharitable and ever ready to put the worst construction upon everything. They are suspicious of evil, not trusting, because of their experience of human weakness. Hence they have no strong loves or hates but go according to the precept of bias. Their love is such as may one day become hate and their hatred such as may one day become love. The temper of mind is neither grand nor generous—not the former because they have been too much humiliated and have no desire to go according to anything but mere appearances, and not the latter because property is a necessity of life and they have learned the difficulty of acquiring it and the facility with which it may be lost. They are cowards and perpetual alarmists, exactly contrary to the young; not fervent, but cold. They are never so fond of life as on their last day. Again, it is the absent which is the object of all desire, and what they most lack they most want. They are selfish and inclined to expediency rather than honor; the former having to do with the individual and the latter being absolute. They are apt to be shameless rather than the contrary and are prone to disregard appearances. They are dependent for most things. They live in memory rather than by hope, for the remainder of their life is short while the past is long, and this explains their garrulity. Their fits of passion though violent are feeble. Their sensual desires have either died or become feeble but they are regulated chiefly by self-interest. Hence they are capable of self-control, because desires have abated and self-interest is their leading passion. Calculation has a character that regulates their lives, for while calculation is directed to expediency, morality is directed to virtue as its end. Their offenses are those of petty meanness rather than of insolence. They are compassionate like the young, but the latter are so from humanity while the old suppose all manner of sufferings at their door. When the orator addresses them he should bear these traits in mind. Elsewhere [29] he says a happy old age is one that approaches gradually and without pain and is dependent upon physical excellence and on fortune, although there is such a thing as a long life even without health and strength.

Thus, on the whole, the Greeks took a very somber view of old age. They prized youth as perhaps no other race has ever done and loved to heighten their appreciation of it by contrasting it with life in its "sere and yellow leaf." Pindar says in substance that darkness, old age, and death never seemed so black as by contrast with the glories of the great festivals and games which every few years brought together all those who loved either gold or glory. Socrates, who refused to flee from his fate and calmly drank hemlock at the age of seventy, and Plato, who lived to be an octogenarian, must, on the whole, be regarded as exceptions, and conceptions of a future life were never clear and strong enough to be of much avail against the pessimism that in bright Hellas clouded the closing scenes of life's drama.

When we turn to Rome, we have, on the whole, a more favorable view. Even in the early stages of Roman life, family and parental authority were well developed and in Roman law the *patria potestas* gave the head of the family great dignity and power. This term designates the aggregate of those peculiar powers and rights that, by the civil law of Rome, belonged to the head of a family in respect to his wife, children (natural or adopted) and more remote descendants who sprang from him through males only. Anciently it was of very extensive scope, embracing even the power of life and death; but this was greatly curtailed until finally it meant but little more than a right of the *paterfamilias* to hold his own

---

[29] *Ibid.*, Book I, Chap. 5.

property or the acquisitions of one under his power.[30]

The Roman Senate was, as the etymology of the word suggests, a body of old men; and as the Romans had an unprecedented genius for social and political organization, the wisdom necessary for exercising successfully administrative functions, which age alone can give, had greater scope. In this respect the Catholic Church later and its canon law were profoundly influenced by and, indeed, as Zeller has shown in his remarkable essay on the subject, derived most of its prominent features directly from the political organization of ancient Rome, also giving great authority to presbyters, elders, and affording exceptional scope to the organizing ability that comes to its flower in later life. Jesus was young and Keim believes that all His disciples were even younger. Those who created ecclesiastical institutions, however, were far older.

In Cicero's *De Senectute* [31] we have a remarkably representative statement put into the mouth of the old man, Cato, as to how aging Romans regarded their estate, and I think the chief impression in reading this remarkable document is the vast fund of instances of signal achievements of old men that are here brought together. This will be apparent from the following brief résumé.

Cato in his old age is approached by youths who want to know what he can tell them about life. He commends their interest in age and tells them he has himself just begun to learn Greek, on which he spent much time in later years. After the first few pages the treatise becomes almost entirely a monologue of Cato. Every state is irksome to those who have no support within and do not see that they owe happiness to themselves. We must not say old age creeps on after manhood, manhood

---

[30] See Black's *Law Dictionary*, 2d ed., 1910.
[31] Cicero, *Cato Major or Old Age*, tr. by Benjamin Franklin.

after youth, youth after childhood, etc. Each age has its own interests—spring for blossoms, autumn for fruit. The wise submit and do not, like the giants, war against the gods. There are very many instances of those who outlived enjoyment and found themselves forsaken, but of more who won notable renown and respect. Perhaps the greatest merit of this book is the instances of noble old age that abound.

Many are great owing to the reputation of their country and would be small in other lands. To the very poor old age can never be very attractive. Think on your good deeds. When Marcus died, Cato long knew no other man to improve by. The four evils charged to old age are: (1) it disables from business, (2) it makes the body infirm, (3) it robs of pleasure, (4) it is near death. He takes these up in detail. The downfall of great states is "generally owing to the giddy administration of inexperienced young men"; and, on the contrary, tottering states have been saved by the old. The young are all ignorant orators. Memory fails in age only if not exercised, and this is true of all abilities. Sophocles wrote his Œdipus to defy those who called him a dotard. Democritus, Plato, Socrates, Zeno, and Cleanthes are cited. Many old men cannot submit to idleness but grow old learning something new every day, like Solon. Although the voice may be low, it may have more command. We should no more repine when middle life leaves us than we do when childhood departs. The adult does not mourn that he is no longer a boy. All must prepare themselves against old age and mitigate its natural infirmities.

The stage delights in weak, dissolute old fellows worthy of contempt and ridicule. Age must support its proper rights and dignities and not give them weakly away. We must recall at night all we have said or done during the day. As to the third, old age being incapable

68

of pleasure, the great curse is indulgence of passion, for which men have betrayed their country. Governments have been ruined by treachery, for lust may prompt to any villainy. Reason is the best gift of heaven, but the highest rapture of feeling makes reflection impossible. Cato then describes with much detail the charm of country life—Cincinnatus, etc. We might well wish our enemies were guided by pleasure only for then we could master them more easily. The old man is dead to certain enjoyments. He does not so much prize the convivium for food as for talk. We must not choose only companions of our own age for there will be few of these left. A talk should turn to the subjects proposed by the master of the feast, the cups be cooling. He says "I thank the gods I am got rid of that tyranny" (venery). He does not want or even wish it in any form.

Far above the delights of literature or philosophy are the charms of country life, and he describes at length the various methods of vine culture, fertilization, improving barren soil, irrigation, orchards, cattle, bees, gardens, flowers, tree planting, etc. The farmer can say, like the ancient Semites when offered gold, that they wanted none for it was more glorious to command those who valued it than to possess it. Then follow many instances of old people who have retired to the country and perhaps even have been called from their farms to great tasks of state. He advises reading Xenophon. An old age thus spent is the happiest period if attended with honor and respect. Old men are miserable if they demand the defense of oratory. In the college of augurs old men have great dignity. Some wines sour with age but others grow better and richer. A gravity with some severity is allowed, but never ill nature. Covetousness is most absurd because what is left of life needs little.

The young should be trained to envisage death. Youth in its greatest vigor is subjected to more diseases than old age. If men too young governed the state, all government would fall. The old have already attained what the young only hope for, namely, long years. No actor can play more than one rôle at once. It takes more water to put out a hot fire than a spent one. The young are more prone to die by violence, the old by over-ripeness. The old can oppose tyrants because these can only kill; and their life, being shorter, is worth far less. The young and old should meditate on death till it becomes familiar and this only makes the mind free and easy. Many a soldier has rushed into the mêlée, with no result, when he knew he would be cut to pieces, and Marcus Atilius Regulus went back to his enemies for certain torture and death because he had promised. There is a certain satiety of each stage of life, and always one is fading as another warms up.

Perhaps, Cato concludes, our minds are an efflux of some universal mind, and there may be an argument for preëxistence. We have not only interest in, but a kind of right to, posterity. The wisest accept death most easily, although it is by no means clear whether we are dissolved or there is a personal continuation.

Roman authors quote "many cases of great longevity," and Onomocritus, an Athenian, tells us that certain men of Greece, and even entire families, enjoyed perpetual youth for centuries. Old Papalius was believed to have lived 500 years and a Portugee, Faria, 300. Pliny tells us of a king who died in his eighty-second year. Strabo says that in the Punjab people lived over 200 years. Epaminondas had seen three centuries pass. Pliny tells us that when, in the reign of Vespasian, statistics of all centenarians between the Apennines and the Po were collected, there were more than a hundred and seventy of them out of a population of three million, six of whom lived over 150 years. According to Lucian, Tiresias lived 600 years on account of the purity of his life, and the inhabitants of Mount Ethos had the faculty of living a century and a half. He tells us of an Indian race, the Seres who, because of temperate life and very scanty food, lived 300 years, while Pliny tells of an Illyrian who lived 500 and the king of Cyprus who outlived 160 years. Litorius of Aetolia was happiest among mortals for he had attained 200 years. Apolonius, the grammarian, outdoes all others and tells of people who lived thousands of years.

Of the condition and status of old people all through the Christian centuries down to the age of authentic statistics we know very little.

Roger Bacon tells us of a remarkable man who appeared in Europe in 1245 and in whom everyone was interested. He claimed that he had attended the Council of Paris in A.D. 362 and also the baptism of Clovis. Bacon's skepticism reduced the claim of this unknown man to 300 years. In 1613 was published at Turin the life of a man who is said to have lived nearly 400 years, enjoying full use of all his faculties; and in the seventeenth century a Scotchman, MacCrane, lived 200 years and talked of the Wars of the Roses. So the lives of the saints are rich in old people—St. Simeon is said to have lived 107 years; St. Narcissus, 165; St. Anthony, 105; the hermit, Paul, 113; while the monks of Mount Ethos often reached the age of 150, as did the first bishop of Ethiopia. Although there are, of course, no vital statistics, there are many reasons to believe that the average length of human life was shorter and that old people in general, although, of course, not without remarkable exceptions, enjoyed little respect. Descriptions of them sometimes appear in miracle plays, more commonly in the form of caricatures, as is often the case on the modern stage, where the personification of old people is often a specialty. There are dotards and fatuities galore and the more dignified figures like King Lear or even Shylock are represented as morally perverse or mentally unsound.

Here should be mentioned the remarkable theory of witchcraft elaborated by Karl Pearson.[32] W. Notestein [33] tells us that by accounting as carefully as the insufficient evidence permits it would seem that "about six times as many women were indicted as men," and also that there were "twice as many married women as spinsters," which is less in accord with tradition. From his account, as well as from the old chapter of C. Mackay on the "Witch Mania" (in his *Popular Delusions*) and also from an interesting study by G. L. Kittredge,[34] it would seem that the first accusations of witchcraft were made against old, middle-aged, and young women almost indiscriminately, while in a later stage of the delusion attention focused on old women, influenced by folklore, which tends to make them hags.

Pearson's theory, developed with great ingenuity, is that witchcraft is a revival of a very old and widespread matriarchate wherein woman not only ruled but society was everywhere permeated by her genius, and paternity was unknown. The key to this older civilization was the development of woman's intuitive faculty under the stress of child-bearing and -rearing. The mother-age in its diverse forms has been a stage of social growth for probably all branches of the human race. With its mother-right customs it made a social organization in which there was more unity of interest, fellowship, partnership in property and sex than we find in the larger social units of to-day. Hence feminists may well look back to this as a golden age, despite the fact that it was in many respects cruel and licentious. It shows that those who talk of absolute good and bad and an

---

[32] "Woman as Witch" in his *Chances of Death*, 1897, vol. 2, pp. 1-50.
[33] *History of Witchcraft in England, 1557-1718*, p. 114.
[34] *Notes on Witchcraft*, Amer. Antiquarian Society.

unchanging moral code may help to police but can never reform society.

Pearson proceeds to argue that certain forms of medieval witchcraft are fossils of the old mother-age and more or less perverted rites and customs of a prehistoric civilization, and even holds that the confessions wrung from poor old women by torture have a real scientific value for the historian of a far earlier stage of life. Primitive woman, thus, once had a status far higher and very different from anything she has since enjoyed. Man as husband and father had no place but came later. Aging women in the matriarchate were depositaries of tribal lore and family custom, and the "wise one," "sibyl," or "witch" passed all this along, as she did her herb-lore. She domesticated the small animals—goat, goose, cat, hen; devised the distaff, spindle, pitchfork, broom (but not the spear, axe, or hammer); and presided over rites in which there were symbols of agricultural and animal fertility and abundant traces of licentiousness and impurity in the sacred dances and ceremonies. "Witch" means "wiseacre," "one who knows," and some were good and some bad dames or beldames. The former brought good luck; the latter, famine, plague, etc. All witches have weather wisdom, and a descendant of the Vola or Sibyl is, in the Edda, seated in the midst of the assembly of the gods and could produce thunder, hail, and rain. Tacitus tells us of men who took the part of priestesses, probably in female attire. Kirmes is a festival lasting several days, primarily for dedicating a church, although it has many features of the celebration of a goddess, who in Christian demonology was first converted into the devil's mother or grandmother and invested with most of the functions of old witches. These, in the witches' sabbath, came more to devolve upon her son. In Swabia the witch stone is an old altar and the ceremonies about it suggest marriage. The devil is a professional sweetheart; his mother, a person of great importance, was supposed once to have built a palace on the Danube, to hunt with black dogs, and to be related to Frau Holda. She watered the meadows in "Twelfth Night" and punished idle spinsters. The devil's mother is only a degraded form of the goddess of fertility and domestic activity and her worship was once associated not only with licentiousness but with human sacrifice. It was these women who were primarily in league with the devil and once a year must dance all night. The hag is the woman of the woods who knows and collects herbs, especially those that relieve the labors of childbirth. The priestess of the old civilization became a medicine woman and midwife, the goddess of fertility being killed in the autumn that she may be rejuvenated in the spring. Thus the witch is a relic of the priestess or goddess of fertility, and the hostility they sometimes exhibit for marriage was because at this stage it was not monogamic but group marriage.

Thus Pearson thinks that Walpurgis customs bring out most of the weak and strong points of ancient woman's civilization, fossils of which lurk under all the folklore of witchcraft. Here we find the rudiments of medicine, domestication of small animals, cultivation of vegetables, domestic and household arts, the pitchfork —which was once the fire-rake—etc. All of these are woman's inventions and were necessary for the higher discoveries. Although he did not invent them, man later made woman use them. The primitiye savage knows nothing of agriculture, spinning, and herbs, but his wife does. It is not he but she who made these symbols of a female deity. The fertility, resource, and inventiveness of woman arose from the struggle she had to make for the preservation of herself and her child. Man was quickened by warfare of tribe against tribe, but that came later. The first struggle was for food and shelter. Thus the father-age rests on a degenerate form of an older group and is not the pure outcome of male domination. He thus believes in a direct line of descent from the old salacious worship of the mother-goddess and the extravagances of witchcraft, and he finds survivals of this even in the licensed vice of to-day. Thus this early civilization of woman handed down a mass of useful customs and knowledge, so that she was the bearer of a civilization that man has not yet entirely attained. If many things in her life are vestiges of the mother age, many in his represent a still lower stratum and the drudgery of the peasant woman in many parts of Europe represents the extreme of the reaction brought about by male dominance.

Otis T. Mason and A. F. Chamberlain have stressed the significance of woman's work in the early stages of the development of the human race, and if it be true that in witchcraft we have a recrudescence of the reactions of man to this preëminence of the other sex, in which woman in her least attractive form—all shriveled, toothless, and as a vicious trouble-maker—is caricatured in the long war of sex against sex, we certainly have here considerable confirmation of some of the views now represented by John M. Tyler [35] that prehistoric woman led mankind in the early stages of its upward march toward civilization. In the eternal struggle of old people to maintain their power against the oncoming generations which would submerge or sweep them away, witchcraft on this view represents the very latest stage of a long and losing struggle of old women for place and influence who in the last resort did not scruple, handicapped though they were by ugliness, neglect, and contempt, to cling to the least and last remnants of their ancient prerogatives.

---

[35] *The New Stone Age in Northern Europe.* New York, Scribner, 1921.

The attitude of children toward old people is interesting and significant, but it is very difficult to distinguish between their own indigenous and intrinsic feelings and the conventionalities of respect and even the outer forms of convention that society has imposed upon them. Many children live with their grandparents and the attitude of the latter toward the former makes, of course, a great difference. Both, especially grandmothers, are prone to be over-indulgent and often allow children greater liberties than the mother would—under the influence, doubtless, of the very strong instinct to win their good-will. But it is very doubtful if the average child loves the grandmother as much as it is loved by her.

Colin Scott [36] obtained 226 reminiscent answers from adults on the question of how as children they felt toward old people and found little difference in the sexes in this respect. No less than eighty per cent expressed negative or pessimistic views; that is, they disliked old people because they could not run and play; because they were sometimes cross, solemn, stupid, conceited; perhaps were thought to envy the young or interfere with childish pleasures, etc.; while not a few expressed points of aversion to wrinkles, unsteady gait, untidiness in dress and habits (particularly of eating), slowness, uncertain voice, loss of teeth, bad pronunciation, etc. Only twenty per cent took a favorable view of old people, regarding them as wise, not only about the weather but about other things; as free to do what they wished; having great power as storytellers; constantly doing little acts of kindness and sometimes interceding with parents in their behalf. For the majority of young children the pleasures of life seem to be essentially over at forty and they look upon people of that age as already

---

[36] "Old Age and Death." *Amer. Jour. Psychol.*, Oct., 1896, vol. 8, pp. 67–122.

moribund. Very often children are overcome by a sudden sense of pathos that old people are facing death, the process of which with lowered vitality seems to them to have already begun. To some, the very aged, even conventionally loved, are inwardly repulsive because their weakness and appearance already begin to seem a little corpse-like; while a few, on the other hand, are animated by the motive to make old people happy because their life seems to them so short or because little things please them so much. It would almost seem from such data as though the modern child was not sufficiently accustomed to grandparents to have fully adjusted to them; and, as everyone knows, there is a very strong and instinctive tendency in children to jeer at and perhaps attempt ludicrous imitations of old age. At any rate, we have here two tendencies evidently in greater or less conflict with each other.

Mantegazza [37] collected very many views from literature concerning old age and death and grouped them in two classes, favorable and unfavorable. The majority of his quotations stigmatize it as repulsive, crumpled in skin and form, perhaps tearful, squinting, with mottled skin, loose, distorted teeth, emaciation sometimes suggesting a skeleton, hardness of hearing, croaking voice, knotted veins, hemorrhoids, tending to drift into an apologetic attitude for living like a beggar asking alms or craving pity, with no strong desires, etc., so that even those who love old people in the bottom of their hearts often do not want them around. These quotations stress the garrulousness, untidiness in table manners, carelessness in dress or toilet, moodiness, exacting nature, and disparagement of present times in always lauding the past. "Old age is pitiable because although life is not attractive, death is dreaded." People sometimes "seem to themselves and to others

---

[37] *Die Hygiene des Lebensalters.*

to live on because the gods do not love them." **Life is** often described as a "long sorrow, the last scene of which is always death." "There are only three events —to be born, live, and die. A man does not feel it when he is born but through life he suffers and death is painful, and then he is forgotten." "Every tick of the clock brings us nearer to death." "We part from life as from the house of a host and not from our own home." "One after another our organs refuse their service and collapse." "All that lives must die, and all that grows must grow old." "Death begins in the cradle." "The harbor of all things good or bad is death." "The elements are in constant conflict with man, slowly demolishing everything he does and in the end annihilating him."

On the other hand, some, like the Stoics, have not only affected to accept death with perfect equanimity but call it the highest good that God has given men. The Epicurean said death was no evil because as long as we live it is not present and when it is present we are not there. Pliny said the gods have given us nothing more to be desired than brevity of life. Others say that the old may have weak bodies but normally have good will and this compensates. Others stress the dignity of age or its steadfastness, its fondness for children and the young. Sometimes the old become epicures in eating and connoisseurs in drinking. Some commend as a laudable ambition the desire of the old to live as long, as well, and as fully as possible. Others think the love of beauty, especially in nature, is greater; still others find a new love of order, better knowledge of self, both physical and mental. He suggests that old age should be almost a profession, as we have to fit to new conditions. It is possible then to take larger views, and he says that of the three attitudes toward death, (1) not to think of it at all, the recourse of the common and the weak, (2) belief in immortality, a very pleasing and comforting delusion, and (3) to face and get familiar with it, the last is by far the highest and hardest. Thus the old must realize that they are as brittle and fragile as glass, cannot do what they once could, become ill from slighter causes and recover more slowly, must especially guard against colds, fatigue, change of habit, and must be always on their guard not to accept others' precepts about keeping themselves in the top of their condition but work out those best for themselves.

In all ages since civilization began we have frequent outcrops of the tendency to divide human life into stages, many or few, more or less sharply marked off one from the other. L. Löw has given us a comprehensive survey of this subject. There has never been, however, any general agreement as to these age demarcations save two, namely, the beginning and the end of sex life, which divides life into three stages. Child life, as we all know, has lately been divided into various epochs—the nursling; the pre-school age; the quadrennium from eight to twelve; puberty; the age of attaining majority; nubility; the acme of physical ability (for example, for athletes *circa* thirty); the beginning of the decline of life, most often placed between forty and fifty, a stage that has many marked features of its own; the development of the senium, marked by impotence, with occasional subdivisions of this stage, as, for example in Shakespeare:

> The sixth age shifts
> Into the lean and slipper'd pantaloon,
> With spectacles on nose and pouch on side,
> His youthful hose, well sav'd, a world too wide
> For his shrunk shank; and his big manly voice,
> Turning again toward childish treble, pipes
> And whistles in his sound. Last scene of all,
> That ends this strange eventful history,
> Is second childishness and mere oblivion,
> Sans teeth, sans eyes, sans taste, sans everything.

79

Our educational curricula are still far more logical in the sequence of their subject matter and their method than they are genetic whereas they should be essentially the latter, as will be the case when the paidocentric viewpoint has become paramount, as it should, over the scholiocentric. We have made much progress since Herbart in determining true culture stages, and while there are very many exceptions to the law that in general the individual recapitulates the stages of the race, this great principle has far wider scope than we have yet recognized. Again, we have made great progress along another line, namely, in distinguishing physiological and especially psychological from chronological age, but here we have little consensus of either method or result beyond the early teens. Yet no observer of life can fail to doubt that there is the same and perhaps even, on the whole, greater average diversity among individuals in mental age as they advance along the scale of years. Some minds are young and growing at seventy while others seem to cross some invisible deadline at forty. But of all this we have no settled criteria and the age of customary or enforced retirement is arbitrary, though very diversely fixed by various industrial concerns, pension systems, etc., without regard to mental age or youth. In fact, the world has so far attempted almost nothing that could be called a curriculum for the later years of life—physical, intellectual, moral, social, or even hygienic or religious, after the very variable period when the prime of life is reached and passed. Happily, however, we do have both vestiges and modern recrudescences of such a view in the field of religion, as may be briefly illustrated in the following paragraphs.

Many have held with DuBuy,[38] that different religions

---

[38] "Four Types of Protestants: A Comparative Study in the Psychology of Religion," *Jour. of Relig. Psychol.*, Nov., 1908, vol. 3, pp. 165–209.

best fitted different ages. He believes that Confucianism, with its stress on respect for parents and ancestors and on the cultivation of practical virtues, best fits the nature and needs of young children; that Mohammedanism, with its passionate monotheism, has a certain affinity for the next stage of life; Christianity is best from adolescence on to the age when the marriage relation is at its apex; Buddhism comes next; and Brahmanism is for old age.

Max Müller [39] says that in very ancient India it was recognized "that the religion of a man cannot and ought not to be the same as that of a child, and that the religious ideas of an old man must differ from those of an active man in the world. It is useless to attempt to deny such facts," and we are reminded that we all have to struggle and have to pass through many stages of clearing up childish conceptions in this field. Most cultivated men come out of these struggles with certain rather firm convictions, but these later may be found to need revision.

But when the evening of life draws near and softens the light and shade of conflicting opinion, when to agree with the spirit of truth within becomes far dearer than to agree with a majority of the world without, the old questions appeal once more like long forgotten friends. The old man learns to bear with those from whom formerly he differed, and while he is willing to part with all that is non-essential—and most religious differences seem to arise from non-essentials—he clings all the more firmly to the few strong and solid planks that are left to carry him into the harbor no longer very distant from his sight. It is hardly creditable how all other religions have overlooked these simple facts, how they have tried to force on the old and wise the food that was meant for babes, and how they have thereby alienated and lost their best and strongest friends. It is therefore a lesson all the more worth learning from history that one religion at least, and one of the most ancient and powerful and most widely spread

---

[39] *The Vedanta Philosophy*, London, 1914, p. 16 *et seq.*

religions, has recognized this fact without the slightest hesitation.

According to the ancient canons of the Brahmanic faith, each man must pass through several stages. The youth is sent to the house of a teacher or Guru, whom he must obey and serve implicitly in every way and who teaches what is necessary for life, especially the Veda and his religious duties. He is a mere passive recipient, learner, and believer. At the next stage the man is married and must perform all the duties prescribed for the householder. But during both these periods no doubt is ever heard as to the truth of religion or the authority of laws and rites. But when the hair turns white and there are grandchildren, "a new life opens during which the father of the family may leave his home and village and retire into the forest with or without his wife. During that period he is absolved from the necessity of performing any sacrifices, although he may or must undergo certain self-denials or penances, some of them extremely painful. He is then allowed to meditate with proper freedom on the great problems of life and death, and for that purpose is expected to study the Upanishads," to learn the doctrines in which all sacrificial duties are rejected, and the very gods to whom the ancient prayers of the Veda were addressed are put aside to make room for the one supreme impersonal being called Brahm. These mahatmas, like some medieval hermit-saints commemorated in the voluminous hagiology of the Bollandist Fathers, were reputed to have often attained very great age and wisdom and to be sought out in their retreats to solve great problems by men still in active life. The bodies of a few of them were fabled to have undergone a subtle process of transubstantiation and thus to have achieved a true mundane immortality.

Thus the religion of childhood and manhood for the

venerable sage is transmuted into philosophy or meditation on the most general problems and the very nature
of not only life but being itself, that Plato described as
the cult of death. The old man, thus, in the classic days
of ancient India directed his thoughts toward absorption. His religion was pantheism, and the theme of his
contemplation was the source of all things and their
return to this source as their goal. Perhaps we might
now say that according to this view, if evolution is the
inspiration of the intellect in its youth and its prime,
involution was its muse in the stages of decline as it
awaited resumption into the One-and-All. Modern
pragmatists, like the best of the ancient Sophists, hold
that the truth that best fits and expresses Me is and must
be held with the completest conviction, and the genetic
idea is that different philosophies and different faiths
fit and express not only different temperaments but
different stages of life, and that, therefore, creeds can
never be fixed and stationary but must be constantly
transformed. There is no absolute or final form of
truth for all save in the dominion of pure mathematical
and physical science, and it is one of the most tragic
aspects of our modern culture that we so often find
mature and even aging men and women arrested in
infantile or juvenile stages of their development in regard to the larger problems of life, for where and just
in proportion as the latter is intense there is incessant
change. Christianity is the best of all religions through
the entire stage of the *vita sexualis* from its inception
to its decline. Its essence is the sublimation of love.
It is the religion of personalization culminating in the
faith in another individual life. It is not the religion
for old men, and the revival of its attitudes, which we
often see in them, is a phenomenon of arrest or reversion
and not one of the advance that senescence should mark

if the last stage of life is to have its complete unfoldment.

Some writers believe that age differences constitute one of the important bases, if not the chief one, in the primitive segmentation of society into layers. It is a common observation that the young tend to be progressive and radical, and the old, conservative, intent that no good thing of the past be lost. Indeed, this is often called the most natural and wholesome basis of division into parties, religious as well as political. In a sense there is eternal war between the old and young, as illustrated, for example, by Turgenev's *Fathers and Sons*. The young are always inclined to brush aside their elders and are psychologically incapable of taking their point of view. So in many a mixed assemblage we have a clash of temperaments that divides fathers and sons, mothers and daughters.[40] In some Australian tribes there is an absolute dominance of the elders, and among some American Indians of the plain there is incessant antagonism between the young braves eager to distinguish themselves in raids against hostile tribes and the older chiefs seeking to prevent a hazardous war. F. Schurtz [41] thinks this antagonism between the older and younger generation, which separates parents from children, forms the germ of classifications of age and is the oldest type of associated groups. Lowie, however, does not think that the kind of age groupings found in such cultures have a purer natural basis but rather that they represent a blending of psychological and conventional factors. It is very hard to transcend the intuitions of one's years. Where these segmentations occur they may or may not be fully organized, but they generally go back to a more primitive social division into boys, bachelors, and married men, very common among

---

[40] R. H. Lowie, *Primitive Society*, 1920.
[41] *Altersklassen und Männerbünde*, 1902.

savages. More elaborated age distinctions probably
arose a little later.

R. S. Bourne [42] also realizes that there is always a
half-conscious war going on between the old and the
young and believes this is a wholesome challenge that
both should recognize to justify themselves. Older men
should not be led captive by the younger and should
neither over-emphasize nor waive their own cherished
convictions, which are the best results of age and experience. To-day the older generation is more inclined
to stress duty and service and to hark back to Victorian
ideals. Perhaps in general they tend a little to over-
individuation but they should choose the golden mean
between insisting upon their own point of view and complete capitulation to youth.

Indeed, we may go much further and say that just
as, despite the love of man and woman, there has always
been a war of sex against sex, so despite the love of
parents and children, there is also eternal war between
the old and young. The small boy loves, reveres, and
obeys his father but often oscillates to the opposite state
of fear and even hate under the law of the so-called
ambivalence of feeling. Each age tends to assert itself
and to resent the undue influence of another age. Youth
pushes on and up and seeks to make itself effective and
to escape or resist control by elders. This is very fully
brought out in the recent literature of psychoanalysis.
In primitive society the boy soon transfers this attitude
toward his parents to the chief of the tribe, and then
perhaps to a supreme being, for all gods are made in the
father image. Indeed, we are now told that the primal,
generic sin in its extreme form is patricide, and one of
the deepest fears is directed against authority. The
pre-Abrahamic sheik was his own priest and king and

---

[42] *Atlantic Monthly,* 1915, p. 385.

that of his tribe. There was no law save his will. Enlarged, perfected, and projected into the sky, the
patronymic sire became a deity. Part of the ancient
reverence for fathers accumulated from generation to
generation was thus transcendentalized into deities and
part of it developed in the mundane sphere as reverence
for rulers, heroes, the great dead, or perhaps into the
worship of ancestors. But one very essential part of
it survives in adult life in the attitude toward authority,
every instrument and bearer of which is thus generically
a father-surrogate. Thus older people feel toward their
deities much as younger children do toward earthly
parents and the greater men in their environment.
There is always a measure of love and dread merging
into each other. Ancient tribes that Robertson Smith
and Frazer describe, after selecting and feeding fat their
rulers for a time, ascribing to them divine prerogatives,
giving them extraordinary freedom in certain respects
while restricting them by severe taboos and in other ways,
finally slew them ritually as sacrifices offered with
piacular rites. All this illustrates the same dual trend
of affectivity within and so does the fate of every deity
who is slain, perhaps with every indignity and torture,
and afterwards resurrected, transfigured, and glorified.

All government in a sense, too, springs from paternal-
ism, and so does all human power, dignity, and prerogatives, so that the French revolutionist and even Nihilist,
who is chronically and constitutionally against all the
powers that be and who feels that every command or
prohibition is a challenge to defy or violate it, only illustrates the extreme of revolt now sometimes designated
as kurophobia.[43]

Of course rebellion against tyranny is commendable.
Many fathers are bad and this cumulative fact has

---

[43] See Le Bon: *The World in Revolt,* 1921.

greatly intensified the instinct of rebellion. In an extreme form this may be expressed in negativism or anti-suggestibility, but sooner or later there is a revolt of all sons against all sires. This, too, acts as a challenge to originality and gives its *élan* to the passion for boundless freedom, which may even degenerate into forms of affectation and a passion for over-individuality. Thus next to hostile nature herself, fathers and what they symbolize have been the objects of man's chief opposition in the world's history. The very words "obey" and "conform" hardly exist in the vocabulary of some recusants. The devil, too, always denies and defies and all through the history of religions has been the typical rebel. The kurophobe is the evil genius of republics and democracies. He prates of rights and has little or nothing to say of duties and on this view he is the product of all the bad fathers in his pedigree.

In many patriarchal and tribal societies the father or chief monopolized the women, whom the sons dared not approach. Hence we are told that they were compelled to seek mates outside, whence exogeny arose. Freudians hold that the son's rancor against the father is rooted in this inhibition of the mating instinct. This doubtless did contribute very much to intensify it as the boy grew to man's estate but it is going too far to say that in the very intricate grammer of revolt, no less complex than Newman long ago showed the grammar of assent to be, other factors did not come in and that there no other social inhibitions of the will-to-live than those of the will to propagate. This rivalry and antagonism, which is probably more deep and multiform than we have yet realized, is seen at every age from early childhood—in the hostility of Freshman and Sophomore, those under and over age for citizenship or for war, in struggles of men in the meridian of life to depose or supplant those a little older, in the countless devices of those who are aging to maintain their power and influence, which perhaps never in history had such an efficient bulwark as when they became secure in the right of testamentary bequest of their property as they wished—and is only mitigated in the case of the very old because they are few and feeble and have already in many ways been superseded and relegated to inefficiency.

Metchnikoff in his essay on Old Age tells us that at Vate the "old men have at least this consolation—that during the funeral ceremonies it is customary to attach to their arms a pig which may be eaten during the feast given in honor of the departure of the soul for the other world." After citing other similar cases, he tells us that civilized people are not unlike savages for although they do not kill superannuated members of the community they often make their lives very unhappy, the old often being considered as a heavy charge, which causes great impatience at the delay of death. This is expressed in the Italian proverb that old women have seven lives and the Burgomasks think that old women have seven souls, besides an eighth soul, quite small, and half a soul besides; while the Lithuanians complain that an old woman is so tenacious of life that she can not be even ground in a mill. He cites the protest of Paris medical students against the decision of the state superseding the law prescribing a limit of age for the professors, saying, "We do not want dotards." A convict in the Saghalien Islands condemned for the assassination of several old men said, "What is the use of making such a fuss about them? They are already old and would die anyway in a few years." In Dostoievsky's *Crime and Punishment* one student declared in a group of his mates that he would kill and rob the cursed old woman without the slightest remorse, and continues, "On the one side we have a stupid, unfeeling old woman, of no account, wicked and sick, whom no one would miss—on the contrary, who is an injury to everyone and does not herself know why she keeps on living and who perhaps will be good and dead to-morrow; while, on the other hand, there are fresh young lives wasting for nothing at all, without being helped by anyone, that can be numbered by thousands." Old men, too, often commit suicide. Prussian statistics show that people between 50 and 80 commit suicide about twice as often as those between 20 and 50, and the same is true of Denmark. "The young and strong adults furnished, therefore, $36\frac{1}{2}$ per cent of the suicides, while the number furnished by the aged amounted to $63\frac{1}{2}$ per cent." Metchnikoff finds that "the desire to live, instead of diminishing tends, on the contrary, to increase with age." "The old Fuegian women, aware that they are destined to be eaten, flee into the mountains, whither they are pursued by the men and carried back home where they must submit to death." "The philosopher in me does not believe in death; it is the old man who has not the courage to face the inevitable." And so it is that old professors rarely wish to abandon their chairs. Nor do they even always renounce the tender passion, a fact illustrated by Goethe, who at the age of 74 fell in love with a girl of 17, proposed marriage to her, and failing in the project wrote his pathetic *Elegy of Marienbad,* in which he said "For me the universe is lost; I am lost to myself. The gods, whose favorite I lately was, have tried me," etc. The weakening of his powers in the latter part of *Faust* and at the end of *Wilhelm Meister* was abundantly shown.

We resume our historical notes with Luigi Cornaro (1464-1566),[44] a wealthy Venetian nobleman, who, as a result of a wild and intemperate life, found himself at

---

[44] *The Art of Living Long,* tr. 1914, 207 p.

forty broken in health and facing death and so radically changed not only his mode of life but his residence and devoted himself, after this crisis, with the "most incessant attention" to the securing of perfect health, studying every item of diet and regimen for its effects upon him. At eighty-three, after more than forty years of perfect health and undisturbed tranquillity, he wrote his *La Vita Sobria,* an essay that was later followed by three others, one written at eighty-six, another at ninety one, the last at ninety-five; the four completing a most instructive life history and one which the most earnest desire and hope of his life was that others might know and follow. He believed that the kind of life most people lead is utterly worthless and emphasized the great value of the later years of life as compared with the earlier ones. His message to the world has been a classic. He hoped that he had made the moderate life so attractive that the attitude of the world toward old age and death would be changed.

In his first discourse he gives many details of how he conceived life in the simple way nature intended it and how we must learn to be content with a little and experience all the joys that come from self-control. When the passions are subdued, man can give himself up wholly to reason. His physicians told him that he must partake of no food save that prescribed for invalids but he found that he must carefully study each article of diet and decide for himself because no general prescriptions avail. By dint of long observations upon himself he started with the belief that "whatever tastes good will nourish and strengthen" and learned that "not to satiate oneself with food is the science of health." He guarded particularly against great heat, cold, and fatigue; allowed nothing to interfere with his rest and sleep, would never stay in an ill-ventilated room, and avoided excessive exposure to wind and sun. At the age of seventy he was severely injured by a carriage accident so that all his friends expected his death and the physicians suggested either bleeding or purging as forlorn hopes. He refused both and trusted to the recuperative effects of his well regulated life. He recovered completely as he, indeed, fully expected to do, although it was thought by his friends to be miraculous. Later, yielding reluctantly to the urgency of physicians and friends, he increased his daily intake of food so that instead of twelve ounces, including bread, the yolk of an egg, a little meat and soup, he now took fourteen ounces; and instead of fourteen ounces of wine, as before, he raised his ration to sixteen ounces. Under this increased diet he grew seriously ill (at seventy-eight). But on returning to his old dietary he recovered.

Hence, he concludes that "a man cannot be a perfect physician of anyone except of himself alone" and that by dint of experimenting he may "acquire a perfect knowledge of his own condition and of his most hidden qualities and find out what food and what drink and what quantities of each would agree with his stomach." "Various experiments are absolutely necessary, for there is not so great a variety of features as there is diversity of temperaments and stomachs among men." He found he could not drink wine over a year old, and that pepper injured but cinnamon helped him, something which no physician could have anticipated. He shows the fallacy of the notion that such a life leaves nothing to fall back upon in time of sickness by saying that such sickness would thus be avoided and that his dietary is sufficient so that in sickness, when all tend to eat less, he has still a sufficient margin, although probably the quantity or quality of food that suits him, he admits, might not suit others. The objection that many who lead irregular lives live to be old he refutes by saying that some have exceptional vitality but that all can prolong life by his method. He tells us that he rides without assistance, climbs hills, is never perturbed in soul, is occupied during the entire day, changes his residence in warm weather to the country which he thinks important, enjoys the society of able, cultivated, and active-minded men, and all his senses have remained perfect.

He tells us that he improved upon Sophocles, who wrote a tragedy at seventy-three, for he has written a comedy; of his seven grandchildren, all offspring of one pair; how he enjoys singing (probably religious incantations), and how much his voice has improved; that he would not be willing to exchange "either my life or my great age for that of any young man," etc. He praises his heart, memory, senses, brain, and is certain that he will die, when the time comes, without pain or illness and hopes to enjoy the other world beyond.

In his later discourses he tells us that although naturally of a very choleric disposition he entirely subdued it. He corrects the notion that the old must eat much to keep their bodies warm; says as old age is a disease we must eat less, as we do when ill; refutes the maxim "a short life and a merry one" and the fallacy that one cannot much prolong or shorten life by regimen; tells us exactly what foods he prefers—soup, eggs, mutton, fowl, fish, etc. At ninety-one he says, "The more my years multiply, the more my strength also increases," and he preaches an earthly paradise after the age of eighty; while at ninety-five he writes that all his faculties "are in a condition as perfect as ever they were; my mind is more than ever keen and clear, my judgment sound, my memory tenacious, my heart full of life," and his voice so strong that he has to sing aloud his morning and evening prayers. He enjoys two lives at the same time, one earthly and the other heavenly by anticipation.

As Cornaro advanced in years he grew very proud

92

of his age, and his four discourses give us the impression that regimen and hygiene were his true religion, although he was very pious according to the standards of his age. His diet, the houses he built to live in for each season, his charities, the public works he instituted, and even the friends he cultivated, like everything else he said and did, were determined largely by what he thought were their effects upon his physical and mental health. No young man or young woman was ever prouder of his youth than he of his age. He gloried in it as manhood and womanhood do in their prime, and no evangelist was more intent on convicting the world of sin, righteousness, and judgment than he was in exhorting men to change their mode of life to make it more sane, temperate, and abstemious—and that in a day and land when gluttony and riotous living were rife. For him a feast, rich repast, or a formal dinner was suicidal; and so were late hours, irregularities, excitement, and every form and degree of excess. So superior is senescence to all the other stages of life that he believed men should be dominated from the first by the desire to attain it as the supreme mundane felicity, because no one can be truly happy but the old. His mission was evidently to be the apostle of senescence.

True, he repeats himself, is often very platitudinous, no doubt, like most old men, greatly overestimates his powers, and if a poor and ignorant man would have been, very likely, a tedious old dotard. But as it is, his treatment of the problem of life is of great and lasting significance.

Lord Bacon [45] was evidently influenced by Cornaro, as he in turn was by the abstemious practices of monks and ascetics. Among the very practical suggestions of his paper we strike many quotations that have become

---

[45] *History of Life and Death.*

familiar to all—Men fear death as children fear to go into the dark, and as that natural fear in children is increased with tales, so is the other; since life is short and art is long, our chiefest aim should be to perfect the arts, and the greatest of them all is that of long life. Diet receives chief consideration. Bacon seems almost to believe that the ancients acquired a mode of putting off old age to a degree that has now become a lost art "through man's negligence." He stresses the power of the "spirits" and its waxing green again as the most ready and compendious way to long life but tells us that it may be in excess or in defect as, indeed, may every other activity; while the middle or moderate way is always to be sought. He discourses on the necessity of sufficient but not too much exercise, which must never be taken if the stomach is either too full or too empty. "Many dishes have caused many diseases," and many medicines have caused few cures. "Emaciating diseases, afterwards well cured, have advanced many in the way of long life for they yield new juice, the old being consumed, and to recover from a sickness is to renew youth. Therefore, it were good to make some artificial diseases, which is done by strict and emaciating diets."

Sleep is an aid to nourishment and it is especially important that in sleeping the body always be warm. Sleep is nothing but the reception and retirement of the living spirit into itself. We must also be cheerful in relation to both sleep and eating and he has many admonitions upon the advantages of pure air, the right affection, hope not too often frustrated, and especially a sense of progress, for most who live long have felt themselves advancing. Old men should dwell upon their childhood and youth, for this means rejuvenation. Hence association of the old with others whom they knew when young is most helpful. Habits, customs, and even diet, must be changed, but not too often or too much. One must constantly observe and study the effect upon himself of all the items of regimen. Grief, depression, excessive fear, lack of patience, are passions that feed upon and age the body. Each must acquire a wisdom "beyond the rules of physic; a man's own observation, what he finds good of and what he finds hurt of, is the best physic to preserve health, and with regard to many things he must wisely and rightly decide whether or not they are good or bad for him, and that independently of all precepts and advice."

Thus in his quaint style, and for reasons most of which science of to-day would utterly discard, he had the sagacity to reach many of the conclusions that are quite abreast of and in conformity with the most practical results of modern hygiene.

Addison,[46] avowedly more or less inspired by Cornaro, after condemning the prevailing gluttony says, "For my part, when I behold a fashionable table set out in all its magnificence, I fancy that I see gouts and dyspepsias, fevers and lethargies, and other distempers lying in ambuscade among the dishes." He delights in the most plain and simple diet. Every animal but man keeps to one dish—herbs are the food of this species, fish of that, and flesh of the third. Man alone falls upon everything that comes in his way. "Not the smallest fruit or excrescence of the earth, scarce a berry or mushroom escapes him." Hence he advises that we make our whole repast out of one dish and that we avoid all artificial provocatives, which create false appetites. He advises, too, that since this rule is so hard, "every man should have his days of abstinence according as his constitution will permit. These are great reliefs to nature as they qualify her for struggling with hunger and thirst and

---

[46] *Spectator,* Oct. 17, 1711.

give her an opportunity of extricating herself from her oppressions. Besides that, abstinence will oftentimes kill a sickness in embryo and destroy the first seeds of an indisposition." He then quotes the temperateness of Socrates, which enabled him to survive the great plague. He finds that many ancient sages and later philosophers developed a regimen so unique that "one would think the life of a philosopher and the life of a man were of two different dates."

Robert Burton [47] thinks old age inherently melancholy, for "being cold and dry and of the same quality as melancholy it must needs come in." It is full of ache, sorrow, grief, and most other faults, and these traits are most developed in old women and best illustrated by witches. The children of old men are rarely of good temperament and are especially liable to depression. He expatiates most fully upon the tragedy of old men and young wives, and gives many long incidents of jealousy and unfaithfulness of women who, although carefully guarded, have made old husbands cuckold. This is often worse in dotards, who become effeminate, cannot endure absence from their wives, etc. On this theme he elaborates for many pages, with scores of incidents from literature and history.

Jonathan Swift [48] describes the *Struldbruggs* or immortals whom he met in a far country. They were distinguished by being born with a red circle over the left eye, which changed in color and grew in size with age. These beings, he thought, must be a great blessing, and he described to those who had first told him of them what he would do were it his great good fortune to be born a Struldbrugg. First of all, he would amass wealth so that in two hundred years he would be the richest

---

[47] *The Anatomy of Melancholy.*
[48] *Gulliver's Travels,* Chap. X.

man in the realm. Next he would apply himself to learning, which in the course of time would make him wisest of all men. Then he would note all events and become a living treasury of knowledge and the oracle of the nation. He would be able to warn rising generations against all impending evils and thus prevent degeneration.

Having heard his ideals, he was told that in fact the state of these immortals was very different; indeed, so pitiful was it that their example mitigated the universal desire to live, so that death was no longer the greatest evil but, on the contrary, undue prolongation of life was a far greater one. The Struldbruggs acted like mortals till about thirty, then grew melancholy until four-score, when they had "not only the follies and infirmities of other old men but had many more which arose from the dreadful prospects of never dying." "They were not only opinionative, peevish, morose, vain, talkative, but incapable of friendship and dead to all natural affection, which never descended below their grandchildren." "Envy and impotent desires are their prevailing passion, but the objects against which their envy seems principally directed are the vices of the younger sort and the deaths of the old. By reflecting on the former they find themselves cut off from all possibility of pleasure, and whenever they see a funeral they lament and repine that others are gone to a harbor of rest to which they themselves can never hope to arrive." "They have no remembrance of anything but what they learned and observed in their youth and middle age and even that is very imperfect, and for the truth or particulars of any fact it is safer to depend on the common traditions than upon their best recollections." "The less miserable among them appear to be those who turn to dotage and entirely lose their memories; they meet with more pity and assistance because they lack many bad qualities

97

which abound in others." If they marry one of their own kind, the marriage is dissolved as soon as the younger comes to be four-score, for they "should not have their misery doubled by the load of a wife."

"As soon as they have completed the term of eighty years they are looked on as dead in law; their heirs immediately succeed to their estates, only a small pittance being reserved for their support, and the poor ones are maintained at the public charge. After that period they are held incapable of any employment of trust or privilege, cannot purchase land or take leases; neither are they allowed to be witnesses in any cause either civil or criminal." "At ninety they lose their teeth and hair, they have at that age no distinction of taste but eat and drink whatever they can get, without relish or appetite." In talking, they forget the common appellation of things and the names of persons, even of those who are their nearest friends and relatives. "For the same reason they can never amuse themselves with reading because their memory will not serve to carry them from the beginning of a sentence to the end. The language of the country, too, is slowly undergoing a change so that the Struldbruggs of one age do not understand those of another but live like foreigners in their own country." They are depised and hated by all sorts of people. When one of them is born it is reckoned ominous and the birth is recorded very particularly, but in general the record is lost after a thousand years. "They were the most mortifying sight I ever beheld, and the women were more horrible than the men. Besides the usual deformities in extreme old age, they acquired an additional ghastliness in proportion to their number of years."

Thus from what the author saw and heard, his keen appetite for perpetuity of life was much abated and he realized that there was no form of death to which he would not run with pleasure in order to escape such a life. He concludes that it is fortunate that his desire of taking specimens of these people to his own country was forbidden by law, and reflects that their maintenance might prove a grievous public charge, for since "avarice is the necessary consequent of old age, these immortals would, in time, become proprietors of the whole nation and engross the civil power, which a want of abilities to manage must end in the ruin of the public."

CHAPTER III

LITERATURE BY AND ON THE AGED

Harriet E. Paine—Amelia E. Barr—Mortimer Collins—Col. Nicholas Smith—Byron C. Utecht—J. L. Smith—Sanford Bennett—G. E. D. Diamond—Cardinal Gibbons—John Burroughs—Rollo Ogden—James L. Ludlow—Brander Matthews—Ralph Waldo Emerson—Oliver Wendell Holmes—Senator G. F. Hoar—William Dean Howells—H. D. Sedgwick—Walt Mason—E. P. Powell—U. V. Wilson—D. G. Brinton—N. S. Shaler—Anthony Trollope—Stephen Paget—Richard le Gallienne—G. S. Street—C. W. Saleeby—Bernard Shaw—A few typical poems and quotations.

As a psychologist I am convinced that the psychic states of old people have great significance. Senescence, like adolescence, has its own feelings, thoughts, and wills, as well as its own physiology, and their regimen is important, as well as that of the body. Individual differences here are probably greater than in youth. I wanted to realize as fully as was practicable how it seems to be old. Accordingly I looked over such literature, both poetry and prose, as I found within reach, written by aging people describing their own stage of life, and by selection, quotation, and résumé have sought, in this chapter, to let each of them speak for him- or herself.

Some find a veritable charm in watching every phase of the sunset of their own life and feel even in the prospect of death a certain mental exaltation. More are sadly patient and accept some gospel of reconciliation to fate. Some distinctly refuse to think on or even to recognize the ebb of the tide. A few find consolation in beautifying age with tropes and similes that divert or distract from the grim realization of its advance.

LITERATURE BY AND ON THE AGED

But perhaps the most striking fact is that so many
not only deliberately turn from the supports offered to
declining years by the Church but have more or less
abandoned faith in physicians, for age is a disease that
their ministrations may mitigate but can never cure.
Men of science find least solace in religion, to which
women are much more prone to turn than men. In most,
love is more or less sublimated into philanthropy and
very often into a new and higher love of nature in all
her aspects. All, with hardly an exception, pay far more
attention to health and body-keeping than ever before
and many evolve an almost fetishistic faith in the efficacy
of some item of food or regimen to which they ascribe
peculiar virtue. They want to prolong life and well-
being to their utmost goal for, with all the handicaps
of age, life is still too sweet to leave voluntarily.

Many old people fortify themselves against the de-
pressions and remissions of old age by familiarizing
their minds with quotations from the Scriptures, hymnology, poetry, and general literature. We have a good
illustration of this in Margaret E. White's volume.[1] It
consists mainly of selections, determined of course by
the author's point of view—that of a liberal religionist
—which has given her, and is well calculated to give
others with her point of view, mental satisfaction. She
wants to have "prisms in her window" to fill the room
with rainbows. As the shadows lengthen she believes
the climacteric should supervene without any break at
all with the prime of life, although there are really two
curves that run a very different course, one of physical
strength and another of experience. When one stands
on the summit of his years, he is buoyed up by great
plans for life; but when he retires, there is nothing
ahead save death and this involves a great and often

[1] *After Noontide,* Boston, 1883, 168 p.

101

critical change. The successful life is one that solves the problems that meet it here without patheticism and without self-delusion.

The author's anthology of quotations and her own reflections are not a cry in the dark but, on the whole, strike a note of courage and her book is of psychological value because it gives us a good idea of how many authors have thought and felt. Most want to be quiet and at home. They console themselves with intimations of a lofty and spiritual, if remote, idealism. Perhaps of all the young people we knew not one will accompany the late survivors. Old age is a benefaction because service to it ennobles all who render it. When wrinkles come in the mind, one sings, the old is ever old; another, it is ever young. One conceives it as the portal to a higher life, while for another it is solely reversionary.

Harriet E. Paine,[2] a retired maiden teacher, had grown deaf and her sight was dim at sixty, when this book was written. Her attitude is one of the very best illustrations of the consolations that are open to those in whom old age is like a summer night, who can maintain their optimism when the senses cut us off from the external world and we have to "economize the falling river" and take in sail. The author has much to say of old people with defective senses and thinks deafness particularly irritating both to the individual and to those about, especially if, as in her case, there is also weakness and diffidence. These impel one to take refuge in the "Great Comrade." Like so many others, she finds great satisfaction in the familiar cases of great things done by old people and thinks that "the higher powers of the mind go on ripening to the last," instancing the remarkable fight made for life by Pope Leo XIII when he was ninety-four, the chief items in whose enlightened policy were inaugurated after he was seventy. Samuel

[2] *Old People*, Boston, 1909, 236 p.

LITERATURE BY AND ON THE AGED

Whittemore, at eighty, killed three British soldiers on April 19, 1775, and then was himself shot, bayoneted, and beaten seemingly to death but had vitality enough to live on to the age of ninety-eight. Sophocles wrote his *Œdipus* at ninety; Mrs. Gilbert acted till over seventy; Mrs. Livermore, Julia Ward Howe, and others furnish examples that hearten her, etc. When the hair grows white it is possible, especially for women, to do many things impossible before.

Being herself in straitened circumstances, she is interested in, for example, the provisions of the New Zealand Parliament in 1898 granting a pension of eighteen pounds per annum to all people over sixty-five of good moral character who had resided in the country twenty-five years and whose income did not exceed thirty-four pounds; and also in Edward Everett Hale's plea for a limited old-age pension bill, whereby a man paying a poll tax for twenty-five years and not convicted of crime should be given a pension of two dollars a week, the state to set aside a part of the poll tax for this purpose. He claimed that the savings to poorhouses would offset the expenditure. But still this author realizes that the old can be happy in comparative poverty if they strive to make their corner of the world brighter. At no time of life are the advantages of culture and experience more precious. She thinks the relations between old and young, so hard to adjust, need special attention. The two can live together only by sacrifices on both sides and this can never be successful unless each is able to take the other's point of view. She rather surprisingly concedes that with true insight the young have more sympathy with the old than the latter, by memory, can have with the young, perhaps because bodily vigor increases love. She would mitigate the stage of criticizing mothers, through which she thinks all girls tend to pass, for old age gives a wisdom that is far harder to acquire and more precious than knowledge.

The very old are very different from the old; for example, an old lady of eighty-nine called on one of ninety-eight and felt rejuvenated. Very few do, when they are old, what they have planned for their old age. The weapon against loneliness is work. "When the world is cold to you, go build fires to warm up." We strive to renew the emotions but find it very hard to do so and feel burned to the socket. In answering the question how far we should let the dead past bury its dead, she deplores the fact that young persons, especially young women, often give to their elders, particularly mothers or fathers, a devotion that involves a complete sacrifice of their own lives and thinks that to accept this is the acme of selfishness in the old. Old age is especially hard, she thinks, for those who have enjoyed the senses most.

Amelia E. Barr [3] says that on March 29, 1911, she awoke early to see her eightieth birthday come in. "I wish to master in these years the fine art of dying well, which is quite as great a lesson as the fine art of living well, about which everyone is so busy." A good old age is a neighbor to a blessed eternity. An English physician said, "If you wish to have a vigorous old age, go into the darkness and silence ten hours out of every twenty-four, for in darkness we were formed." "Never allow anyone to impose their pleasures upon you; if you have any rights, it is to choose the way you will spend your time." "On the margin gray, twixt night and day," the author finds special comfort in the lines

There is no death.
What seems so is transition.
This life or mortal breath is but the suburb of the life elysian
Whose portal we call death.

---

[3] *Three-score and Ten.* Dedicated to Chauncey Depew.

It is a sin, she says, to become so mentally active that we are unable to keep quiet and go to sleep. The Greeks knew little of insomnia and the English have been great sleepers and dreamers, holding perhaps with Wordsworth that "our birth is but a sleep and a forgetting," etc.

This author is an astrologist and tells us that nine insane rulers were born when Mercury or the moon, or both, were affected by Mars, Saturn, or Uranus, and five people of genius were ruled by the same planets and became insane. She really mourns less for what age takes away than what it leaves behind.

The tone of her work differs radically from that of Miss Paine. The latter seeks and finds compensations so satisfactory to herself that she ventures into print with them, apparently for the first time, hoping that she may thereby help others to live out their old age better; while the former indulges her literary instincts to produce another book and is far more inspired by the muse of Death than that of Life. The kismet motive, which is expressed in her recourse to astral fatalism, manifests not a *pis aller* resource first found when she was old but one that had long been with her, and it is an interesting recrudescence of the same psychological motivations that in the East made fatalism and among Calvinists made the doctrine of divine decrees and foreordination so attractive.

At the age of eighty-three she worked six hours a day instead of nine as formerly, avoided routine, tried to give her mind new thoughts, and thought this mental diet kept her strong. She took two cups of coffee in the morning and more at night, persisted in lying abed ten hours although she slept but seven, eschewed all preserved fruits, etc. She had a constant sense of the Divine and her whole standpoint is very different from that, for example, of Burroughs.

SENESCENCE

Mortimer Collins [4] looks back on a prolonged life with calm philosophic poise and concludes that length of life is wholly dependent upon ideas. The theory of Asgill that it is cowardly of man to die appeals to him. Sylvester calculated the lives of nine mathemeticians with an average age of 79, but Collins finds nine literary men whose average age was 85, and so concludes that "imagination beats calculation." We are islands in an infinite sea; only the instant is ours. The soul makes the body. He holds that in England there is no mode of life healthy enough to secure longevity, either in the city or country, while London is a slow poison. He wants a Utopia, but without religion. He would have a journal kept in every locality noting length or brevity of life, with the causes thereof, as a kind of *vade Mecum* for the inhabitants. All should live in the open, with plenty of water and hills, enough sleep and good food. Marriage should be congenial and love a liberal education; in short, marriage should be completion. Parents early spoil their children and later fear them. Politics should be eschewed for it shows only the worst side of human nature. We should have books telling us how to enjoy summers, the secret of which even the English gentleman has not yet found. Literature, especially the classics, helps to longevity, and in old age people should do that which they most love, that is most natural and that gives greatest freedom to the play instinct—not that which pays best. Gardening takes us into partnership with God and he prescribes country walks with the sun and the sea. The country gentleman should live an almost Homeric life. The large number of octogenarians in Westmoreland, the lake region of Wordsworth, which has often been noticed, is very significant. The laziest man usually lives longest, but lazing is an art.

---

[4] *The Secret of Long Life,* London, 1871, 146 p.

The style of this author is in places almost lapidary, his views are quaint and abrupt and the reader is impressed with the idea that he is supremely satisfied with old age as he has found it. His radicalism is good-natured and his love of paradox suggests an affectation of originality that does not, however, much impair his fundamental sincerity. He illustrates a type of precocious maturity that finds pleasure in ideas not very well matured.

Colonel Nicholas Smith [5] is a homely philosopher of old age who has brought together a vast body of items to hearten the old and to support the thesis that all can greatly prolong their lives if they will. He thinks that as years advance the average brain does more work, and the body less. With remarkable industry he has gathered records of scores and hundreds of old people living, or recently dead, who have maintained their vigor and remained "invincible children," who never became wholly sophisticated but still dream, wonder, and believe. He almost seems to agree with Emerson that a man is not worth very much until he is sixty.

Most of his book consists of brief records of men who maintained their activity to a great age. Many of these are familiar enough but we sample a few. Mommsen, for example, frail and small, lost his library by fire when he was sixty, a calamity that all thought would end his career. But he did much of his best work later, toiling on his *History of Rome* nearly to his death in his eighty-sixth year. George Ives, when his friends congratulated him on attaining his hundredth year, was found at work in the field and said that even if he knew he were to die the next day he should "carry on" as if he were immortal. Mrs. H. W. Truex on her 96th birthday in 1904 finished a quilt of nine hundred and seventy-

---

[5] *Masters of Old Age*, Milwaukee, 1915, 280 p.

five pieces and during the previous year had completed six such. Sir Joseph Hooker, the botanist, worked almost up to his death at 87, holding that rich natures develop slowly. Carlyle published the last volume of his *Frederick the Great* at the age of 69; Darwin, his *Descent of Man* at 62; Longfellow wrote his *Morituri Salutamus* for the fiftieth anniversary of his graduation; W. C. Bryant published his translation of the *Odyssey* at the age of 76; O. W. Holmes wrote his "Guardian Angel" at 70 and "Antipathy" at 76, while the "Iron Gate" was for a breakfast given in honor of his seventieth birthday; George Bancroft at 82 published his *History of the Foundations of the Constitution of the United States;* Frances Trollope, failing in business at the age of nearly 50 and a stranger in this country, turned to a literary career, and between the ages of 52 and 83 wrote upwards of a hundred volumes, mostly novels of society; Humboldt, at the age of 74, began his *Cosmos,* the fourth and last volume of which was issued the year before his death, in 1858, at the age of ninety; Cervantes published the last part of his *Don Quixote* at 78; Goethe wrote till he was 80 and finished the second part of *Faust* only shortly before his death; Victor Hugo wrote his *Annals of a Terrible Year* at 70, and his *Ninety-Three,* which some regard as his best story, at the age of 72; Mary Sommerville kept up her scientific activities and at 92 said she could still read books on the higher algebra four to five hours in the forenoon; Weir Mitchell wrote his *Hugh Wynne* at 66 and *Constance Trescot,* a very remarkable psychological study of a woman, when he was 76. A deposed minister began the study of medicine at 72 and practiced for several years, dying in the harness. A. J. Huntington was acting professor of classics till he was 82. Mrs. A. D. T. Whitney published her twenty-seventh volume at the age of 80, etc.

LITERATURE BY AND ON THE AGED

There are two views of age. One is Hogarth's picture—a shattered bottle, cracked bell, unstrung bow, signpost of a tavern called the "World's End," shipwreck, Phoebus's horses dead in the clouds, the moon in her last quarter, the world on fire. It only remained to add to this the picture of a painter's palette broken. This was his last work and he died at 67. Over against this we might place E. E. Hale, who late in life said his prospects cast no shadow and became very anxious to see the curtain rise. When he was 80 he published his *Memoirs of a Hundred Years* and at 82 was chaplain of the United States Senate. Gladstone locked every affair of state out of his bedroom and said that when we sleep we must pay attention to it, for a workless is a worthless life.

This author agrees with J. H. Canfield, who protested that the old should stay in the harness and not step out to give the young men a chance, for they never had a better chance than to work with their elders, as colts are best broken in with old horses. As we grow old we see that nothing, after all, matters as much as we had thought. Smith finds comfort in the fact that, according to the census of 1900, one in every two hundred becomes an octogenarian and that out of a population of 36,800,000 there were 176,571 reputed to be 80 years of age or over.

He finally gives us his own empirical observations about foods and concludes that three-fourths of all the poor health in the country is due to dietary errors or to "carrion and cathartics." The old should eat no meat, take no drink with meals, avoid starch, recognize the error in the belief that they need stimulants, and should not try to be fat but realize that progressive emaciation is normal. Appetite should be our guide although we should eat only about half what we want. He, too, praises laziness as a concomitant of longevity and recognizes a vast difference in dietary needs. He would never use laxatives but depends upon two glasses of water half an hour before breakfast and two in the afternoon, and would never mix cooked vegetables nor fruit.

The popularity and wide sale of this book must have been extremely gratifying to the author as not only showing wide and deep interest in the subject but as also supplying, by copious data and illustrations, the kind of encouragement the old often sorely need. The author makes no pretenses of being scientific and accepts cases of reputed great age with no critical scruples.

Byron C. Utecht [6] thinks the day is dawning when one hundred and fifty years will be the usual span of life. He gives many statistics to show that the average age is slowly increasing, particularly in Switzerland, where in the sixteenth century it was 21.2 years whereas in the nineteenth it was 39.7. He quotes Finkenberg of Bonn, who concludes that "the average length of life in Europe in the sixteenth century was 18 years and now it is 40," the average in India being now about 23.6 years as against 19, two hundred years ago. These figures, it should be noted, however, are little more than conjectural.

Utecht, like Colonel Smith, has collected data about many people who have reached the age of 100, some of whom he photographs. He believes man not only lives longer but is more vital than formerly. He seems to accept without proof that a Montana Indian lived to be 134; an Oregon woman, 120; and a Mrs. Kilcrease of Texas, 136. He tells us of one Arkansas woman who reached 112 years, keeping a large garden almost to the end of her life, who at the above age walked six miles and back to see her great-great-granddaughter

---

[6] "When Is Man Immortal?" *Technical World,* March, 1914.

married. She claimed her age was due to clean, honest living, plenty of work, a desire to help, keeping busy, and caring for others. A. Goodwin of Alabama (106) walks five miles a day and works several hours in his garden. He eats what he likes, reads without glasses, and is the head of one of the largest families in the country, their reunions being attended by more than eight hundred persons. He had been a hunter and still uses his rifle and ascribes his longevity to interest in out-of-door sports as a young man. He has been so busy he can hardly realize he is old, wants fifty years more of life if possible and feels that he is going to have it. He has been temperate, sleeps much and regularly, and has a horror of worry. Mrs. Mary Harrison of Michigan celebrated her hundredth anniversary and did not seem as tired as any of her two hundred guests. She had been a humorist and would never look on the dark side of things. An Ohio lady of 91 who has been devoted to a motorcycle cannot bring herself to give up her joyrides, although she now has a young man to guide the wheel. She has always lived in the country and worked hard and ascribes her longevity chiefly to her rides.

Utecht has collected perhaps two-score more instances of people well over ninety and concludes that all of them were, in their prime, more or less athletic—at least none were weaklings. He thinks the longest-lived people are average men and women who have a good hygienic sense. None were intemperate, few were highly educated, and most were inured to hardships and even drudgery in youth, so that the study of all their lives practically tells the same story of simple life in the free air, with enough but not too much work and with exemption, for the most part, from worry.

It would be interesting to know if a more critical study of the actual age of many of these and other quoted centenarians would substantiate their claims. No such investigation, however, has ever been made into the many cases reported by this and the preceding author.

I append a few special records that seem peculiarly challenging. The first is that of James L. Smith,[7] a veteran of the Civil War. Twenty years ago he weighed two hundred and twenty pounds, was warned against excitement, and his friends and physician were horrified when he proceeded to run his flesh off. It was a great effort for so heavy a man but in six months he had reduced his weight to one hundred and ninety and was running more than six miles a day, his daily work being the directing of two hundred district messengers. Yielding to the protests of his friends he ceased his exercise, because he was told that he could not punish his heart and lungs thus and not suffer and was liable to drop dead. Growing fleshy again, with increased shortness of breath, he began to run again daily, reducing his weight once more to a hundred and sixty and developing a physique and complexion like that of a far younger man. At seventy he ran never less than five and often ten miles a day, holding that senility is a disease of the mind and that youth and its vigor can be maintained if one only believes in himself. He has raced in many parts of the country and has a standing offer to run any ten survivors of the Civil War in relays of one to a mile, he himself running the whole ten. His offer used to be accepted; it is so no longer. The day he was seventy he "covered a half mile faster than a roller-skating champion," and at seventy-three ran half a mile in 2 minutes and 44 seconds. On a dirt road he has run ten miles in 1 hour, 13 minutes, and 48 seconds, exactly the same time in which he ran the same distance in the

---

[7] "A Physical Marvel at Seventy-three," *Amer. Mag.*, Dec., 1917.

Grand Army marathon at Los Angeles six years before, and says that he finished in fine condition.

Still more interesting, although perhaps not more authentic, is the autobiographic record of Sanford Bennett.[8] At the age of fifty he was broken in health and had to give up his position because of a feeble heart and dyspeptic stomach. After trying various cures he, like Smith, developed one of his own, consisting chiefly of very manifold exercises taken, for the most part, in a recumbent position to lessen the arterial strain upon his weak heart, and with little and finally no apparatus. By persistent adherence to this regimen the circulatory and digestive functions were slowly recuperated and his muscles underwent remarkable development in bulk and power. Many photographs of himself, with only a breech-waist, show him to have acquired a symmetry and fulness of physical development of which any young athlete might well be proud. Under self-massage wrinkles of face and neck disappeared, the growth of the hair on his head was somewhat increased, and its grayness was more or less modified. His spirits and the courage with which he faced life and reëntered business showed a rejuvenation of mind and feelings no less remarkable than that of the body. By more or less systematic methods he strengthened his eyes; improved the condition of his liver and kidneys; freshened the skin; greatly bettered the varicosities (photographed) of the veins of his legs; and materially improved the action of his heart, all the while recognizing the influences of the unconscious mind upon his physical condition. He has entirely overcome his tendency to adiposity, strengthened his voice, increased the girth of his chest and his respiratory capacity, etc.

It is impossible to con this book and its untouched

---

[8] *Old Age: Its Cause and Preservation,* The story of an old body and face made young, New York, 1912, 309 p.

photographs without the conviction, which has been strengthened by my own correspondence with the author, that he has undergone a remarkable physical transformation. We have already enough such instances to suggest that senescence normally releases in healthy natures new motivations for the conservation of health and that if these are given their due expression and if all aging men and women came to realize that as the decline of life sets in they must be, more and more, not only their own hygienists but their own physicians, far more might be accomplished in many if not most cases than the world at present suspects.

This suggests the lesson that Charles Francis [9] has drawn from his life, namely, that exercise is the chief cause of his vigor at seventy. His life in connection with his vocation as a printer has been extremely active and arduous and he ascribes his present condition to athletics and his exceptional fondness for dancing. He insists that next to this comes the avoidance of worry and thinks that every normal old man develops a more or less full creed of hygienic Do's and Don'ts. Charles Cliff thinks the way to eighty is to work hard in youth and then gradually take it easy.

Many modern writers, like Cicero's Cato, ascribe great efficacy to the accumulated examples of old men who have achieved exceptional success late in life, not only in business, arts, and letters but in the greatest art of all, that of conserving health and youth. We can easily conceive of a new temple of fame to immortalize those who have mastered the art of deferring senility and death.

Captain G. E. D. Diamond [10] claimed to be 103 and in his book tells us how he lived—no sweets, meats,

---

[9] "Young at Seventy," *Am. Rev. of Revs.*, vol. 57, p. 415.
[10] *The Secret of a Much Longer Life and More Pleasure in Living It*, 1906.

stimulants, tobacco, tea, or coffee; had never married; found a panacea in olive oil taken internally and with which he once or twice daily rubbed his body; found great virtue in a cup of hot water at breakfast, grapefruit at luncheon, bread buttered with olive oil; used milk, and fish. He discants at length upon the kinds, purity, and mode of application of his panacea and is a polemic vegetarian.

The late Cardinal Gibbons [11] thinks no one ever died of hard work and says that he almost never had an idle moment. He forced himself to lie in bed at least eight hours and did not worry if he did not fall asleep. The foundations of health are laid in youth and he laid the greatest stress upon plenty of regular exercise suitable to one's age, moderation in eating and drinking, plenty of sleep, an occupation, and avoidance of worry.

John Burroughs [12] said, in 1919, that he was better than thirty years before. Old age is no bugaboo but is a question of cutting out things, as he did with tea, coffee, eggs, raw apples, pastry, new bread, and alcohol, never having used tobacco. He was better by leaps and bounds when he omitted eggs, a suggestion he derived from Professor Chittenden. Malnutrition is the door through which most of our enemies enter. He retired at nine, rose at six in the winter and with the sun in summer, walked three hours in the forenoon, read from seven to nine in the evening, was much out-of-doors, and thought he wrote more and better in the last three than in any other three years of his life. And yet he did not come of a long-lived ancestry.

Rollo Ogden [13] thinks that in the first call the old man

[11] "Why I am Well at Eighty," *Ladies Home J.*, April, 1919.
[12] "How I Came to Be Doing More Work at Seventy-Seven than at Forty-Seven," *Ibid.*
[13] "Viewpoint of a Sexagenarian Contributor," *Unpartizan Rev.*, July, 1920.

meets to take himself out of the way there is generally more pity than anger but he is too proud to accept pity. Nobody is so impetuous as an old man in a hurry. Vain longings for the sensations of youth make life after forty often a dangerous age, as physicians know. He believes there are many intellectual hazards and thinks it a delusion of the old that the young are different from those they knew in their youth. In judging the rising generation we oldsters must, at any rate, admit that they did well in the war. The old must make a serious effort to penetrate the secret of youth; they must put no end of questions to it even though they are not able to find answers to them. There must be a reorganization of life and a reorientation; and also, what is perhaps often harder, a new subordination. The old are, on the whole, more curious about the young than afraid of them.

Another suggestion arises from an autobiographic volume of a retired clergyman, which is dedicated to his grandchildren.[14] The book is unique in that it gives few details of his life but stresses certain strong impressions derived from early boyhood, school days, his first experience with death, gropings to solve the problems of life and of the choice of a vocation, etc. He confines himself, for the most part, to experiences that made the deepest and most lasting impression upon him, the mysteries that have haunted his soul, self-criticisms, the rest and other cures he has tried, friendships made, and the great causes he has espoused. On laying aside his ministerial duties he realized that we must not retire within ourselves but draw closer to kindred humanity, and felt at liberty to enjoy literature, art, nature, and travel, realizing that there were many powers that had not been vented in his vocation. He found himself tak-

---

[14] James M. Ludlow, *Along the Friendly Way,* Reminiscences and Impressions, New York, 1919, 362 p.

ing sober and broader second thoughts of even religion, here discovering a new sense of freedom, as he believes retired lawyers do in reflecting on the differences between their own sense of absolute right and duty to their clients. He was glad, he says, that he could "now break with some of my past notions, go squarely back on some former, cocksure declarations," and he realized that "I did not know a lot of things I once thought I knew." There is a wonderful exhilaration in standing at the opening of views from which one has been previously barred by constitutional preoccupation and engagements. He realizes that "courtesy to the cloth leads most men to treat ministers as they would treat women—the seamy side of life is not shown them." It is easy, as one grows old, to retain abstract knowledge and the ripe fruits of philosophy, history, and even science; and age, too, has its recreations.

Perhaps the chief suggestion of this book is that every intelligent man, as he reaches the stage of senescence, should thus pass his life in review and try to draw its lessons, not only for his own greater mental poise and unity but for the benefit of his immediate descendants, for whom such a record must be invaluable. Thus the writing of an autobiography will sometime become a fit hygienic prescription for a rounded-out old age.

Brander Matthews [15] says that when a man is in sight of Pier No. 70, as Mark Twain called it, he should take down sail and examine his log-book. He must not feel that young people are wanting to brush him aside but should realize that he can help them. He gives a very full account of his own experiences as a magazine writer and deplores the fact that many of our twentieth-century editors are newspaper men, whereas formerly they were literary men. The most serious lesson he draws

[15] "Confessions of a Septuagenarian Contributor," *Unpartizan Rev.*, July, 1920.

SENESCENCE

from his own experience is that young writers should take only subjects in which they are profoundly interested and "not take down the shutters before they have anything to put in the shop windows." He rejoices that he has never accepted a dictated subject but has always labored in fields attractive to him and so, in short, followed an inner calling.

Ralph Waldo Emerson [16] says the dim senses, memory, voice, etc., are only masks that old age wears. There are young heads on old shoulders and young hearts. The essence of age is intellect. "He that can discriminate is the father of his father" and Merlin as a baby found in a basket by the riverside talks wisely of all things. Is it because we find ourselves reflected in the eyes of young people that we feel old? "The surest poison is time." Age is comely in coach, chairs of state, courts, and historical societies, but not on Broadway. We do not count a man's years until he has nothing else to count. One says a man is not worth anything until he is sixty. "In all governments the councils of power were held by the old—patricians or patres; senate or senes; seigneurs or seniors; the gerousia, the state of Sparta, the presbytery of the church, and the like, are all represented by old men." Almost all good workers live long. The blind old Dandolo, elected Doge at 84, storming Constantinople at 94, and afterward recalled again victorious, was elected at the age of 96 to the throne of the empire, which he declined, and died Doge at 97. Newton made important discoveries for every one of his 85 years. Washington, the perfect citizen; Wellington, the perfect soldier; Goethe, the all-knowing poet; Humboldt, the encyclopedia of science—all were old.

"All men carry seeds of all distempers through life

[16] *Old Age.*

118

latent and die without developing them." But if we are enfeebled by any cause some of these sleeping seeds start and open. At fifty we lose headache and with every year liability to certain forms of disease declines. Now one success more or less signifies nothing because reputation is made. Success signifies much to a client but nothing to the old lawyer. Again, another felicity of old age is that it has found expression. Things that seethe in us have been born, so that the throes and tempests subside. "One by one, day by day, he learns to cast his wishes into facts." We set our house in order, classify, finish what is begun, close up gaps, make our wills, clear our titles, and reconcile enemies. Thus there is a proportion between the designs of man and the length of his life. In February, 1825, Emerson called on John Adams, who was nearly 90, just as his son had been elected President at the age of 58, nearly the same as that of Washington, Jefferson, Madison and Monroe.

Oliver Wendell Holmes [17] discourses in his clever, self-conscious, and desultory way upon old age, concerning which he says many smart, studied, and even quotable things that add, however, no new standpoint or idea. He personifies old age, for example, as first calling on the professor and leaving his card, that is, a mark between the eyebrows; calling again more urgently; and at last, when he is not let in, breaking in at the front door. He seems to feel that death is a sort of disgrace and ignominy and compares the child shedding his milk teeth with the old man shedding his permanent ones. He would divide life into fifteen stages, each of which has its youth and old age. As we enter each stage we do so with the same ingenuous simplicity. Nature gets us out of youth into manhood

---

[17] *The Autocrat of the Breakfast Table,* Chap. VII, and also in *Over the Teacups,* p. 26, *et seq.*

as old sea captains used to shanghai sailors. Habits mark old age but we should begin new things and even take up new studies. He gives an imaginary newspaper report of the address of Cato on Old Age, and several times lapses into poetry. He feels that he has less time for anything he wants to do, realizes neglected and postponed privileges, tells of the great charm he feels in rowing on the Charles, and gives us all the data for estimating that he is very proficient in the exercise. He praises walking but says saddle leather is preferable, though more costly. He is very grateful that he does not need eyeglasses.

In *Over the Teacups* he says that at sixty we come within the range of the rifle pits and describes the nine survivors of his class, which graduated fifty-nine members. But here he is most impressed with the amazing progress he has seen—the friction match, the railroad, ocean steamer, photography, spectroscope, telegraph, telephone, phonograph, anesthesia, electric illumination, bicycle, etc., telling us that all his boyish shooting was done with a flintlock and all his voyaging on a sailing packet. He has a tingling sense of progress that amounts to a kind of pity for his own youth; and although he cannot conceive how it is possible, he has a faint hope that progress may go on at the same rate. The thing to be avoided is automatism, which is habit gone to seed. We must be sure and take in sail betimes. In deciding between duties and the desire to rest, many have actually welcomed the decay of powers in order that they might rest. He bitterly condemns conservative religious dogmas, which have done so much to disorganize our thinking powers, and recognizes the happy tendency to soften and then throw off creeds as one grows old as if in order to return to the source of life as ignorant and helpless as we came from it. He ends with a meager array of facts to indicate that poets are

not short-lived and that although their powers may
wane, some of the best poems have come from people
of advanced age.

The late Senator G. F. Hoar [18] thinks young people
contemplate old age and death from a distance, as
Milton's "Hymn on Morning" was written at midnight.
"I would indite something concerning the solar system
—Betty, bring the candles." Old age is a matter of
temperament and not of years. In some, old age is
congenital. Lowell says, "From the womb he emerged
gravely, a little old man." John Quincy Adams fought
the House of Representatives at 83; Josiah Quincy
attacked the "Know-Nothings" at 85—said the bats
were leading the eagles. He broke his hip at 92 and
when Dr. Ellis called, he was so charmed that he forgot to ask him how he was and went back to do so.
Quincy said, "Damn the leg." Gladstone, aged 83, faced
a hostile government, House of Lords, press, aristoc-
racy, university, and perhaps a hostile queen, and said,
"I represent the youth and hope of England. The solution of these questions of the future belongs aright to
us who are of the future and not to you who are of the
past." There are certain functions especially assigned
to age, for example, the magistrate passes upon things
after the controversy is over. Senators by law must
be at least thirty but the average age of them is nearly
sixty. Methuselah's days must have been stupid. Age
should cultivate unripe fruit. The greatest penalty of
growing old is losing the friends of youth, dying in the
death of others. But a large capacity for friendship
atones. General Sherman's friendship was like being
admitted to an order of nobility or knighted. His circle
of friends grew throughout the country although no
one was more choice in his selection or more outspoken

---

[18] *Old Age and Immortality,* 1893.

in his opinions. Of old, age was marked by splendor in dress and punctilious stateliness in manner, and art often thus represents it.

Each generation, as it passes, gets from its successor much more criticism than sympathy; the heir is not on good terms with the king. "Crabbed age and youth cannot live together." No English monarch ever built a tomb for his predecessor. We should thank God that Abraham, Isaac, and David are well dead.

It is young men who deal most courageously with the doctrine of immortality; old men have made no contribution to it. They are silent or do not wish to be suspected of cant or hypocrisy, or perhaps fear striking their heads against a stone wall. If there is no immortality it is the great souls who will be most disappointed and the world will be "only the receptacle of a compost heap of the carcasses of an extinct humanity." A cruel Highland chief shut his rebellious nephew in a dungeon, fed him on salt meat, then let down a cup which on opening contained no water, and left him to die of thirst. The Divine treats us this way if there is no future. Old men develop individuality. They reason less and less about the future and trust reason less. But "beside the silent sea I wait the muffled oar," assured that "no harm from Him can come to me on ocean or on shore."

W. D. Howells [19] said at eighty that he was less afraid of dying than when he was young. Virtues may become faults, for example, thrift may make a miser, his love of gold being more tangible than of greenbacks. It is, indeed, a shame to die rich. We are often young in spots, for example, on a spring morning. Slight acclivities seem to grow up into hills. After too long sitting, for example, in the theater, we realize that we have over-rested. The golden age, he thinks, is between fifty

---

[19] "Eighty Years and After," *Harper's*, 1919. p. 21.

and sixty. Those who have made themselves wanted are still so. Our utmost effort is less. We are not dull, as the young think us because we seem so to them. A reader has exhausted most of the best literature and yet of rereading old books and reading new ones we never tire and have our favorite passages. We should interest ourselves in public questions. It hurts to be always told how young we look. We forget names we were most familiar with and recall them by their uses or perhaps by their foreign equivalents. He thinks old women, however, do not forget words. Tolstoi said that memory is hell and a future state that recalls all would be a bore. Titian outlived 99 and painted to the end. His masterpiece, the bronze doors of the sacristy at St. Mark's, was done when he was 85. When tired he withdrew to a dark, warm place. John Bigelow in the nineties gave a charming lecture on Dumas. Versus the solitude of old age, the young do often seem dull. We do not help other old men enough. Woman's sympathy goes far to bridge this interval. Some grieve that they cannot help with their own self-support. Howells says he is a great dreamer and forgets where he puts things, for example, his spectacles.

H. D. Sedgwick [20] thinks Harvard seniors more disposed to answer questions than to ask them. Youth may be worth living, but is old age so? Young men know nothing of youth; they cannot realize it objectively, for they despise it and want to hurry on. The "kid" would be a Freshman. He feels at first just outside the door of something delectable. The boy does not enjoy himself so much as the old man looking on "for such is the kingdom of Heaven." The young are individualists absorbed in self. They form cliques excluding hoi polloi. They over-praise their own

---

[20] "De Senectute," *Atlantic,* 1913, p. 163.

college, but their ego is always the center. It is really
the spectator in the theater that gets the most out of
it. Youth is exclusive in its foolish divisions. The old
do not dwell on differences but common qualities. The
old man finds no solace in isolation but in community.
He loves humanity; seeks a refuge for self; passes
lightly over differences of speech, clothes, and customs.
Perhaps this is due to the slow approach of night, which
makes all draw together for the warmth of friendship.
The old man snuggles to the breast of humanity and
is less prone to lose himself in random interests. If he
cannot get about in space, he turns to the essential truth
of the universe. The gods do not know the words
"great" or "small." The old see wonders in the iris.
Youth seeks the top of the mountains because it cannot
see the wonders in what is common and what is right
about. The old are more religious and less subject to
emotional crises. They do not see God in the fire or
smoke but can see Him in the commonplace, and find
beauty in cloud, flower, and tree; while youth is too busy
with its own emotions and their tyranny. The records of
earth tell of bestial cruelty. The globe is cooling and
youth resists it like Prometheus. To youth the energy
of the world is inexplicable. All is the product of brute
force. Out of the dust came the eye and the brain and
the mind, and all the turmoil is like labor-pangs to produce love, beauty, and happiness. Everything is full of
aspiration. Out of the universe will come God, who
is slowly evolving from the material without. If the
matter of life has produced the passions of humanity,
it is charged with potential divinity.

Walt Mason [21] says that until his system falls apart he
will stay on deck, with his coat-tails in the air, refusing
to be relieved, even though he may require overhauling

---

[21] "I Refuse to Grow Old," *Amer. Mag.*, Sept., 1919.

LITERATURE BY AND ON THE AGED

every few days. When he was young he was careless in dress, but as he grew older he became very fastidious and was inclined to turn a new leaf in dress every day and give the best imitation possible of a young man. But we who were born during the Van Buren period cannot look like little Lord Fauntleroys. He studied old men and found that one did not believe in adding machines while most hated innovations in general. An old man who criticises anything present is always very unpopular and when he praises it, the attitude of everyone changes toward him. The young hate ancient history and want to lay it away in moth-balls. Eternal vigilance is the price of eternal youth.

Edison at the age of seventy-two said he worked eighteen hours a day and that it was hard for him to take a week-end off. When Colonel Death comes around the corner and says "Time's up," Mason says he wants him to find him in a hand-to-hand conflict with his trusty lyre. Every town has a coterie of "old boys" who are against everything; they write letters to the press, etc. Now, idleness is the worst thing for an old man and for his disposition. If he retires at 50 kindly, he will grow impossible by 70. The old are always blaming and brooding over the final showdown. It is always possible that the next cold or bit of rheumatism may break down the carburetor, but why worry?

E. P. Powell,[22] a Florida clergyman, cannot conceive old age for young Sidis and others like him. Charity should not help people to get rid of work but conceive a haven of rest. A workman damns epitaphs readable a few years hence. Humanity must not be loaded with a mass of pensions. Old age must not be a luxury. Good sleep should renew the world. Rev. Tinker improved sweet corn, Rev. Goodrich, potatoes. Worry is

---

[22] "The Passing of Old Age," *Independent*, Jan., 1914.

one road to the cemetery and idleness is another. The working problem is more important than that of diet. The author writes his sermons lying on the floor and spinning a top. A Florida June morning, he says, is far better than a month in Paradise. He does not care for heaven because he is more interested in the divine earth. The family should include four generations. We should all strive for perpetual youth. "Few children but better," should be our motto. Premature old age is reprehensible. The world is full of half dead men. We shall never abolish death. Present society is death-hastening and life-wasting. Fisher would prolong by (1) eugenics, (2) personal hygiene, (3) public, (4) what might be called domestic hygiene.

U. V. Wilson [23] says that the seasons or nature were never so pleasant. He has the leisure that he toiled for all his life. Every year seems shorter (being now only one-seventy-third of all) so that he feels he is approaching the infinite point of view. Religionists tell us that it is hard for the Lord to save an old man but now that the days and years shrink we approach eternity. Seventy-three is the age of his physical being but he is really centuries older. His circle of friends is narrow but closer. He had a fad for hunting and fishing and photography and his sense of youth remains forever. He dreads decrepitude and helplessness and hates to see his body tumble down, like a man in a dungeon seeing the world only through a very small window. Second childhood suggests that if the eye fails, there are glorious things beyond it can see; that if the ear fails, there are inner harmonies. He feels like a youth shut up in an old body. Infirmities are forerunners of immortal health. So he does not fear death because it only removes barriers between him and the fullness of life.

---

[23] "At Seventy-Three and Beyond," *Atlan.,* 1914, p. 123.

D. G. Brinton [24] says "that old age is synonymous with wisdom is a comical deception which the gray-beards have palmed off on the world because by law and custom they hold most of the property and want most of the power as well." "As we grow old, we cease to obey our finer instincts" (Thoreau). "The experience of youth serves but to lead old age astray, and this is nowhere so plain as when an old man pretends a zest for the pleasures of the young. No fool like an old fool." "Every age has pleasures sufficient which are appropriate to it, and these alone should be sought after." If youth respects the laws of nature, old age is very tolerable. It brings many compensations for losses, and although not likely to be so happy as the best of middle life, it should be and often is superior in this respect to youth. "Probably it would generally be so were we more willing to learn the lessons appropriate to it."

One writer says no man can be happy till he is past sixty, and another, "He who teaches the old is like one who writes on blotted paper." A long life is the desire of all, and old age, which all abhor, is the hope of all. "It alone justifies a man to himself and before others." "The sage is he whose life is a consistent whole and who carries out in his age the plans which he made in youth." "The Jews of Frankfurt average ten years more of life than the non-Jewish citizens because they avoid unsanitary avocations and observe wiser rules of diet." At seventy-five exposure to cold is thirty-two times more dangerous than it is at thirty years of age. "The sorrows of age are usually the returns of the investments of youth, these proving of that sort which levy assessments instead of paying dividends. A short life and a merry one is the maxim

---

[24] *The Pursuit of Happiness*, 1893.

of many a youngster. The hidden falsehood at the core
of this philosophy is the belief that happiness belongs
to youth alone." "The admiration of the early periods
of life is one of a common class of illusions." "He who
would work securely for his own welfare will not be
led astray by the belief that any one period of life contains solely or in any large measure the enjoyments of
life as a whole. He will, therefore, not eat to-day the
bread of to-morrow. He will guard the fires of youth
that he may not in age have to sit by the cold ashes
of exhausted pleasures." The price of so doing is premature senility, loss of zest in life due to the early
exhaustion of irrational enjoyments. "The only malady
which all covet is the only one which is absolutely fatal,
old age." No passion is so weak but that a little pressed,
it will master the fear of death. "He who is haunted
by the dread of dying makes himself miserable for fear
he cannot make himself miserable longer."

Few modern writers have written more sagely on old
age than N. S. Shaler, late professor of geology at
Harvard.[25] He attaches great importance to the interval between the end of the reproductive period and
death, which in lower creatures is very brief if it exists
at all. In domesticated animals there is hardly any
normal old age and they do not seem to know a climacteric. There is a great variation among different races
in this period of senescence, which is so peculiar to man.
This interval is very brief among savages. But with
the beginning of speech all the relations of the individual to his group change. If old animals live on,
they do so to themselves and not for the benefit of their
kind. But in man the old individual becomes a store-
house of acquired or traditional knowledge, and wisdom
has, for the first time, a distinct value in organic associa-

[25] *The Individual: A Study of Life and Death,* 1910, especially Chap. 13,
"The Period of Old Age."

tion. It was in this way that the reproductive period was shortened, or perhaps we had better say that life was prolonged beyond it. In civilized society the old are still members of the species, not aliens or enemies. When a people begins to have a literature or a religion and a large body of mores as social inheritance develops, the value of old age increases.

The old have to maintain a more dignified demeanor. They are readapted and can go on with life as before, especially as they now have eyes and teeth preserved. The best attitude toward the old is one that assures a broader view of life and better sense of values and marks the modern passage from the earlier division of men into ranks and occupations, in which women, youth, and old men were once separated from the active and militant class. Thus the position of the aged is now bettered by keeping in close relation with their fellows.

The growth of wealth has helped democratic individualization and thus helped old age. "The presence of three or four generations in the social edifice gives to it far more value than is afforded by one or two." They "unite the life of the community and bridge the gap between successive generations." "As the body of the tradition which makes the spirit of a people becomes the greater, it is the more difficult to effect the transmission of it from stage to stage in the succession." Despite the volume of printed matter, including history, there is a spirit of society that cannot be preserved in books. Who can doubt that if veterans of our Civil War had been more numerous and influential, we should have plunged into the late war with Spain. There would have been more men who really remembered what war meant and its lessons, for the new generation lacked the true sense of what conflict was and went about it light-heartedly. So the need of strict military discipline generally has to be relearned with each war. The same is true of hygienic policies in the army. There are, thus, many political, social, and even business follies that would have been avoided had the wisdom and experience that only old age can bring been more dominant. Thus we could make our historic records not only more effective and more complete in regard to its matter but also more perfect as regards the lessons it conveys. History is often written by men who are separated from the times they chronicle and the best way to bridge the gulf is to keep in touch as long as possible with the generation that was making history.

But the endeavor to retain the aged is not merely an effort to preserve the lives of the old but part of the problem of avoiding premature death for everyone. Thus since man came there seems to be a sudden loss of longevity if we measure it solely in terms of the period of growth. If this really has occurred, it may be that the term is less fixed than we should expect it to be if the institution were of more recent date.

Anthony Trollope [26] tells us of a small republic, Britannula, situated somewhere in the South Pacific and which had freed itself from England, that had been induced by its leader, Mr. Neverbend, who was deeply impressed with the sufferings and dangers of old age, to pass a law that at a fixed period, which after much discussion was fixed at 67½ years of age, everyone in the colony should be taken with great honor to a college beautifully situated five miles from the capital city and there spend a final year, at the end of which he was to suffer euthanasia at the hand of the chief by being placed under an opiate and bled to death. Details are given of the many discussions that led up to this legislation, with the justifications for it and descriptions of the college. When the law was passed, there was no

---

[26] *The Fixed Period*, New York, 1881.

one in the community of great age. Deposition or rele-
gation to the college was to be a matter of much pomp
and dignity, with bells, banquets, and processions, and
life within the walls was to be made attractive by every
means.

The first to reach the required age, Crasweller, ten
years the senior of the founder, was a man of immense
vitality and wealth, the most efficient proprietor of a
very large estate, and when the day of his deposition
drew near he dismayed the founder by insisting that he
was a year younger, although all knew his age, which
was to be tatooed upon the skin of everyone. Meanwhile, an interesting love episode is described between
his daughter and the son of the founder. There was
much bitterness and recrimination and it is realized that
it will never do to compel the withdrawal by force of
the first victim, who was to set a high example to all
others; and so finally the year falsely claimed is allowed
to pass and then Crasweller is taken in state to the college itself, which another citizen was growing weary
of tending because it was untenanted. There were many
criticisms of its new and unfinished state and of the
proximity of the cremation furnaces, which were said
even to smell of the bodies of the animals that had been
consumed in them.

Meanwhile, as the others were drawing near to their
term, support of the plan passed over into covert and
then overt opposition, and just as the first victim with
his escort entered, an English man-of-war appeared—
in response, it afterwards became known, to a petition
of the citizens to stop such a proceeding, which thus
cost the colony its independence. Thus Crasweller was
freed and Neverbend, the founder, retired to England,
where his musings at last convinced him that the world
was not yet quite ready for his great reform. It might
work if and when men were philosophers but it would

SENESCENCE

doubtless have to be postponed at least during the lives
of his grandchildren, and perhaps indefinitely. Thus
the women, who had always opposed it, and the populace,
who welcomed it when they were young but condemned
it as they grew old, had their will and its realization
is yet to come. The reasons that led to the scheme were
that the misery, uselessness, troublesomeness, and often
obstructiveness of old age still remain and are ever increasing in force, so that something like this must surely
sometime be.

Stephen Paget [27] gives us an excellent description of
what he thinks a typical state of mind of old age, but
which I deem an excellent illustration of senile degen-
eracy. The old man, he says, wonders at his own
existence, is bewildered at the feel of the pen in his
hand, at the taste of his food; that he is alive when so
many millions are dead or unborn; at a funeral is fascinated by someone's whisper or the contour of a face
or some other irrelevancy; is smitten with momentary
surprise that he is or that it is it; finds an apocalypse
on looking in the glass; is oppressed by a sense of mystery that is very far from philosophic contemplation; and
realizes that when others observe him thus, they reflect
that there is no speculation—"No speculation in those
eyes that thou dost glare wtih"; finds himself growing
out "of the world, of life, of time"; feels it not unreasonable to consider the one, the all, the infinite, if his mind
drifts that way. His mind wanders while he wonders
whether heaven lies about him in his second infancy.
Perhaps it all brings the kind of smile we call wistful.
He may go crazy over a human eyebrow or a breath of
air; common things seem novel; the dull things fas-
cinate. One enjoys a vagabond ease on the street; is
irked at fine manners; is fond of news. The old prob-

[27] *The Man in the Street,* 1907, 405 p.

lems of politics and religion lose their charm and in place of pure art we turn to that of the street. He says we old are thus a sentimental lot and for the sake of economy live on our emotions, which cost nothing. This point of view he deems more or less philosophic, etc.

This state of mind the psychologist would call dissociative, if not dissolutive. It is the dementia præcox of old age and can mean nothing but disintegration and befuddlement. True, childhood is often lost in wonder at items of experience that later are synthesized into wholes and become commonplaces. But this goes with a keen rapport with the environment, which the senses are developing, while this author's musings reveal a falsetto last look before we are melted or diffused into the cosmos. Such reveries are letting go, not taking hold of life. They are the decadence of the philosophic spirit and belie the normal tendency of old age, which is to knit up experiences into synthetic wholes, to draw the moral of life, and to give integrity to the soul.

Thus Mr. Paget seems to be the victim of a kind of senile Narcissism, revering its chief traits in his symptoms, yielding himself with a kind of masochistic pleasure to any chance impressions that present themselves. He has ceased to strive and to will, and there is no justification of his point of view, that his state is akin to that of certain transcendentalists who have fallen into deep puzzlements over what Bronson Alcott called "the whichness of the what."

Old age is neither helped nor understood by the cheap and chipper paradoxes about it of those who tell the old that they are not so save in years and that these do not count, or who affect to marvel at the passion to look and seem young. One writer [28] even tells us that the old are beautiful and thinks it is a perverse precept of social

---

[28] Richard le Gallienne, "Not Growing Old," *Harper's,* 1921.

condition to think of chronological age at all. "We should say eighty years young;" "properly speaking there is no old age," etc. All this is really the state of mind of a mental healer who does not wish old age, disease, or death, and so denies their existence and turns his back upon reality. It is the state of mind mythically ascribed to an ostrich, although the best observers deny that it ever buries its head in the sand from fear of danger. Such cajolery of the old is like baby-talk to children, which only infantilism or advanced second childhood relishes. It suggests infirmary wards and is itself a product of the type of psychic invalidism and valetudinarianism that is interesting to the psychologist because the appetite for it suggests the dreamy state of mind in which delusions become factual if they embody our desires. The old should be beyond attitudinizing or affecting a youth that is gone, for this is to live a lie, which is dangerous not only to their serenity, for old age should be the age of truth, but to health and even life.

G. S. Street [29] refutes the statement that of late, especially since the war, there is a great and growing gap between the young and the old, who speak a different language mutually unintelligible; that the old can no longer understand the young; etc. This has found frequent expression in recent literature. The rising generation is said to have its own interests, ideas, and even language, to have broken away from the old, and even to have developed a new poetry and art. A generation ago there was such a gap. The grown-ups were Olympians and there was little attempt of either young or old to understand each other. There was little friendship between dons and students but we have now a popular cult not only of childhood but of adolescence.

---

[29] "Young and Old," *Nineteenth Century*, June, 1920.

It is said that psychoanalysis is becoming a cult of the young generation but Freud himself was not born yesterday. A very few soldiers have complained bitterly of the selfishness and stupidity of their elders who sent them into the trenches, safely staying at home themselves. There are, of course, aging politicians and diplomats who are little in touch with the future as represented by the sentiments and aspirations of the young.

But, on the whole, the war has brought old and young nearer together. The old have given up their foolish airs of superiority and the young have been matured by their experience. To be sure, these oldsters often criticise the young generation, that it is aggressive and free of speech or conduct; and there are young people who, under the illusion of new ideas, are aggressive. But such a gulf as has existed between the old and the young has always been mainly the fault of the old, and the qualities of the young give them less excuse for this attitude than they ever had before. Perhaps the world is a little too much in the hands of people who are a little too old, but this is being rapidly remedied.

C. W. Saleeby, M.D., [30] says that young children never worry and youth does so almost entirely for the future, while the worries of old age are chiefly retrospective and may take the form of regrets. If young people feel these, it is only for a brief space, for they are resilient and soon react. In middle life the struggle for existence is keener and the "might-have-beens" cannot always be dismissed, although those in good health can usually soon surmount them. But this is more difficult in old age unless, indeed, it is "a lusty winter, frosty but kindly." Wordsworth describes old age as it should be in this respect in "The Happy Warrior":

[30] *Worry and Old Age,* 1909, Chap. 14.

SENESCENCE

Who not content that former worth stand fast
Looks forward persevering to the last,
From well to better daily self-surpassed.
Who, whether praise of him must walk the earth
Forever and to noble deeds give birth
Or he must fail, to sleep without his fame
And leave a dead, unprofitable name—
Finds comfort in himself and in his cause
And while the mortal mist is gathering, draws
His breath of confidence in heaven's applause.
This is the Happy Warrior, this is he
That every man in arms should wish to be

. . . . . .

A being breathing thoughtful breath
A traveler between life and death,
The reason firm, the temperate will,
Endurance, forethought, strength, and skill.

There is a vast difference between old age as commonly seen and as it should be. The average type
of humanity is undergoing a change. Civilization means
city-fication and this involves a state of mind very different from that of the rustic. Worry has become the
disease of the age as it was not formerly when man's
vegetative nature was stronger. It is a *maladie des
beaux esprits*. We are no longer content to eat, sleep,
and sit in the sun. The old always and greatly need
grandchildren and it was never so hard to provide occupation for them, for their temptation now is to become
self-centered, which is perhaps most common in women.
It takes a different form in men superannuated by some
automatic rule. Pitiful is the state of those who withdraw from occupations that have required and developed
great mental activity.

The young, on the other hand, are less tolerant than
formerly of the foibles and frailties of age. We live
at such a high speed that it seems slow, if not stupid,
and lack of sympathy adds to its burdens. The very

idea of the family is declining and there is little left of the old sentiment for the patriarch, so that "the faster we move, the wider must become the gap between the young and those who, like the aged, have ceased to move." Indeed, old age "is probably less tolerated and less tolerable to-day than ever in the past," for the old were never so out of it. It might be expected, as death draws near, that religious anxieties would increase, but the contrary is true. Youth was never so unable to apply the principle *Tout comprendre c'est tout pardonner* or to make allowances. So it is the young who worry most about religious matters. "Absence of occupation is not rest. The mind that's vacant is a mind distrest."

If the man who has lived solely for sport is ill prepared to meet old age, he who has lived solely for business is still less so. He has had no time to cultivate his more human tastes but has developed his potentialities in only one direction and when superannuation comes his soul is bankrupt. He generally now has money as well as time to spend and so devotes himself to increasing his material comforts in a way that beckons death, because high living is no substitute for high thinking. He should discover the least atrophied of his powers and devote himself to their eleventh-hour development. The man of the modern nervous type should lay up treasure that age cannot corrupt. Herbert Spencer said the purpose of education was to prepare for complete living.

One of the most beautiful and normal attributes of old age is interest in the young, without which age is lonely and life becomes, as the preacher said, "vanity of vanities." "If old people are confined to the company of other old people, they hasten each other's downward course." There was "even a certain psychological truth symbolized in the old idea that the company of a young

girl was the best means for the rejuvenescence of an
old man." "Never was the tendency to abandon old
age to its own devices so strong as it is to-day." Spencer
thought the care of the aged by their dependents was
the fit complement for the care that in earlier years had
been devoted to them and regarded the imperfection of
this return the great defect of our practical morals.
Indeed, the author doubts "whether the aged were ever
so much to be pitied as they are to-day." The psychological needs of old age are greater than ever.

In his *Health, Strength, and Happiness,*[31] he gives an
earnest, practical caution for all, but especially for the
aged, to eat less; and particularly so in warm weather.
"We dig our graves with our teeth." Fat is hardly a
part of the body at all. Flesh is really muscle, so that
the fat man should be said to be losing flesh. "The
whole secret of prolonging one's life consists in doing
nothing to shorten it." The writer profoundly believes
in government by the elderly in years and thinks that
the really greatest works in many of the most difficult
fields have been done by them. He stresses the fact that
there is a certain kind of wisdom that nothing but age
can bring. He sees the chief cause of senile degeneration in the hardening of the arteries, due to the necessity
of disposing of superfluous fat. A man is really as old
as his mind and he doubts whether we are producing
more really living elderly men and women than did the
ancient world. He is bitter in his condemnation of the
common phrase, "Too old at forty."

Bernard Shaw [32] thinks mankind is headed straight
for the City of Destruction and can be saved not by
eugenics or by a new and better education, as H. G.
Wells opines, but by prolonging human life to *circa*

---

[31] London, 1908.
[32] *Back to Methuselah: A Metabiological Pentateuch,* New York, 1921,
400 p.

three hundred years. If the length of life were reduced to one-half or one-quarter of what it now is we may assume that our culture and institutions would decline because children could not direct them. It is exactly the equivalent of this that has actually happened, only instead of life being shortened to half or a quarter of its span the problems of life have doubled or quadrupled in magnitude and difficulty so that present-day man is not grown up to them. Trained only to run a motor truck, he is now since the war called on to be an air pilot, and this requires a long and arduous training with a great deal of preliminary selection or weeding out. Thus man must now simply either live a great deal longer or the race will go under.

This can be done and Shaw tells us how. It is simply by wishing and willing it intensely enough and for generations. Lamarck, the first creative evolutionist, devoted his life to the "fundamental proposition that living organisms changed because they wanted to." They wanted to see and so evolved eyes; to move about and so grew organs of locomotion; the forbears of the giraffe wanted to browse on taller and taller tree-tops and so grew long necks, etc. All this was done by the same phyletic impulsion as now impels us to talk, swim, skate, ride a wheel, etc. We strive at it long and persistently and by and by, presto! the power comes from within because we will it, and it is never lost. In this same way man can and will acquire the power of living several times longer than he does now. As he does so he will put away his present occupations and interests, sports, amusements, party politics, religious dogmas, ceremonies, and indeed most of the things that now interest the populace, and come out into a new adulthood with vastly enhanced powers and a far wider horizon. Those who do this first will become pilots of mankind, which at present seems doomed for want of more wisdom and better leaders. Darwin and especially the Neo-Darwinians who believe in "circumstantial evolution" launched the world on a career of egoism in morals and mechanism in life that has brought it to its present pass and made it forget that all true evolution is from within, vitalistic, and voluntaristic.

Shaw's drama opens in Eden, where Adam, oppressed by the conviction that he must live forever, first faces the fact of death in finding the putrefying body of a fawn. The gorgeously hooded serpent explains to Eve how she is to renew life by offspring from her body, and because of this she and Adam are assured that they need live only a thousand years. In the next scene Cain the Killer justifies his vocation.

In the second part, which opens in our day, two brothers, one a liberalized clerical and the other a biologist, agree that life is too short to be taken seriously and that neither of them is within a hundred and fifty years of the experience and wisdom they have been sincerely pretending to. To be a good clergyman or biologist requires several centuries. Man now dies before he knows what life or what science is. Indeed, life is now so short that it is hardly worth while to do anything well. Then a past and present prime minister, obviously caricatures of the two most famous men who have lately filled that position in England, enter and try —each according to his method and hobbies—to interest the brothers in one popular cause after another, but in vain; and are finally plainly told that they have not lived long enough to outgrow personal and local prejudices or to see things in their true perspective. The statesmen, failing to find campaign material serviceable for the next election in this new Gospel of the Brothers Barnabas, then ask for a prescription that will prolong their lives and, failing to obtain either, cease to be interested. It does not seem practical to found a Longevity Party and it might be dangerous to let everyone live as long as he wanted to. The statesmen are finally told that as they are incompetent to do God's work He will produce some better beings who can.

In Part III, A.D. 2170, The thing Happens. An archbishop, now 283 years old, is convinced that "mankind can live any length of time it knows to be absolutely necessary to save civilization from extinction." Such lengthening may now happen to anyone and when he is convinced that he is one of these elect everything changes. A well preserved lady who appeared in a former part as a parlormaid but who is now 224 years old enters and discourses sapiently on the traits of the short-livers and complains that there are so few grownups. "What is wrong with us is that we are a non-adult race." Her own serious life began at 120.

In Part IV we are transferred to the year A.D. 3000. An Elderly Gentleman, attired in very pronounced fashions that have not changed from our day, comes from Bagdad, now the British capital—London being only a park and cities being for the most part abolished. He is an amateur student of history and comes to revisit the home of his remote ancestors but finds it now tenanted only by long-livers who regard him as a child and chaperone and instruct him as such. At first he loquaciously vents his own opinions on a great variety of subjects with the utmost confidence but finally, under the tutelage of a Primary and a Secondary, and at last from contact with an awful Tertiary (for thus those in the first, second, and third century of their lives are known and labeled) he loses confidence, becomes more and more depressed at finding so many things he cannot understand, and has a serious attack of the "discouragement" that is generally the doom of all short-livers who visit these parts. In the end the aged Briton is so confounded by the wisdom that he cannot comprehend that life loses all its attractions and he finally dies of exhaustion at the feet of the Oracle. Napoleon also swaggers and boasts upon the stage, but his ideals, too, are shown to be only characteristic of the short-livers and he is completely subjected.

Part V of this Pentateuch is dated A.D. 31,920. Children are now born from eggs, clamoring to get out when about as mature as our youth are at seventeen, so that there are no children in our sense. They are grown-ups, according to our standard, at three or four. Art and science, after incredible labors, are at last able to produce two homunculi, a male and a female. They represent the consummation of circumstantial or mechanical evolution. They appear, talk, will, feel, apparently not as the reflex mechanisms and automata they are but as completely human. They have, however, almost incredible powers of destruction which they turn first against their own fabricator. So dangerous are they that they have to be destroyed because not truly human since they lack the creative urge from within.

This amazingly bold projection of Shaw's imagination into the void is elaborately wrought out and needs very careful reading to be rightly appraised. Almost every reader will agree that he goes much too far in disparaging about all that modern man has done or cared for so far in the world as childish doll-play. This is its pessimism. Its optimism, which lies in the hope of vastly increased longevity and wisdom, will be thought to compensate, or to fail to do so, according to the temperament of the reader. The new dispensation, which is to come when man has grown up, for in the last part it is seen that he may live even 700 or 800 years, will be ushered in by those individuals who are most perfectly convinced of the desperate state into which man has now fallen but nevertheless profoundly believe both that he is worth saving and that he can be saved. George

Eliot's way of prolonging life by giving to moments the significance of days will not do because great events often have no power to speed up but must evolve very slowly. The best type of old age as we know it is still too puerile to expect very much from.

Shaw's conceptions of the old are neither attractive nor constructive but priggish because presuming on their years to demand respect for a wisdom that is no-where in evidence. There is almost no suggestion that they have done anything to improve the material or psychic conditions of human life. No great inventions are suggested unless telephonic communication by tuning forks. These Ancients seem to derive their greatest pleasure from disparagement of their own youth and, what is far worse, of youth in general. The long-livers are cynical, addicted to sneering, rebuke, criticise, and do not inspire, construct, achieve, or even teach; in fact they only make the gestures and show the affectations of sagehood. They are divided in their counsels whether to exterminate the short-livers or to leave them to natural selection. Thus they are a class apart and we have almost no hint as to the stages by which they evolved. Now we are told that they are "elected" to longevity or achieve it as "sports," while in the Preface it is insisted that it comes by a long series of persistent efforts.

On the whole, happy as was his choice of scene, fascinating as are these almost actionless conversations, the whole thing is a *jeu d'esprit,* with no message of practical import to our age or to the aged unless it be to slightly encourage the hope in the latter that by willing to do so more and more intensely they may add somewhat to their length of years. Shaw's Ancients are simply a board of censors to carry out his own whims and who have grown arrogant as their powers increased. Altogether they are so unlovely that the reader would hesitate whether he would prefer to be a bloodless Ancient or to take his chance of being exterminated by them as a short-liver. The two Ancients in the fifth book of the Pentateuch, 700 and 800 years old respectively, are chilly, loveless, almost clotheless, sleepless, hairless creatures, happy in enjoying a wisdom of the nature of which we are given very few hints. They teach that all works of art from rag dolls to statues, and even to homunculi, are needless, and the intimation is that they are well on the way to becoming independent of the body, which they have subjected and which has lost all its attractions. We are not even told how the gigantic eggs from which the race is born at adolescence are produced. The final verdict of Lilith, the androgynous mother of our first parents in Eden, is that in giving Eve curiosity, which was still impelling the race to conquer matter and then resolve itself back into bodiless vortexes and energies, she had made no mistake for the Ancients are ever gaining in wisdom to comprehend the universe and, despite the slow decay of their bodies, are likely to attain the goal of achieving real but immaterial truth, beauty, and goodness all in one, so that she need not exterminate man and produce in his place a new and higher race of beings. Thus Shaw's Ancients are the direct antithetes of Nietzsche's supermen.

The poets of all times and climes have had something to say of old age, and vastly more of death. The latter has always been one of the chief themes of Christian hymnology and both its gruesome horrors and its consolations have found expression in countless tropes—sleep, harvest, crossing the river, and many others that are fairly burned into the consciousness of all who have come into contact with the church. Hymns have given the Western world ideas of death that the scientific descriptions of it show to be utterly false to fact, for the dying almost never face death consciously, so that its terrors are generally quite unknown to those who meet it; while the cajolements that the Great Enemy has really been conquered in his stronghold and the supreme fear of the world banished, which, as I have elsewhere shown,[33] came to its most ecstatic affirmation at Pentecost, are no less fallacious. Thus along with its anodyne Christianity has invested death with a new horror of hell unknown to the pagan world. Moreover, it has always been taught. as something exogenous or as a graft upon a more primitive stock and it is the latter that the psychologist chiefly seeks to know. Thus, excluding the more artificial reactions that have come to it from this source, I have reduced my first numerous selections to a very few that express the natural spontaneous repercussion of the three chief attitudes of mind regarding it.

The first is the death thought that always and everywhere tends to find its first expression in ingenuous youth and this has never been more fully and normally portrayed than in Bryant's "Thanatopsis," [34] which is familiar even to school children and which was written by the author in his ripe adolescence. This might have been composed in ancient pagan Hellas or even by a Buddhist as well as by a Christian, so generic and germane is it to human nature as it evolves. Tennyson's "Crossing the Bar," [35] while it shows vestiges of the same youthful *appercus* that lingered into the author's maturer years, is far more specific, more funereal, and really the farewell address of a dying soul to survivors. The euthanasia motive is far less pronounced in it.

The second attitude is illustrated by Matthew Arnold

---

[33] See my *Jesus, the Christ, in the Light of Psychology*, New York, 1917, Chap. XI, p. 694, *et seq.*
[34] See the end of the last chapter.
[35] *Ibid.*

and by the lugubrious phase of Walt Whitman, both written after decrepitude had begun. Poems written in this spirit arouse the question whether old age is intrinsically pessimistic or perhaps even pathological. Should senescents express or repress the inexorable and progressive limitations and weaknesses senescence brings in its train, or strive to ignore if they cannot be oblivious to them? Are not such abandonments to pathos, in their deeper psychological motivation, a cry for pity, to which strong souls feel it unworthy to appeal? Are they perhaps atavistic vestiges or echoes of a time when the old were more cruelly treated? Why spend time and energy in mourning for what old age takes away rather than in finding "joy in what remains behind" and which no other stage of life can give? Hysterical symptoms are often only an appeal for sympathy by those who crave, perhaps subconsciously, more attention and service, which only selfishness would think lacking. Psychopaths and paranoiacs have often made literary capital of their aberrations, as have adolescents out of the ferments peculiar to their age. All this has its place but should, in my opinion, always be known as what it is, namely, abnormal and aberrant and thus belonging entirely to science and not to literary art.

The third or reminiscent type expresses the inveterate instinct of the old to look back upon life, to illumine and interpret its memories by such philosophy as experience brings, in some measure, to all who can reflect. It is a happy circumstance that senile amnesia always begins with the loss of recent recollections, while those of early life are only later and very rarely effaced. This resource is always open to the aged, who can relive the most interesting stages of their early and adult lives, unify them, and draw the moral of them as a whole. The world owes much and, as it grows old, will owe ever

more to the autobiographic impulse of those who achieve
normal senectitude.

The following is Matthew Arnold's "Growing Old":

> What is it to grow old?
> Is it to lose the glory of the form,
> The lustre of the eye?
> Is it for beauty to forego her wreath?
> —Yes, but not this alone.
>
> Is it to feel our strength—
> Not our bloom only, but our strength—decay?
> Is it to feel each limb
> Grow stiffer, every function less exact,
> Each nerve more loosely strung?
>
> Yes, this, and more; but not
> Ah, 'tis not what in youth we dream'd 'twould be!
> 'Tis not to have our life
> Mellow'd and soften'd as with sunset-glow,
> A golden day's decline.
>
> 'Tis not to see the world
> As from a height, with rapt prophetic eyes,
> And heart profoundly stirr'd;
> And weep, and feel the fulness of the past.
> The years that are no more.
>
> It is to spend long days
> And not once feel that we were ever young;
> It is to add, immured
> In the hot prison of the present, month
> To month with weary pain.
>
> It is to suffer this,
> And feel but half, and feebly, what we feel
> Deep in our hidden heart
> Festers the dull remembrance of a change,
> But no emotion—none.

147

SENESCENCE

It is—last stage of all—
When we are frozen up within, and quite
The phantom of ourselves,
To hear the world applaud the hollow ghost,
Which blamed the living man.

From Walt Whitman I quote the following four extracts:[36]

THANKS IN OLD AGE

Thanks in old age—thanks ere I go,
For health, the midday sun, the impalpable air—for life, mere life,
For precious ever-lingering memories, (of you my mother dear—
    you, father—you, brothers, sisters, friends,)
For all my days—not those of peace alone—the days of war the
    same,
For gentle words, caresses, gifts from foreign lands,
For shelter, wine and meat—for sweet appreciation.

A CAROL CLOSING SIXTY-NINE

Of me myself—the jocund heart yet beating in my breast,
The body wreck'd, old, poor and paralyzed—the strange inertia
    falling pall-like round me,
The burning fires down in my sluggish blood not yet extinct,
The undiminish'd faith—the groups of loving friends.

QUERIES TO MY SEVENTIETH YEAR

Approaching, nearing, curious,
Thou dim, uncertain spectre—bringest thou life or death?
Strength, weakness, blindness, more paralysis and heavier?
Or placid skies and sun? Wilt stir the waters yet?
Or haply cut me short for good? Or leave me here as now,
Dull, parrot-like and old, with crack'd voice harping, screeching?

AS I SIT WRITING HERE

As I sit writing here, sick and grown old,
Not my least burden is that dulness of the years, querilities,
Ungracious glooms, aches, lethargy, constipation, whimpering
    ennui,
May filter in my daily songs.

[36] By permission of, and special arrangement with, Doubleday, Page & Co.

148

LITERATURE BY AND ON THE AGED

Longfellow strikes a less pessimistic note:[37]

MORITURI SALUTAMUS

Ah, nothing is too late
Till the tired heart shall cease to palpitate.
Cato learned Greek at 80; Sophocles
Wrote his grand Œdipus, and Simonides
Bore off the prize of verse
From his compeers
When each had numbered more than four-score years.
And Theophrastus at four-score and ten
Had but begun his characters of men.
Chaucer at Wadstock, with the nightingales,
At sixty wrote The Canterbury Tales.
Goethe at Weimar, toiling to the last,
Completed Faust when eighty years were past.
These are, indeed, exceptions, but they show
How far the gulf stream of our youth may flow
Into the Arctic regions of our lives
Where little else but life itself survives.

.   .   .   .   .   .

Whatever poet, orator, or sage
May say of it, old age is still old age.
It is the waning, not the crescent, moon,
The dusk of evening, not the blaze of noon.
It is not strength but weakness, not desire
But its surcease, not the fierce heat of fire,
The burning and consuming element,
But that of ashes and of embers spent.
In which some living sparks we still discern,
Enough to warm but not enough to burn.
What, then, shall we sit idly down and say
The night hath come; it is no longer day?
The night hath not come; we are not quite
Cut off from labor by the failing light.
Something remains for us to do or dare,
Even the oldest tree some fruit may bear.
Not Œdipus Colonus, or Greek Ode,
Or tales of pilgrims that one morning rode
Out of the gateway of the Tabard Inn.
But other something would we but begin,

---

[37] By permission of, and special arrangement with, Houghton Mifflin Co.

149

SENESCENCE

For age is opportunity no less
Than youth itself, though in another dress,
And as the evening twilight fades away
The sky is filled with stars invisible by day.

I also append the following quotations:

At sixty-two life is begun,
At seventy-three begins once more;
Fly swifter as thou near'st the sun
And brighter shine at eighty-four.
    At ninety-five
    Shouldst thou arrive
Still wait on God and work and thrive.

It has been sung by ancient sages
That love of life increases with years
So much that in our later stages,
When bones grow sharp and sickness rages
The greatest love of life appears.

Hard choice for man to die or else to be
That tottering, wretched, wrinkled thing you see,
Age then we all prefer; for age we pray;
And travel on to life's last lingering day,
Then sinking slowly down from worse to worse,
Find Heaven's extorted boon our greatest curse.

Many a man passes his youth in preparing misery for his age,
and his age in repairing the misconduct of his youth.

It is easy to die but difficult to die at the right time.

The danger of shipwreck is less in mid-ocean than near to shore.

Time wears out masks; the old show what they are.

The misfortunes of life are that we are born young and become
old.

Grow old along with me!
The best is yet to be,
The last of life, for which the first was made!

LITERATURE BY AND ON THE AGED

What I aspired to be,
And was not, comforts me.
BROWNING: Rabbi Ben Ezra.

What is age but youth's full bloom
And retiring, more transcendent youth?

Old men must die or the world would grow mouldy, would only breed the past again.—TENNYSON: Becket.

Youth is a blunder; manhood a struggle; old age a regret.—DISRAELI: Coningsby.

See how the world its veterans rewards!
A youth of frolics, an old age of cards.
POPE: Moral Essays.

Alonso of Aragon was wont to say in commendation of age, that age appears to be best in four things—old wood best to burn, old wine to drink, old friends to trust, and old authors to read.—BACON: Apothegms.

Dr. Clara Barrus, who for many years has labored in the closest personal contact with John Burroughs, has kindly sent me, along with much other information, the notes he made during the last months of his life for an article that he never lived to complete on Old Age. The quotations and *appercus* that he collected and that most impressed him were such as the following:

As men grow old they grow more foolish and more wise.

Young saint, old devil; young devil, old saint.

A man at sixteen will prove a child at sixty.

When men grow virtuous in their old age they only make a sacrifice to God of the devil's leavings.

Nobody loves life like an old man.

An old young man will make a young old man.

151

SENESCENCE

Old age is a tyrant who forbids men, under pain of death, the pleasures of youth.

Reckless youth makes rueful age.

Young men think old men fools and old men know young men to be so.

The evening of life brings with it its lamps.

A youthful age is desirable but aged youth is troublesome and grievous.

To me the worst thing about old age is that one has outlived all his old friends. The past becomes a cemetery.

It is characteristic of old age to reverse its opinions and its likes and dislikes. But it does not reverse them; it revises them. If its years have been well spent it has reached a higher position from which to overlook Life; it commands a wider view.

Old Age may reason well but old age does not remember well. The power of attention fails, which we so often mistake for deafness in the old. It is the mind that is blunted and not the ear. Hence we octogenarians so often ask for your question over again. We do not grasp it the first time. We do not want you to speak louder. We only need to focus upon you a little more completely.

I probably make more strenuous demands upon him who aspires to be a poet than ever before. I see more clearly than ever before that sweetened prose put up in verse form does not make poetry any more than sweetened water put in the comb in the hive makes honey. The quality of the man makes all the difference in the world. A great nature can describe birds and flowers and clouds and sunsets and spring and autumn greatly.

We in our generation have become so familiar with a universe so much larger than that known to the Ancients that we naturally wonder how the wise men of Greece and Rome and of Judea could have had or seem to have had so little curiosity about the earth upon which they lived and of which they were so ignorant.

LITERATURE BY AND ON THE AGED

Cicero found that age increased the pleasure of conversation. It is certainly true that in age we do find our tongues if we have any. They are unloosened, and when the young or middle-aged sit silent the octogenarian is a fountain of conversation. In age one set of pleasures is gone and another takes its place.

The old man reasons well, the judgment is clear, the mind active, the conscience alert, the interest in life unabated. It is the memory that plays the old man tricks.

Names and places with which one has been perfectly familiar all his life suddenly, for a few moments, mean nothing. It is as if the belt slipped and the wheel did not go around. Then the next moment away it goes again. Or shall we call it a kind of mental anesthetic or paralysis? Thus, the other day I was reading something about Georgetown, S. A. I repeated the name over to myself a few times. Have I not known such a place some time, in my life. Where is it? "Georgetown." "Georgetown." The name seems like a dream. Then I thought of Washington, the Capitol, and the city above it, but had to ask a friend if its name was Georgetown. Then suddenly as if some chemical had been rubbed on a bit of invisible writing, out it came! Of course it was Georgetown. How could I have been in doubt about it; I had lived in Washington for ten years.

CHAPTER IV

STATISTICS OF OLD AGE AND ITS CARE

I—Numbers of old people increasing in all known lands where data are available—Actuarial and other mortality tables—Expectation of life and death-rate at different ages—Longevity and fecundity—Death-rate in different occupations—Irving Fisher's ideas on longevity—The population problem—Longevity in ancient Egypt and in the Middle Ages—Diversity of statistical methods and results.

II—Growing need of care for the indigent old—Causes of improvidence—Ignorance and misconception of what old age is and means—Why the old do not know themselves—Old age pensions in Germany, Austria, Great Britain and her colonies, France, Belgium, United States—Industrial pensions and insurance, beginning with railroads—Trades unions—Fraternal organizations—Retiring pensions in the army and navy—Local and national insurance — Teachers' pensions — The Carnegie Foundation—Criticism of pension systems—Growing magnitude, urgency, and diversity of views and methods—The Life Extension Institute—"Borrowed Time" and "Sunset" clubs—Should the old organize?

BEFORE discussing the nature and functions of old age, which chiefly concern us in this volume, we must in a brief, summary way answer two preliminary questions: (1) how many old people are there in the registration areas of the world to-day as compared to earlier times and to the total population; and (2) what is done for them publicly and privately. Each of these topics has a copious literature and experts of its own. On the first or statistical problem there is still great diversity of methods and results, which I simply present and make no attempt to harmonize, for this would be premature. As to the second point, of care, I have also attempted only a bird's-eye view and avoided details.

154

STATISTICS OF OLD AGE AND ITS CARE

I

The population between the ages of 65 and 74 in various countries (1900)[1] is as follows: United Kingdom—1,418,000 (including England, Ireland, Scotland, Wales, of which England and Wales have 1,076,000; Scotland, 151,000; Ireland, 191,000); Germany—2,003,-000; Prussia—1,185,000; France—2,246,000; Italy—1,435,000; United States—2,186,000.

The percentage of the population 65 and upwards in various countries is: United Kingdom—5 per cent (in England, Wales, and Scotland the percentage is 5 per cent, and in Ireland 6 per cent); Germany—5 per cent; France—8 per cent; Italy—6 per cent; United States—4 per cent.

Allyn A. Young[2] gives a table bringing out the following facts, taking the population of continental United States in 1900 as 75,994,575 as a basis:

Age	POPULATION			
	Native White	Foreign White	Colored	Total
70	123,818	66,941	18,213	208,972
75	79,214	40,886	10,061	130,161
80	42,095	19,559	6,995	68,649
85	17,271	7,059	2,854	27,184
90	4,551	1,796	1,190	7,539
95	833	430	766	2,029
99	195	168	255	618

Solomon S. Huebner[3] says a mortality table is a picture of a generation of individuals passing through time. He takes a group of them and traces their history year by year until all have died. The American Experience

[1] From Webb's *New Dictionary of Statistics*, 1911, p. 471.
[2] *A Discussion of Age Statistics*, Rept. 13, Bull. Bur. Census, 1904.
[3] *Life Insurance*, N. Y., 1915.

tables, almost exclusively used for computation by the old insurance companies, contain the following and are based on 100,000 individuals:

AMERICAN EXPERIENCE TABLE OF MORTALITY

Age	Number Living at Beginning of Designated Year	Number Dying during Designated Year	Age	Number Living at Beginning of Designated Year	Number Dying during Designated Year
70	38,569	2,391	83	8,603	1,648
71	36,178	2,448	84	6,955	1,470
72	33,730	2,487	85	5,485	1,292
73	31,243	2,505	86	4,193	1,114
74	28,738	2,501	87	3,079	933
75	26,237	2,476	88	2,146	744
76	23,761	2,431	89	1,402	555
77	21,330	2,369	90	847	385
78	18,961	2,291	91	462	246
79	16,670	2,196	92	216	137
80	14,474	2,091	93	79	58
81	12,383	1,964	94	21	18
82	10,419	1,816	95	3	3

In a table headed "Actuaries' or Combined Experience Table of Mortality"[4] we have the following, taking 100,000 persons of ten years of age as the basis:

Age	Probable Number of Persons Living	Expectation of Life
70	35,837	8.54
75	24,100	6.48
80	13,290	4.78
85	5,417	3.36
90	1,319	2.11
95	89	1.12
99	1	.50

In a very valuable state report[5] collating data from many sources for convenient use by the legislature it

[4] *World Almanac*, 1921, p. 438.
[5] *Report of a Special Inquiry Relative to Aged and Dependent Persons in Massachusetts*, 1915.

appears that the total number of persons 65 or over in Massachusetts by the census of April 1, 1915, was 189,-047. It is generally supposed that during recent years the ratio of the aged to the total population has increased, but the tables show that in Massachusetts this did not hold true for the forty years ending in 1915. Mortality rates in most localities have fallen, but improved conditions of life have not affected the ratio of the aged to the total. Still, the duration of life has continuously increased, owing to medical and sanitary science and improved standards of living; and while the younger element of the population has been chiefly affected, the span of life of the aged has also been somewhat prolonged. Hence if this tendency continues the need of pensioning would increase.

A. Newsholme[6] presents a table giving the annual death rate, per million persons living, from a few prominent diseases, showing that there is a falling off in the death rate from old age. The author adds: "If this were a real falling off, it would not be an indisputable advantage as most people would prefer to die of old age. The decline under this head, however, is chiefly due to an improved specification of the causes of which the old die." He gives copious statistics on the causes of death. He also gives an interesting table (p. 237) on the basis of 100,000 of each sex, showing graphically the steady decline in death liability and that the percentage of death is least at 12 and the early teens and soon after begins slightly to increase, falling somewhat more rapidly after 40 and then becoming a little less rapid after 70; while at 90, only 2,000 of the original 100,000 remain alive.

Director Sam L. Rogers of the Bureau of the Census published tables of vitality statistics[7] to show expecta-

---

[6] *The Elements of Vital Statistics,* Lond., 1909, 326 pp.
[7] "Death Rate and Expectation of Life," *Science,* vol. 43, 1916.

tion of life at all ages for the population of New England, New York, New Jersey, Indiana, Michigan, and the District of Columbia (these being the mortality death registration states) on the basis of the population in 1910 and the mortality for three years. They are like life tables of insurance companies with the exception that they are based on the whole population. According to these tables the average expectation of life for males at birth is 49.9 years; for females, 52.2. Expectation of white males reaches its maximum at the age of 2 (57.7 years). At the age of 12, it is 59.2 years; at 25, 39.4; at 40, 28.3; at 50, 21.2; at 60, 14.6; at 70, 9.1; at 80, 5.2 years. During the first month of life the death rate of native white boys is nearly 28 per cent higher than that for girls. The twelfth year seems to be the healthiest for the native whites and thereafter there is continuous increase in the death rate. Expectation of life is not the same as saying that a man has an even chance of living that number of years, because expectation represents the average remaining length of life at any given age in a stationary population. A native white male child at birth has one chance in two of reaching sixty. At the end of his first year he has more than an even chance of reaching sixty-four. At forty-two he has an even chance of attaining seventy. At all ages women live longer than men and expectation in the country at all ages is distinctly greater than in the city.

R. Henderson's work[8] sets forth the theoretical relations with reference to the duration of human life, describing those mortality tables that have had the greatest influence on the development of the science of life contingency and its applications in this country. The author establishes a connection between mortality tables and mortality statistics and tells how to interpret the latter.

[8] *Table of Mortality Statistics.*

The methods of constructing mortality tables from census and death returns and from insurance experience are then taken up. The writer deals only with life contingencies and not at all with monetary applications and gives us a new table. "The present value of a sum of money payable at death cannot be properly calculated in assuming it to be payable at the end of a definite period equal to the expectation of life." Nor can the present value of a life annuity be calculated by assuming it to be certainly payable for that period.

W. S. Rankin[9] tells how he applies vital statistics to sick towns or cities in a way to first restore consciousness by telling them just where they stand relatively with regard to death rates and second to bring about reforms. He has various charts and diagrams. The opinion of prominent people in every community is, in general, that their health conditions are good, but when asked what the death rate is they can give no answer. One community compelled a railroad to build and maintain an expensive overhead bridge at a cost of $1,500 a year to prevent one death and the aldermen appropriated only $150 to prevent fifty deaths. The first thing in treating sick social organisms is to restore consciousness.

Alexander Graham Bell[10] in the study of a family which is almost classic found that the average duration of life was 34.6 years; 35.2 per cent of these persons died before they were 20 years of age, and 7.3 per cent lived to be 80 or older. A second danger period was found in adolescence, ending at 23. Both sexes showed an increase of deaths during adolescence. More females than males lived to be 95. But the fathers, on the aver-

---

[9] "The Influence of Vital Statistics on Longevity." Address at the sixth annual meeting of the Association of American Life Insurance Presidents, Dec., 1912.

[10] *The Duration of Life and Conditions Associated with Longevity:* A study of the Hyde genealogy (dealing with 8,797 persons) ending, for the most part, with the year 1825.

age, lived longer than the mothers and the children born between four and eight years after the marriage of their parents lived longer than those born later. Those who live to be old come from long-lived parents. The long-lived seem to inherit disease-resisting qualities and also are more fecund than the short-lived. He says[11] that in this family mothers who lived to extreme old age had, on the average, larger families than those who died earlier in life, for example, those who died before forty had, on the average, only three to four children apiece. The long-lived proportion is practically doubled when one parent lives to be old and quadrupled when both parents do so. The people who lived to be old represented the disease-resistant strain of their generation and on account of their superior fecundity this quality is distributed largely throughout the population. "A very large proportion of each generation is sprung from a very small proportion of the preceding generation; namely, from the people who lived to old age. The members of the short-lived group come from the short-lived parents. The children of the long-lived parents are on the average stronger, more vigorous, and longer-lived than the children of others, and there were more of them per family."

Scott Nearing[12] says that the years from 45 to 60 or 65 should be the most valuable ones from the social point of view. He reminds us that if the average length of life were doubled the population would in a generation double without any increase in the birth rate. The average length of life in the leading countries of the world varies much. In Sweden, for males it is 53.9; France, 45.7; England and Wales, 44.1; Massachusetts, 44.1; India, 23.0. Men born in America of native white parents live on the average only 31 years; those born

[11] "Who Shall Inherit Long Life?" *Nat. Geog. Mag.*, June, 1919.
[12] *Social Adjustment*, New York, 1911.

of foreign white parents, 29.1 years. Men in the modern cities die when they are one score and ten. There is a great difference in occupations: for shoemakers the death rate per thousand is 8.7; farmers, 11.02; tailors, 13.65; cigar and tobacco makers, 21.67; servants, 21.78; and laborers, 22.3. Such figures suggest the dangerous occupations. As to the length of the working life, from 15 to 65, out of every one thousand males living at the age of 15, 440 will survive to the age of 65, while the rest will have fallen out for some cause. So society has lost more than half its working force at the end of the working period. In the 16th century the average length of life he estimates at 21.2 years; in the 17th, 25.7; in the 18th, 33.6; and in the 19th, nearly 40 years. Finkenberg thinks that in the 16th century it was between 18 and 20 years; at the close of the 18th, over 30; while to-day it is from 38 to 40. We have no data for the United States as a whole that are of any value. Among males in England the average length of life is increasing at the rate of 14 years per century; France, 10; Denmark, 25; Massachusetts, 14. Although these figures are only approximations, Nearing thinks life is probably twice as long as it was a few centuries ago.

Irving Fisher[13] says in Europe the span of life is double that in India. The death rate in Dublin is twice that of Amsterdam and three times that of rural Michigan. Life is probably twice as long as it was three or four centuries ago and is increasing more rapidly now than ever. The rate of progress is very variable in different countries, the maximum being in Prussia. Improvement is most in females and the rate of increase is accelerated perhaps four years a century on the whole, although during the last three-quarters of the nineteenth century Fisher thinks it has increased nine years. At

[13] "Report on National Vitality," Bulletin of the Committee of One Hundred on National Health, July, 1909, No. 30.

least fourteen years could be added to human life by eliminating preventable diseases, which would be the equivalent of reducing the death rate about 23 per cent. In a table he shows that seven of the ninety causes of death are responsible for over one-half of the shortening of life. He gives us a diagram that shows where the saving of life has been and might be greatest. The area between the curves shows that from 1855 to 1897, 550,-000 years were saved for a supposed group of 100,000 persons, or 5.5 years per person. The addition of 12.8 years to the lifetime of each of 100,000 persons might be divided into three groups, namely, that of preparation, the working period, and the decline. The chief cause of prolongation is found in new hygienic ideals.

Metchnikoff thought that the lengthening of human life would at once decrease the burden on the productive period, which is some 55 per cent of the total years lived —assuming the working period to be from 17 to 60— and that the latter limit would shift forward. As life becomes complex and as knowledge increases the period of preparation should be prolonged. Men should graduate later. Life should be lived on a larger scale, with more utilization of accumulated experience and less disastrous immaturity. Now we have to force young men into positions prematurely because of their vitality. Metchnikoff says "Old age, at present practically a useless burden on the community, will become a period of work valuable to it." Human life will become much longer and the par value of old people will become much more important than it is to-day.

Willcox thinks the death rate in the United States is at least eighteen per thousand. Moreover, we have some three million persons always on the sick list, more among the old than the young since morbidity increases in age. But at least one-third are in the working period. The loss by consumptives alone is figured at sixty mil-

lion dollars. Now, it costs no more to raise a man
capable of living eighty years than it does to grow one
who has the capacity of living only forty. Health means
increased vitality and makes life, in Mallock's phrase,
better worth the living, for health is the first wealth.
We can do much to raise American vitality.

Fisher adds[14] that in the United States the general
death rate has steadily fallen for several decades, as is
common in all civilized countries. Many think this
means a gain in national vitality. This may be true
for the younger age but the "gain has served to mask
a loss of vitality at the older age periods. This latter
phenomenon, a rising mortality in elderly life, is something almost peculiar to the United States." In other
lands this fall in death rate has been due not solely to
the reduction of mortality in infancy and adult life, for
most countries have improved their mortality at every
age period. Probably this is due to "some unknown
biologic influence or to the amalgamation of the various
races that constitute our population. It must be ascribed
in a broad sense to lack of adaptation to our rapidly
developing civilization." The American decreases in
younger ages are not as great as in England and Wales
and they change into increase at about the age of forty-
five and continue to increase thereafter, while in England and Wales the decline occurs at all ages. In 1900
or thereabouts the death rates in the middle ages of life
were heavier in the United States than in Prussia,
France, Italy, and Sweden. Since then death rates in
the United States at these ages have grown even greater.

Better hygienic methods, according to Fisher,[15]
started with Pasteur, who said it was within the power
of man to rid himself of every parasitic disease.
Hygienists have followed this clue. The Roosevelt Con-

---

[14] *How to Live,* New York, 1915, Section 7.
[15] "The Extension of Human Life," *Sci. Am. Sup.,* May 4, 1916.

servation Committee in its report on national vitality and the summary of European life tables show that human life lengthened during the 17th and 18th centuries at the rate of only 4 years per century, while during the first three-quarters of the 19th it lengthened almost twice as fast and since that four times as fast, or about 17 years per century. If we could continue to increase life seventeen years a century, the world would soon be peopled with Methuselahs. We are witnessing a race between two tendencies, the reduction of the acute infections, such as typhoid, and an increase of the chronic or degenerative diseases, such as sclerosis, Bright's disease, etc. The degenerative tendency appears more in evidence here than elsewhere. In Sweden the expectation of life increases at all ages. Even the nonagenarians have more years to live than did those of former days in the United States. We are freer from germs than our ancestors but our vital organs wear out sooner. And this degeneration of our bodies follows that of our habits. In England, where these diseases are not increasing, individual exercise out of doors probably has something to do with it. In Sweden individual hygiene is better cultivated than anywhere else in the world. It is the only land where public health includes private habits and touches the life of the people, especially through the school. The best statistics show that a large number of our young men and women suffer from diseases of heart, kidneys, lungs, and circulation, with impairment enough to consult a physician, that is, over half of our young men and women in active work and presumably selected for their work as fit, are found, although unaware of the fact themselves, to be in need of medical attention; while 37 per cent are on the road to impairment because of the use of too much alcohol, tobacco, etc. Now, a stitch in time saves nine. Thus the lesson to all of us is obvious.

STATISTICS OF OLD AGE AND ITS CARE

I. M. Rubinow [16] says the problem of poverty among the old is connected with inability to find work because productive power has waned forever. American experience in tables of mortality shows that of 100 persons at the age of 20, 53 will reach 65; 12, 70; at which time the average expectation of life will be $8\frac{1}{2}$ years. If we take 100 people at the age of 30, 53 will live to 65; 48 to 70. But this table was compiled half a century ago, although it is still used—to the great profit of insurance companies as expectation has greatly increased. Ten to fifteen years of life over sixty-five are assured to more than half all wage workers. In 1880 the percentage of persons 65 or over was 3.5; in 1890, 3.9; in 1900, 4.2; in 1910, 4.3. The number over 65 per 1000/15 increased from 54 to 60 in 1890, and to 63 in 1910. Employed males over 65 per 1000/15 constituted 50 in 1890; and in 1900, 47. Thus the production of old men is increased while the proportion of old men is declining. In 1880, of all old men over 65 years of age, 73.8 per cent were gainfully employed; in 1900, only 68.4 per cent. The total number of men over 65 in 1900 was 1,555,000. Thus economic progress in ten years meant an additional hundred thousand thrown out of employment. In agriculture, 6.1 per cent of the men employed are over 65; in the professions, 5.5 per cent; but in manufacture and mechanics, only 3.5 per cent; and in trade and transportation, 3 per cent. Thus old men are either thrown out or shifted to unskilled occupations. What does the "iron law" of the increase of old age dependency under a system of wage labor mean? It is wrong to seek the cause in exceptional misfortune or in psychological or ethical feeling. The author of "Old Age Dependencies in the United States" says after sixty men become dependent by easy stages—property,

---

[16] *Social Insurance*, New York, 1913, Chap. 12, "The Old Man's Problem in Modern Industry."

friends, relatives, and ambition go and only a few years of life remain, with death final. The wage-earner is swept from the class of hopeful, independent citizens into that of the helpless poor.

As to the population problem, Raymond Pearl has studied the ratio between births and deaths in France, Prussia, Bavaria, and England and Wales from 1913 to 1920 [17] and finds that, in general, the birth ratios rose during the war—in England to the 100 per cent mark—and that immediately after the war was over the death-birth ratio began to drop rapidly in all countries. Vienna suffered perhaps more than any other city but made the best recovery, showing how promptly the growth of population tends to regulate itself back toward the normal after even so great a disturbance. Thus the war, which was the greatest depopulator since the epidemic of the Middle Ages, caused "only a momentary hesitation in the steady onward march of population growth." If we take any given land area of fixed limits, there must necessarily be an upper limit to the number of people it can support, but this limit will be approached asymtotically and the most rapid rise will be midway between the upper and lower limit, namely, at that point where half the possible resources of subsistence have been drawn upon and utilized. The statistician must approach this problem as the astronomer does in calculating the complete orbit of a comet, that is, he must construct his curve from a limited number of specific data. If we study the curve of growth of population in this country, we find that we have long since passed the most rapid rate of increase. If we compare this with that of France, which is an old country and much nearer the upper limit than ours, which started near the lower asymtote only a century and a

---

[17] "The Biology of Death," *Sci. Mo.*, March-Sept., 1921, *incl.*

half ago; or compare it with that of Serbia, which is intermediate, all the statistics available conform with singular accuracy to the theoretic curve.

Professor Pearl concludes that this country has passed the point of most rapid increase, that this rate began to decline about April 1, 1914, when our population was 98,637,000, and that our upper limit will be reached about the year 2100, when the population will be 197,274,000 or nearly double what it is now, with about 66 persons per square mile. Our population will be then far less dense than in many other countries, but the latter are not self-supporting. He even estimates how many calories, vegetable and animal, each individual will require daily and compares this with the agricultural possibilities of the future. Such considerations lead him to stress the importance of birth control. This had long been practiced in France before the war, where the birth- and death-rate nearly balanced, so that industrial development simply raised the standard of living. Germany, on the other hand, encouraged the increase of her population by every means and her scheme was, when the pressure became too great, to facilitate the overflow of her surplus population elsewhere. "A stationary population where birth-rate and death-rate are made to balance is necessarily a population with a relative excess of persons in the higher age groups, not of much use as fighters, and a relative deficiency of persons in the lower age groups where the best fighters are. On the contrary, a people with a high birth-rate has a population with an excess of persons in the younger age groups."

In his discussion of life tables Pearl starts with that of Glover based on the registration area of the United States in 1910. If we assume an original hundred thousand starting together at birth we note that at the beginning of the second year of life only 88,538 survive.

In the next year 2446 drop out; the year following, 1062. At forty about 30,000 have passed away and the line descends with increasing rapidity until about eighty, when it drops more slowly till soon after the century mark all the original hundred thousand have passed away. Expectation of life is the mean or average number of persons surviving at a stated age. Pearl's diagrams show that the expectation of life of those born in Breslau in the seventeenth century was very much lower than that of an individual born in the United States in 1910, the difference amounting to 18 years. At the age of ten it has sunk to 12; at twenty, to 10 years; at fifty, to 4. But the individual of eighty in Breslau in the seventeenth century could expect to live longer than the individual of the same age now in the United States. The same result is found if we compare United States tables now with those of England in the middle of the eighteenth century, where expectation was also less before and greater after eighty. Pearson's study of Egyptian mummy cases two thousand years old shows that expectation there was far lower yet through all the early stages of life, although after seventy those who survived had a greatly increased expectation. Thus either man to-day is constitutionally fitter to survive or else he has made himself better conditions up to about the seventh decade. The reason why expectation increased after that period is because conditions were so unfavorable that all but the very most rugged succumbed earlier in life and the proportion of those who reached advanced age was far less than now. In Rome, during the first three or four centuries of the Christian era, the expectation was less yet until nearly sixty, after which it rose, and it is significant that expectation of life was far less under the conditions then prevailing for women than for men at all ages of life, which is the reverse of conditions now prevailing. In the Roman provinces, however, expectation was greater than in the Eternal City. In the Roman-African population, although there was greater mortality to about forty, expectation of life was superior after that age in the early part of the Christian era to what it now is.

In considering life tables that give the number óf deaths occurring at each age, which give an S-shaped curve falling very rapidly before the end of the second year and reaching its highest subsequent point at seventy, Karl Pearson finds in this S-shaped curve five components which he typifies as five Deaths shooting with different weapons and with differing precision as the procession of human beings crosses the Bridge of Life. The first Death is a marksman of deadly aim and unremitting diligence who kills before as well as after birth. The second, who aims at childhood, has a very concentrated fire. The third, who shoots at youth, has not a very deadly or accurate weapon but one rather to be compared with a bow and arrow. The fire of the fourth marksman is slow, scattered, and not very destructive, as if from an old-fashioned blunderbus. The last Death plies the rifle, which none escape. Pearl justly criticises this conception because "no analysis of the deaths into natural divisions by causes or otherwise has yet been made such that the totals in the various groups would conform to these frequency curves." Thus he holds that Pearson's concept of the five deaths does not represent any biological reality but only demonstrates, as any other equally successful curve would do, that deaths do not occur chaotically but instead "in a regular manner capable of representation by mathematical function in respect of age."

SENESCENCE

II

Let us glance briefly at the public and private provisions in different lands for the care of the aged, another large topic with a literature of its own. Here, too, we find great diversity of method and theory which it would be premature to attempt to harmonize. Indeed, so limited is our present knowledge of old age that the available data here also open rather than close most of the great questions about it, although we do seem to be at the beginning of a new era regarding this stage of life. If on the one hand, the length of life is increasing, as we have seen, on the other the intensity of modern life and industry is steadily reducing the age of maximal efficiency so that we feel the handicap of years earlier in life than formerly. The pressure of the advancing upon the retiring generation is ever-growing and if the manual laborer lives longer, he feels the impairment of age sooner. In fact, society is coming to a clearer realization, on the one hand, that youth must be served and conserved and, on the other, is just beginning to see that the same is true of old age.

Not only is the average length of human life increasing as civilization advances but so is the relative and absolute number of old people. Although under the harder conditions that once prevailed those who reached advanced years did so by inherent energy of constitution as the choicest products of natural selection (even though relatively fewer in numbers), it is fortunate that those who now attain 60, 70, 80, etc., are on the average far more comfortable, as well as more numerous than ever before. Not only is eyesight conserved, loss of teeth made good, and many of the ailments of the aged mitigated by modern medicine and hygiene, but by homes, pensions, etc., their lot is made far easier.

Youth tends to live in and for the present and middle

life is too absorbing; while the decrepitude of old age seems so remote and its attainment so uncertain that the masses of mankind are still far too improvident of the future. It is somewhat as if our race had developed in tropical abundance where there was little need of providing food, clothing, and shelter, and had not adjusted even to a more northern climate, still less to the complexities of modern civilization and least of all to the increased chance of attaining old age with its infirmities. Still, great progress has been made in foresight and futures play an ever greater rôle in human calculations. The impulse to accumulate possessions itself always has a protensive factor and we cannot amass property without thinking of its safety and its use, and so we lay by, insure and bequeath.

Nevertheless, under the conditions of life in the modern city, and especially since the Industrial Revolution and the employment of masses of women and men at wages that always tend to gravitate toward a minimum, it is impossible for many to save and also to rear families, while intemperance and vice always furnish their quota to the classes that outlive their serviceable years in dire poverty and, as old age advances, become increasingly dependent not only for subsistence but also for personal care. There are still a few students of the social and economic questions here involved who urge that all the aged, even the latter group, should, if possible, be cared for in their own homes by their children and grandchildren and that to remove them to institutions, public or private, not only robs them of interest in life but weakens filial piety and is detrimental to the interests of the family and to the instincts upon which it rests. They urge that all children owe to all parents this return for the care that was bestowed on them during their early, helpless years and that such ministrations are essential for a true and complete home, etc. But even if we grant all this, there still remain the childless old and poor who are alone in the world. There are also the vicious, toward whom their children, with too much reason, feel that they owe nothing, that their own very existence was due to the accidents of passion, and that they were not only unwelcome guests but were made the victims of cruelty, want, etc. Then there are the sick who cannot be properly cared for at home and each additional mouth always means less food for all the rest.

The old most of all need personal provision and suffer most from mass treatment, for they are not a class but are hyperindividualized. Not only do some become old while they are yet young in years, and vice versa, but there is the greatest diversity in food, regimen, and in most bodily and psychic needs. To say nothing of disposition, diathesis, or temperament, the old often develop what seem to others senseless idiosyncrasies that are really expressive of essential traits and require not only kindly consideration but careful study. It is hard for them, most of all for old women, to be deprived of contact with the young and to be confined to intercourse with only those of their own generation. It is also hard on them to be denied the privilege of privacy at will, of having certain things all their own, with a secure place accessible to them alone in which to keep them. For myself I am convinced that the so-called moroseness of old age is largely due to the inconsiderate treatment it receives. Its real instinct is to serve no less than to conserve. Even in the best appointed homes for the aged that I have visited the great need seems to me to be occupation with things felt to be useful and individual exemptions from rigid rules mechanically enforced for all. All have their own tastes, aptitudes, habits, as well as mementos and keepsakes, which should always be respected, and every possible facility should be given not only for visits and correspondence but for current reading in order to maintain a larger surface of contact with the world without. The old thus constitute, in a sense, a privileged and even a new "leisure class," which Veblen omitted to characterize. The very fact that they have survived means that they have borne the burden and heat of life's trying day better than those who have died. In a large over-all sense, thus, they survived because they were the fittest and even though they may have wrought solely with an eye to their own personal benefit they have, nevertheless, helped on the world's work. Our streets, buildings, machines, farms, mines, goods, produce, means of transportation—all these are, in a sense, the bequest of vanished and retiring to future generations, and even whatever stamina their children have is more or less due to their virtue, while their very longevity is perhaps the best of all they have transmitted to their offspring for, as A. G. Bell has shown, fecundity and long life go together.

Again, as the young and middle-aged most often show the energy that impels to migrations, it is often inferred that newly settled lands contain the lowest percentages of old people. This, however, seems to be true only for a very limited period and indeed the reverse may soon come to be the case, for the very vigor that impels the emigrant is a trait of those who will also live long; whence it often comes that after a few decades new territories have relatively more aged people than are found in older communities from which the more viable have emigrated and the less viable been eliminated by death. This is, on the whole, fortunate, because the wisdom that only years bring acts like a balance wheel to regulate the impulsions of youth, which always need to be more or less controlled. Thus, in our Western communities we often observe, along with the most advanced ultra-modern steps in material progress and the newest political devices, a certain conservatism in social mores, creeds, etc., which show not only a stagnation but a regression of culture that is typical of progressive senescence and its psychic retardation.

We do little to fit for old age and so come to it unprepared and uninformed. The senses fail, but usually so gradually that we rarely realize the full extent of our loss; at any rate, we have time to become adjusted and perhaps reconciled to it. The muscles very gradually atrophy, so that all efferent energy declines and we can do ever less. Indeed, in a new and quite scientific fashion we can speak of old age as the "great fatigue," for Hodge, Dolley, and Richardson and Orr have shown that the changes in brain cells are almost identical in both. Loss of memory for recent events disorients the old from their environment. They forget names and their vocabulary contracts as the brain shrinks. The mental pace slows down. Their feelings and emotions are less intense, while control over them is often diminished. The friends of their youth are dead; their authority is gone; they are not consulted where once they had everything to say. And so they come at last by slow degrees to realize that they belong to a generation that is passed and the little world about them of which they were once so vital a part is neglecting if not actually crowding them aside. If they come to see that things go on very well without them, both they and their environment are fortunate; but alas! for both if they gravitate toward the conviction that as they withdraw all goes wrong.

Nearly every civilized country to-day makes some provision for the aged poor. While they are often cared for along with the infirm and sick in hospitals, or with paupers in poor- and workhouses, or allowed to beg on the street, etc., there are now many charitable funds and pensions, public and private, provided especially for the aged. Most funds for all the dependent classes can also be used for their benefit at home or in institutions; and social and philanthropic work, where it exists, is always ready to consider helpless age, which has its own appeal to sympathy and benevolence. The number of such cases is almost everywhere increasing and so are the provisions for them. As charity has always been praised as a virtue, it is now becoming also a science, and the peculiar nature and needs of old age are being better understood, although there is yet very much to be done in studying this stage of life which has in the past been so neglected and misunderstood. We are now far more ignorant of senescence than of adolescence, childhood, or middle age, but it is quite as unique, on the whole, and more apart than any of these other periods. There is a sense, too, in which those in each stage of life know least of it. The child knows little of childhood, which had to be discovered in this "century of the child." The second childhood of old age often knows itself only little better. The child cannot, the old will not, realize their age for what it is and what it means.

Our conspectus is as follows:

The first German Old Age and Invalidity Insurance Law dates from 1889 and has been modified since by various supplementary acts so that it is now very comprehensive. These acts were due to the social democratic agitation that prompted Bismarck to set a backfire and thus allay the discontent of the working classes. Old-age insurance has been obligatory since 1889 upon practically all laborers and officials paid under $500 a year and the right to insure voluntarily is extended to others. The employer is held responsible for the insurance of everyone and deducts the workman's share of the premium from his wages. In 1910 some 14,000,000 out of a population of 60,000,000 were thus insured.

The obligation to insure begins with the 17th year and a percentage of the wages must be paid for 1200 weeks. The Empire and the employer also contribute—the former a fixed annual sum of $11.90. There are five wage classes and a special postal service with insurance stamps. It is, however, impossible to obtain from German reports much data for old age alone, which is almost always classed with invalidity and often with accident, sickness, etc. As in every country, there was at first much discussion whether such social insurance should be compulsory or voluntary, contributory or non-contributory, universal or partial, etc., and different countries and agencies have decided these questions differently.

Austria since 1906 had a limited system of old age insurance for certain salaried employees of the middle class. But a sweeping change in the bill in 1908 was intended to include nearly 10,000,000 of the population. Old-age pensions could be paid at 65 to those insured for a period of thirty years. The scheme was worked out in very great detail but, as in other German lands, was a distinctly political measure provoked in Austria by the Socialists, who, as elsewhere, at first hesitated to adopt a measure that gave the Government, to which they had been opposed, the prestige of having realized so many of their own ideas by these measures. The movement soon won many supporters, however, from their ranks. As a political *coup* it was a great success and most Socialists could find no alternative but to accept it, at least in principle, although criticism of the small and inadequate funds received by the pensioners is common.

H. J. Hoare [18] best describes the British Old Age Pension Acts 1908-1911, the scheme of which is as fol-

[18] *Old Age Pensions: Their actual working results in the United Kingdom,* London, 1915, 196 pp.

lows: Both sexes, married or single, over 70, of British nationality, who for 12 years out of the last 20 were residents, and whose yearly income does not exceed 31 pounds and 10 shillings, are eligible for pensions. They make no contributions, the money coming from the state. The scheme is worked jointly by the Civil Service and local authorities; and only inmates of workhouses, asylums, inebriates' homes, prisons, and those who have habitually failed to work are disqualified. The pension cannot be charged or assigned and if the pensioner is bankrupt, the pension cannot pass to a trustee or creditor. The receipt of such a pension deprives of no franchise or privilege and subjects to no disability, as is the case with those who accept the poor rates. In 1913, 363,811 men and 604,110 women were pensioners, 62.5 per cent of all being women. Where the yearly means of the pensioner does not exceed 21 pounds, he or she receives 5 shillings a week; if between 21 and 23 pounds 12s. 6d., 4 shillings a week; and so on through 6 classes, those whose income is between 28 pounds 7s. 6d. and 31 pounds 11s. receiving one shilling a week. As a matter of fact, however, 94 per cent of the pensions are at the full rate. The expense of administering this system is less than half of one per cent of the total amount of pensions.

In 1920, 920,198 old men and women received pensions.[19] The chief grievances the old find against this system are: (1) that it does not begin at 65; and especially (2) that it is so little, for, of course, no one can begin to exist to-day on 5s. a week. Both these limitations cause very acute complaint among the beneficiaries themselves.

Practically every other European country has adopted

---

[19] Edith Sellers, "From the Old Age Pensioners' Standpoint," *Nineteenth Century*, Jan., 1920.

some form of old age relief.[20] Denmark in 1891 put in operation a scheme of outdoor relief for the deserving aged poor. This, too, was done as a political move to reconcile radicals and liberals. Its pensionable age of 60 years is, I believe, the lowest anywhere found. The amount of the dotation is not fixed; local authorities decide it in each individual case. It must be, however, "sufficient for support." Communes and the state bear the expense equally.

Belgium's Old Age Pension Act of 1900 is a comprehensive scheme of assisted insurance and non-contributory pensions. It aims, first, to encourage workers to save; and, second, to help the aged by special grants. It has its own superannuation fund bank. Annuities rarely exceed $72 and are payable at 65. The pensions are graded according to the age of the insured, and at last accounts nearly a million, or one-eighth of the population, benefited.

France has a voluntary, contributory old-age insurance system administered through a national bank with a state guarantee, which goes back to 1850 but has been much perfected by subsequent legislation. It differs only in detail from the Belgian scheme. The amount of the insurance is not less than $12 or more than $48 a year and may be given in money, hospital service, or provisions. The permissible pension age in France is now 65.

Since 1898 Italy has had a system of voluntary, contributory insurance, subsidized by the state, which provides annuities after the age of 60 if the recipient has paid his dues for 25 years.

The chief British colonies have adopted very wise and comprehensive systems of old age pensions. New Zealand provides a maximum pension of $130 a year

[20] *Report of the Massachusetts Commission on Old Age Pensions, Annuities and Insurance,* Jan., 1910, 409 pp.

in monthly installments to those of 65 who are "of good moral character and have led a sober, reputable life." Each pension is only granted for a year but is renewable upon request.

The Australian colonies, one after another, enacted old-age pension laws near the close of the first decade of the present century. These grants are made "as a right and not as a charity," and the commissioner determines the amount of the pension within limits according to what he deems the needs of each case. A special investigation is made for each applicant.

The Canadian system (1908) differs widely from that of Australia. Its preamble states that it is to promote thrift and to encourage individual provisions for old age. The Minister of the Interior may contract with any Canadian for the sale of an annuity, between the limits of $50 and $600, although none can be payable under the age of 55. If the purchaser of an annuity dies before it becomes payable, all of it with compound interest is returned to his heirs. As this system is voluntary, very vigorous efforts were made by organizers and lecturers to bring it to the attention of, and make it attractive to, the people, and these thrift campaigns have been highly educative.

Francis A. Carman[21] tells us that the Canadian scheme, like most others, was to alleviate the universal dread of the poorhouse. It was adopted to circumvent the growing demand for the support of old age by the Government. Its unique features are: no forfeiture in case payments are interrupted or ceased, and the annuities cannot be mortgaged, seized for debt, or anticipated. Admirable as is the scheme, there have been less than two thousand to enjoy its full benefits. It has not reached the day laborer but, for the most part, only clerks and teachers.

---

[21] "Canadian Government Annuities," *Polit. Sci. Quar.*, 1915, p. 425 *et seq.*

SENESCENCE

The United States is the only nation that has no retiring system or provision for old age, even for its employees, save for soldiers and for judges of the Supreme Court, who may retire after ten years of service or on having attained the age of 75 on full salaries. Military pensions go back nearly to the Revolutionary War. There has been much legislation since. In 1908 there were no less than 951,687 pensioners who received more than $153,000,000, the survivors of the Civil War constituting 65 per cent of all. There are also retirement pensions for officers and enlisted men in the regular Army. Officers at the age of 64 must be retired, with no option, on three-fourths pay.

No American state has established any system of old age pensions, although many Southern states provide for Confederate veterans; but many states or cities have provided for firemen, policemen, teachers, and certain other public employees.

Mabel L. Nassau [22] personally studied the history of one hundred poor old people in the very heart of New York city and observed them as a neighborhood study, dividing her cases into those wholly or partly self-supporting, and wholly or partly dependent upon their families or upon charity. She stresses the fact so abundantly illustrated that it was impossible for most of these destitute individuals to put by money for their old age. The lives of most of them had been spent in the direst poverty, with low wages, almost no industrial training, long intervals of non-employment, illness often due to malnutrition, not to mention the really not very common effects of drink and vice. They often have little experience in buying and have all their lives been cheated and imposed on. Very many have the finest sensibilities, although this is often not suspected because

---

[22] *Old Age Poverty in Greenwich Village*, 1915, 105 pp.

they lack education to express their feelings. In this stratum of society, although the young are often underfed and the middle aged overworked, the old have the hardest time. The burden of the aged falls hardest upon the children, who must get a work certificate as soon as possible to help feed their grandparents. The old generally have a horror of going to an institution; and many of these are so managed as to justify this dread, separating married couples, imposing senseless rules, providing poor food and perhaps no recreation, and greatly restricting liberties, so that life is hopelessly monotonous, with no incentive for personal effort. The inmates generally have no private place, even a locked drawer, to keep personal effects, so that they can really own nothing. Mills' hotels seem nearer the ideal. Many systems to help the old involve conditions that amount to dominating their lives. Old age is really a risk to which all are liable and self-respect and thrift require us to give more attention to it. It should be no more of a disgrace to accept a pension for old age than for service in war. State aid assumes that the old have added to the health and power of the state by their work, and recognizes this.

The Baltimore and Ohio Railroad established the first pension system in this industry in 1884 and in the last two decades many corporations, mercantile houses, banks, etc., have established such systems. The above Massachusetts Report supplies many details of fifty of these systems. In the modern business world the problem of dealing with aged employees is increasingly difficult. The use of machinery, specialization, and the modern efficiency ideals have made it increasingly hard for the old to keep the pace and the universal demand now is for younger men, so that many firms actually refuse new men over thirty-five. Men wear out fast. To carry the incapacitated on their payroll is not only not economic but discouraging to the working force and it is not humane to turn them adrift. The general scheme adopted in view of these facts is either voluntary or compulsory retirement at a certain age, with weekly or monthly allowances, the amount of which depends upon the length of service and the wage, the expense of the system being borne by the employer with help from the employee. The economic motives, of course, have been more potent than the humanitarian. It has been good business policy, for it not only prevents the waste of using worn-out men but it stimulates loyalty on the part of the working force. Voluntary retirement is generally at 60 and compulsory at 70, but this varies greatly, as does the time of service upon which aid is conditioned, which is usually from 10 to 30 years. Often the allowance is one per cent of the average wage during the last 10 years; for example, an employee who has worked 40 years at an average wage of $50 a month would receive $20. The system is generally administered by a board composed of both employers and employees. Some firms expressly repudiate all contractual rights.

Inquiry was made in Massachusetts of over a thousand employers but only three hundred and sixty-two replies were received; and of these only four had regular systems of retirement pensions, although often special grants were made. This was a very delicate inquiry and the excuses for the absence of any pension system usually were that the business was itself too insecure or that the working force was too unstable and transitory.

Many fraternal organizations have old-age benefits. But the early history of this movement is strewn with financial wrecks, because the rates were too low and philanthropic impulses outweighed scientific methods. Very few of these organizations had anything that can

be called old-age pensions or benefits, although some of
them are now coming to do so.

A few trade unions have superannuation features,
particularly the International Typographical Union and
the Amalgamated Societies of Engineers, also carpen-
ters and joiners. But here, again, benefits are small.

Industrial insurance is really life insurance for small
amounts and is designed for wage earners, with premiums payable weekly, collected from homes by agents,
and the premiums graded in multiples of five cents.
This method really began in London in 1854 and despite
initial errors the movement has grown rapidly, so that
there are now many millions of industrial policies in
force in that country. But only very recently have they
attempted specific insurance against old age. Here the
premiums usually cease at 65 and the annuity is rarely
over $100.

The Krupp Company at Essen had, before the war,
one of the most elaborate systems of age insurance,
conducted solely for the benefit of the employees and
to which the Company contributed largely. The scheme
is complex and was often interpellated in the *Reichstag*,
especially on the point of forfeiture of payments of
members who leave the firm. Each workman pays 2½
per cent, which is deducted from his wages. The
system is chiefly for those who do not earn over 2000
marks a year. Retirement is permissible after 20 years
of service or on reaching the age of 65. After 20 years
the workman receives 40 per cent of his earnings, increasing yearly by 1½ per cent up to a maximum, after
44 years, of 75 per cent. If he dies, his widow receives
half his pension, and each child 10 per cent. If the
mother dies, each child receives 15 per cent. The total
membership varies from 30,000 to 40,000, and the
average pension is 683 marks. A number of other large

German industrial concerns have adopted certain features of this scheme.

Most of the Friendly Societies of Great Britain make provision for old age insurance but only to a limited extent, insuring at the same time against sickness, unemployment, providing death benefits, etc. The germ of all such work is found in the medieval trade guilds, and the necessity of it was immensely enhanced by the development of the factory system and what is called the Industrial Revolution.

After 20 years of discussion, the Sterling-Lehlbach Act, passed by Congress and which went into effect in August, 1920, provides federal civil-service pensions for all classes of employees upon retirement. It is contributory and compulsory, requiring each to contribute 2½ per cent of their salaries. The minimum age of retirement is 65; all must retire at 70; and 15 years of service are required for eligibility to an allowance, the annuity running from a minimum of $180 after 15 years of service to a maximum of $720 after 30 years. The scheme takes no account of the amount of salary at the time of retirement and certainly $720 is no inducement to a man receiving $2000 to resign.

In recent years there has been a growing conviction not only that the salaries of teachers must be increased, "but some kind of retiring allowance provided for all public school teachers, if teaching is to become a profession." [23] These are provided by nearly every country of Western Europe; and in 1916, 32 states in this country had made some provision for the retirement of teachers, most of them contributory systems where teachers insured themselves against disability.

Our country, however, is still far behind others in

---

[23] Joseph Swain, "State Pension Systems for Public School Teachers," *Bureau of Education Bull.*, 1916.

this respect.[24] The first city-school system to provide retirement funds was in Chicago in 1893, followed two years later by a New Jersey mutual-benefit plan, and there are now eight or nine types of state, county, and city pension systems in the country. The peculiar difficulty here is found in the fact that one-fourth of our 720,000 school teachers leave teaching every year, making the average term of service four years and causing 185,000 new inexperienced teachers to begin each year. Thus few expect to benefit from such a system and so long as it is voluntary it is utterly inadequate. "While pensions and tenure help to secure and hold good teachers, they also make it possible to free schools with social justice and dignity from superannuated and incapacitated teachers. This is almost as great a benefit as the others to the schools, the children, and society."

There are two volumes[25] which, as Professor H. S. Pritchett well says in an able article on pension literature (*Fifteenth Annual Report of the Carnegie Foundation,* 1920) "mark the close of one period in the history of pensions and the beginning of a new scientific one." The most difficult question is the method of calculating the amount of superannuation benefits. If the basis is the flat rate, this is simple; but if it is the average of the salary given during the last five or ten years, or during the whole period of service, the difficulty in determining the amount of actual contributions to yield the prospective benefit becomes very great. Teachers' salaries are, especially now, very unstable. A pension system based on anticipated pay leaves too much in suspense. It is difficult to provide pensions on a subsistence

---

[24] "Report on Teachers' Pensions," *N. E. A. Proc.,* 1919, vol. 57, p. 145 *et seq.*

[25] See Paul Studensky, *Teachers' Pension Systems in the United States,* New York, 1920, and the companion volume of Lewis Meriam, entitled *Principles Governing the Retirement of Public Employees,* New York, 1918.

basis, which also bears some relation to final salary. If
the pension is too high, there is temptation to retire too
early; if it is too low, to retire too late. Ultimately, too,
teachers must be able to migrate without loss or change
of status and this would involve reciprocity between
different cities and even states. In New York, before
the new system went into effect in 1921, there were
2,000 different rates; and in Pennsylvania, 86. The new
system of New York, which developed because the old
one had settled into bankruptcy, although optional for
teachers appointed before 1921 is compulsory for those
appointed after and the pension is to consist of half the
average salary during the last five years; the payment
is not to exceed $800 and this will be paid after 25 years
of service. The old view which held that the very word
"pension" suggested a cripple and real manhood would
compel everyone to lay by for old age, and which flattered those who entered their profession in youth with
the hope that in old age they "might be permitted to
sun themselves on the veranda of a state poorhouse,"
has entirely passed away. But pensions are no longer
considered as a form of charity or a form of paternal-
ism, or even as a reward for service. They only demand
of the teacher the same thrift as do savings and their
proper function is to secure efficiency of service and they
should be regarded "as a condition of service just the
same as a salary." Most of even the best recent systems,
like that of the District of Columbia and the Y. M. C. A.
officers' pension plan, which is just about to go into
operation, are a compromise between the old and the
new ideas. The same is true of civil-service pensions in
New York state and city.

The Carnegie Foundation for the Advancement of
Teaching in 1920 had a total fund of $24,628,000 and
its retirement allowances for that year were $875,514.04,
with allowances then in force to 555 individuals, or an

average to each of $1,568.77. The fund was originally administered solely in the form of gifts but the unexpected number of applicants made it necessary to gradually change to a contractual plan involving very moderate contributions from the institutions benefited, which now include those of Canada as well as of this country. It is one of the most wise and beneficent gifts of the great philanthropist who founded it and its influence in giving permanence in the sense of security to active professors still efficient, and relieving institutions of those past their usefulness to make way for younger men, is unquestionably for good.

The President of the Foundation has grappled with the whole subject of industrial pensions. It was at first planned that the same principles should be applied here as those in the more stabilized professions but this is impossible because of the labor turnover each year, which amounts to 100 to 200 per cent of their employees in some industrial establishments. It is one of the functions of the pension system to reduce the turnover and to secure continuity of service and avoid migrations. Many systems do not provide for the return of the employee's contributions in the cases of withdrawal or dismissal, or for the use of such contributions for other purposes, so that the fund accumulated would soon, in some cases, run into millions. It does not follow, however, that the opposite tendencies now manifest to seek a solution of the problem in a non-contributory scheme are sound, for this would still encounter the opposition of labor unions, who see in all such schemes a return to feudalism or an attempt to make labor stick to its job by the use of vague promises, to the fulfillment of which the employee himself contributes in the long run in the form of depressed wages. The Metropolitan Life Insurance Company, however, seems to have found a way out and has proposed to "write annuity contracts maturing at the age of 65 under which the pension is purchased each year in small units representing either flat rate or a percentage of salary. The employer, the employee, or both, make a contribution each year toward the pension to fall due on the retirement of the employee," who receives a bond each year that assures him a pension when he retires, each bond being complete in itself. This scheme costs little to administer and it meets the objection against a non-contributory system, that although pensions defer pay only the employee who survives in the same service until retirement receives the benefit promised, by the provision that this bond is given each year and becomes his property, to be realized at a fixed age in later years.

Frederick L. Hoffmann[26] gives us one of the sanest and most compendious summaries of the negative views on this whole subject. Present systems have not eliminated poorhouses or the pauper's grave. Of the 1,981,208 individuals in the United States over 70, according to the census of 1898, a great majority would welcome a pension; and of all legislation this is most irreversible. On the contrary, old beneficiaries constantly agitate for more. State pension systems, too, do not materially reduce the cost of charitable relief, whether indoor or outdoor. Only in a last resort should the state attempt to do what can be done by private institutions or by private individual foresight and nothing should discourage voluntary thrift of any kind. Where pensions have caused the removal of beneficiaries from asylums or almshouses, the results have generally been unfavorable. Pensions are chiefly of benefit to those not within the scope of poor law administration or private charitable aid. It is just this class which pensions would help that is now most efficient in

---

[26] "Problem of Poverty and Pensions in Old Age," *Amer. J. Soc.*, vol. xiv, 1908-9, p. 282 *et seq.*

helping themselves. If the family is at all kept up to its ideal, the young will help the old as they have been helped by them. This is not charity but mutual aid based upon mutual obligation for service rendered and there can be no substitute for this. It is this class that forms the backbone of a nation and which, by even moderate foresight, could provide for a modest support in their old age. The billions of dollars that they have invested in savings banks and in insurance institutions of various kinds show that they are not unmindful of the future. Legislation is needed to stamp out fraudulent enterprises designed to attract small savings on the plea of large returns; therefore, security should be the first consideration in such investments. The prevailing wages should make it possible for the masses of wage earners to provide the support necessary for their old age, at their own cost and in their own way, if they are given sufficient intelligence and motive and could feel sufficient security. To take an example, 5 per cent of a wage of $900 per annum, or $45, commencing with the age of 30 and continuing to 65, would produce an annuity of $450. Of course, the earlier in life the periodical payment begins, the smaller would be the annual amount required to be paid. The fact is that parents who have done well by their children seldom come to grief in their old age, except by special misfortune. Nothing must be done to weaken the virtues here involved. The view that old-age pensions should be given as a right and not as an act of charity is one-sided, because wage workers have not spent their lives in behalf of the state but have sought to aid themselves in their own way and sold their services to the highest bidder.[27]

---

[27] See Spender, *Treatise on State Pensions in Old Age,* London, 1892; G. Drage, *The Problems of the Aged Poor,* London, 1895, 375 pp.; Metcalf, *Universal Old Age Pensions,* London, 1899, 200 pp.; Booth, *Pauperism and the Endowments of Old Age,* New York, 1906. For extended inquiries

L. W. Squier[28] tells us that of the 18,000,000 wage earners in the United States, about 1,250,000 reach the age of 65 in want and are not sufficiently supported by public or private charities which, in round numbers, cost the country $250,000,000. Of the 2,000,000 non-fatal accidents Hoffmann estimates per year, the old, to be sure, have somewhat less than their share. The United States Bureau of Labor lately estimated that $220,000,-000 per annum is the average the laborer has to pay for medicines alone, not including doctors' bills, and about 79 per cent of those in almshouses are either physically or mentally defective. Our total pension outlay for the War of the Revolution, that of 1812, the Indian wars, Mexican, Civil, and Spanish, in regular establishments and unclassified, he estimates at $4,230,-381,730. Despite the world unrest there are probably ever increasing numbers who look forward to a quiet old age, and we must depend more and more upon inculcating thrift wherever possible and encourage all to earn more than a living wage.

Present-day man, at his best, is certainly far below the standard, for nowhere among wild animals do we find so many with defective teeth, vision, tonsils, bowels, flat foot, etc., and the rejection of nearly one-third of the drafted men for physical unfitness was a most significant fact. The trouble is men will not take pains to prolong life and still shrink from medical examinations at all ages. Some tell us that old people do so most of all, fearing to know the truth about their condition.

This very cursory sketch must suffice to show the increasing interest in and the growing magnitude of the economic problem of old age. But before closing this

see *The Report of the Royal Commission on Old Age Pensions* by the Commonwealth of Australia, 1906; also, William Sutherland, *Old Age Pensions in Theory and Practice*, London, 1907.

[28] *Old Age Dependency in the United States*, New York, 1912, 361 pp. a masterly book.

chapter let us glance at the efforts of the new Life Extension Institute to prolong life and increase efficiency. It is said to be "five per cent philanthropy," and all those whose lives are insured are to make a definite effort to avoid sickness and defer death. Members are inspected gratis and all others can be for a moderate fee. A regular system of examination for repairs is provided for, just as all manufacturers do for their machines, with a written report to the person's family physician. At the start the Postal Life Insurance Company turned over to the new organization its well established system of examinations for policy-holders and the Metropolitan Life made an agreement for periodic examinations. The company's conservation policy leads an impaired man to consult a physician before it is too late, and this, we are told, has reduced the death rate among those examined. They plan to extend this over the whole country. Two-thirds of the profits beyond 5 per cent are to go toward increasing the further usefulness of the Institution. Judge W. H. Taft is chairman of the Board of Directors while Irving Fisher is chairman of the Committee of One Hundred on Hygiene.[29]

In the *Nation* of January 8, 1914, commenting on the hygienic reference board of the Life Extension Institute the writer tells us that they will even tackle such problems as ventilation, how to clothe and feed the body, etc. Some have advocated compulsory annual examinations for all. This the *Nation* condemns. There is the danger of false diagnosis as to degree or kind of defect. An ailing man might be injured by knowing the seriousness of his trouble. It might detract from the joy of life and to compel it would be an undue invasion of liberty, for it is not like vaccination and similar measures necessary for all.

---

[29] *The Survey*, vol. 31, 1914–15, p. 483.

What the old need is an occasional examination of sight and hearing, of respiratory, circulatory, digestive, and perhaps sexual system, each by an expert, with hygienic and therapeutic suggestions based upon these results. This the Life Extension Institute does not attempt to furnish and it is perhaps too much to expect yet.

A few other voluntary organizations for the benefit of the old should be mentioned here.

The "Borrowed Time Club" of Oak Park, Illinois, dates from the year 1900 but was reorganized in 1911, and in 1920 had 294 names on its roster. It admits only those of seventy years of age or more and has clubrooms of its own in which it holds weekly meetings. One of its most impressive customs is an annual meeting devoted to the memory of the brethren who have died during the year, with a service at which a floral tribute is laid upon each vacant chair placed in a line on the platform by younger members of the families of the deceased. Political and religious questions are barred. There are no fees but a voluntary offering once a month, and any citizen of whatever creed or race, whether rich or poor, is eligible. Fraternal sympathy and companionship are fostered. There is music and a prayer at most of the meetings, illness of members is reported on, current events discussed, and a program usually provided. "The main purpose of the organization is to bring happiness to others." There are perhaps a hundred and fifty associate members. This club has several branches, and others of similar name and character have been established in other cities.

To the writer, the name of the club seems unfortunate in assuming the Biblical limitation of life at three-score-and-ten, as if we were incurring indebtedness and living on by the special indulgence of Father Time if we surpass that age. Why are we debtors after more than before this age, when the fact is we are living on capital accumulated or inherited and in no sense on credit? The religious features that seem to characterize every program are well and no one could have anything but commendation for the interest displayed in sick members or in the annual tributes to the dead. But the thanatic outlook from the "west window" should not predominate and the discussion of current events and interest in vital problems should be kept most lively to offset the attitude of patheticism to which the old are only too prone.

The Sunset Club, at present largely composed of women over sixty, has little organization although it has many branches in various parts of the country. Its purpose is not only to have old people help and be helped by others to useful occupations but to supply reading matter, chaperones, etc. Anyone can start a club anywhere, intellectuals can get together, the rich can help those in need, those with unoccupied time can help those who need sympathy and companionship, those with happy homes may occasionally open them to the homeless, or they can simply form good cheer circles. There are no dues but volunteer funds have sufficed for this "silver-haired sisterhood," which has often provided friends for the friendless and employment for the unoccupied. Many women of the more or less leisured class have thus found spheres of usefulness which they preferred to bridge, gossip, "kettledrum or kaffee-klatsch." Some branches of the club have an exchange where members can send things that they make for sale. Young couples, especially brides, are often aided in starting homes.

In Kilmarnock, Ayrshire, Scotland, is a beautiful public park with an avenue of old trees under which the old men of the district who were come to the resting time of life used to foregather "for a crack and a smoke." Then a kind man, remembering the frequent rainy days there were, presented them with an old railway carriage as a shelter where this group could meet in shower or shine. Later the park was extended and a public-spirited man erected a pretty little dwelling for the club, red tiled, with a veranda all around. Here are games and books and here the club meets at will. Provision has also been made for a yearly summer holiday for the members.

Stroudsburg, Pennsylvania, boasts an octogenarian society, the last annual meeting of which on September 29, 1921, witnessed a gathering of twenty-one members.

A sagacious and venerable correspondent has suggested to the writer that the time is ripe for some kind of a senescent league of national dimensions which should, of course, establish relations with all existing associations of the old but should slowly develop a somewhat elaborate organization of its own, with committees on finance, on the literature of senescence, including its psychology, physiology and hygiene, etc. If such an organization under any name were founded, it should certainly have an organ or journal of its own that should be the medium of correspondence, keeping its members informed to date upon all matters of interest or profit to them, perhaps keeping tab on instances of extreme longevity or unusual conservation of energy, with possibly a junior department eventually for youngsters of fifty. It should concern itself with the phenomena connected with the turning of the tide of life, which so often occurs even in the fourth decade. It would be interesting to know how such an organization would appeal to intelligent old men and women. That it might do great good is hardly to be doubted.

CHAPTER V

MEDICAL VIEWS AND TREATMENT OF OLD AGE

The self-knowledge that doctors give—Insidious approach of many diseases—Medical views of the old age of body and mind (senile dementia) —Charcot—G. M. Humphry—Sir James Crichton-Browne—H. M. Friedman—H. Gilford—H. Oertel—A. S. Warthin—W. Spielmeyer— I. L. Nascher—Sir Dyce Duckworth—Robert Saundby—Arnold Lorand —T. D. Crothers—C. G. Stockton—W. G. Thompson—M. L. Price— G. S. Keith—J. M. Taylor—C. W. Saleeby—C. A. Ewald—Raymond Pearl—Protest against the prepotence of heredity in determining longevity.

By an instinct that is very deep and strong most old people shrink from realizing just what their stage of life is and means, although most are ready enough to discuss such symptoms as are forced upon their consciousness. Disguise it as we will, old age is now only too commonly a hateful and even ghastly thing. Even those most garrulous and pessimistic about their infirmities are often prone to an almost fetishistic focalization upon certain symptom-groups of their own to the neglect of others by the same mechanism by which general anxiety may come to a head on a single phobia, which is thus exaggerated, because all the affectivity of their more general state finds an outcrop in some special fear. This mechanism is the same, too, as that by which love may find a vent for itself in some amatory fetish. Few, indeed, are the old men, and perhaps fewer still the old women, who do not seek to seem to others younger than their real physiological age, and all even to their innermost selves are prone to dwell more on what the great

195

deprivator leaves behind than on what he has taken away. Childhood and youth long forward, old age longs backward.

Wishing to really know myself as old, I subjected myself upon my retirement to the examination and tests of some half dozen medical experts for eyes, ears, heart, lungs, digestive tract, kidneys, and even sex, but was surprised to find how hard it was to do so. A strong minority of my impulses preferred the ignorance that is often bliss. There are no mental tests of generally recognized validity above the teens, so that we have no criteria for determining psychological age for even the elderly, while psychoanalysts refuse on the express authority of Freud to take on patients over forty. When it was well over I was glad, for most organs and functions were found to be in fair condition, although one was in need of some special care. I realized anew, however, that there are no gerontologists, as there are experts for women, children, etc., and that barring acute attacks I must henceforth, for the most part, be my own physician and that I must give far more attention than ever before to keeping well and in condition. Body-keeping for the old is a very personal and pressing problem requiring much time and attention, and the methods that are successful differ so widely that the diet and regimen good for one might be dangerous, if not fatal, for another. But my chief interest for months centered in rather voracious medical and psychiatric literature upon senility and its disorders till my friends thought me in danger of growing morbid and predicted and feared hypochondria. Gruesome and depressing as it all was, it had nevertheless a certain grim fascination to know what a cohort of disorders encamp about and prey upon the aged, any group of which is liable to assail and perhaps take the citadel of life by storm. Evasion of these enemies gives a new sense of heroism.

Rheumatism, lumbago, varicose veins, calcified arteries, compensated for by enlargement of the heart, its valvular leaks and weakness, high abnormal blood pressure, adiposity or progressive emaciation, shaking palsy, cramps, bronchitis, asthma, shortness of breath, gout, stone, Bright's disease, diabetes, constipation, piles, hernia, prostate troubles, tuberculosis, cancer, dyspepsias, flatulence, nausea, vertigo, flaccid and atrophied pudenda, feeble voice, defective sleep, failing eyesight and hearing, weakness of muscles, gaps in dentition, rather more hygienic than the complete edentate state; and beyond all these and many more the certain prospect of death just ahead or around the corner, liable to come from many of these causes or from any one of them already so well advanced that to know is no longer to prevent it—these are the things the old face if they have the courage not to flee from real facts. One or more of these maladies is sure to strangle, starve, bleed, poison, or paralyze us suddenly or slowly, and that ere long. Some of us will die from the top down with dementia more or less developed, while for others some vegetative organ will collapse and drag down with it all the rest of our powers, which might otherwise go on for a decade or two. These are the things that often make the old pessimistic. They are the secrets of age that must be kept from the young lest they interfere with their joy of life and which religion and philosophy have done their best from the beginning of history to mitigate. Thus the soul of the old, when it confronts the sternest of all facts at close quarters, grows more and more prone to seek diversion than consolation, for the former in fact is the chief resource of senescence although, as I shall indicate later, modern science is slowly evolving a third and better one.

Meanwhile, since medicine is far from having yet developed any systematic or coherent gerontology, although it has marshaled many facts and given us many hints toward such a science, it has seemed to me that in the present state of knowledge I can serve the reader better by epitomizing, without any attempt at systematization that would be certainly premature, the *aperçus* and the standpoints of those who seem to me in recent years to have written more wisely than others upon this theme, as follows.

The only attempt at a history of what medicine has done for old age that I can find is in an old book by Charcot[1] in which he attempts to list and characterize the far too few studies of any importance made upon the subject up to that date. He urges that medical science should give far more attention to it.

Dr. G. M. Humphry[2] gives us a memorable study of five hundred old people of over eighty years of age, including an equal number of males and females. He stresses the fact that the descending changes of development are just as orderly as its earlier ascending phases and that civilization enables us to see far more of the natural processes of senescence than was possible when the conditions of life were ruder, for we can now promote the powers of self-maintenance to a degree impossible before. "The chief requisite for longevity must clearly be the inherent or inborn quality of endurance, of steady, persistent, nutritive force, which includes recuperative power and resistance to disturbing agencies and a good degree of balance between the several organs." That is, each must be sound in itself and have due relation to the strength of other organs. "If the heart and digestive system are disproportionately strong, they will overload and oppress the other organs, one of which will give way."

His findings indicate that both men and women of

---

[1] *Clinical Lectures on Senile and Chronic Diseases,* Lond., 1881, Lecture I.
[2] "Old Age and the Changes Incident to it," *Brit. Med. J.,* March 9, 1885.

average size and stature live longer than those much larger or smaller. He thinks, too, that there must be some trait associated with the development of the tubercle bacillus, "which is not only not incompatible with longevity but is not infrequently associated with it"; and this condition he found in eighty-two of the cases he studied. Most of them belonged to long-lived families, had enjoyed good health, appetite, and digestion, had taken little medicine, eaten little meat, been only very slightly addicted to alcohol, had been good sleepers, and rarely suffered from long or exhausting diseases. Most had been much out-of-doors. The average number of teeth in all these subjects was six for men and three for women, and only fifty-seven were entirely without them. The upper or alveolar part of the jaw tended to be absorbed and only the later, firmer growth of the lower part of it to be retained. In primitive man probably loss of teeth would materially shorten life. The skull, which generally becomes lighter, may also sometimes become heavier and increase inwardly as the brain shrinks. The rate of the heart varies very little as age advances. From eighty to ninety years he found it averaged 73-74 beats per minute in men and 78-79 in women. Respiration was 19-20 times per minute and, like the heart, was very slightly accelerated, although the respiratory change might be due to the prevalence of bronchitis in old people.

He found little tendency to senile dementia and many of even the very aged had their mental faculties intact and took a keen interest in passing events, possessed clear judgment, and were full of thought for the present and future welfare of others. "It is no less satisfactory to find that the active, even severe and long-continued intellectual activity of the matured brain seems in no way to impair its enduring qualities, and that good, earnest, useful employment of the body and mind are not only compatible with but even conducive to longevity."

Of 157 of the males who replied, only six had ever had diseases of the prostate or bladder, so that in general he thinks that "the aged body does not seem to be, on the whole, prone to disease." Few of his returns indicate the presence of any special malady. "We know that even cancers, when they attack old people, often make slow progress in them and sometimes fail to make way at all, remaining stationary or even withering, and the susceptibility to contagious disease appears to decrease from infancy to old age. Quite as remarkable is the fact that recovery from wounds, fractures, or operations, seems to be quite as rapid, and sometimes more so than in middle age. Indeed, wounds in the old heal very quickly provided they do not slough, indicating two opposite tendencies." He also finds evidence of greater vital energy in parts nearest to those diseased provided they are able to live at all, as if nature had recuperative processes of stimulating parts adjacent to lesions. He chronicled few more surprising results than the infrequency of sclerosis.

Sir James Crichton-Browne's long article[3] is a classic and is based on very comprehensive statistical and other studies. He tells physicians that it should be their great aim to grow old themselves and to be the cause of old age in others. The marked increase in the duration of life in recent decades has been almost entirely confined to its early stages. After 45 the decline in the death rate has been insignificant; and after 65, as we have elsewhere seen, it has actually increased. Thus the proportion of men ripened by experience has in fact declined. What carries off the old? Not fever, smallpox,

---

[3] "Old Age," *Brit. Med.,* Oct. 2, 1891.

or phthisis chiefly, as was once the case, but the following in order of frequency: cancer, heart diseases, nervous troubles, and kidney complaints, and these are all degenerative diseases due not so much to intemperance as to the new strains of modern life, which are less felt in the country and less by women.

Society needs to have life lengthened instead of abbreviated at its extreme end but men and women to-day are growing old before their time. We often have deaths reported to be from old age between 45 and 55. Indeed, atrophy and debility often come prematurely. The long-sightedness of old age seems to begin earlier than it used to do and the increased number of those who wear glasses cannot be entirely explained by better diagnosis. It is quite clear that those who live in hot climates show these optical symptoms of old age earlier than Europeans. The teeth, too, are certainly degenerating earlier than formerly, and early baldness is probably increasing still more. Senile insanity or atrophy of the brain is certainly more common and appears earlier. It abounds in our metropolitan asylums where human wreckage accumulates. Very many enter the outer circles of melancholia without proceeding to dementia and still fewer proceed to suicide, the rate of which is also rapidly increasing after 45. Touches of this kind of depression are very often felt at the turning point of life or soon after, perhaps at the first discovery of gray hairs, and many are tormented in private and perhaps in the silent watches of the night by the realization that youth is leaving them. Such, however, is the law of nature, for even the stars and planets grow old, as we know by their spectra. The voice is not normally shrill or quavering but may be very strong unless the crop of wild oats, which always ripens in later years, is too rank. Conscience may awaken near the turn, especially if too many dregs have accumulated in the cup of life or the machinery has been overstrained. The fact is, the infirmities often attached to age may, each of them, in single cases be absent, so that typical old age is rare, and any one of them is far less prevalent than is generally supposed.

Our life is made up of a series of evolutions of a group of different functions that develop serially, beginning at different age epochs, reaching their maximum vigor, and then declining. The hyaline cartilage dies of old age when bone is formed of it, as the milk teeth do. The thymus gland has completed its growth at the third year and slowly atrophies with every sign of age. The nervous system has the most sustained evolution. The infant, child, youth, are learning higher coördinations, and the psycho-motor system is not completely evolved till the end of the teens. The hand and arm centers continue their development and do not attain their perfection before thirty. The writer studied workmen in various factories and found that in many cases proficiency in manipulation grew for a decade and then became stationary at thirty, beyond which it could never be increased, and later declined. This decline took place sooner in highly specialized than it did in more general movements. In some artists, however, manual skill may increase to a great age.

In the brain centers that preside over language there is continuous development, so that it has been carefully estimated that our powers of expression culminate between 45 and 55. Demosthenes' *De Corona,* his masterpiece, was delivered at the age of 52; Burke's impeachment of Hastings, when he was 58; and many authors have thought their vocabulary and command of language at its best during this decade. After this, faint symptoms of aphasia and amnesia begin to show themselves. But it is in the frontal lobes, in which it is now believed

MEDICAL VIEWS AND TREATMENT

that the powers of attention, reason and judgment are located, that the acme of development comes still later, perhaps in the decade ending at the age of 65. Indeed, Moebius and others have shown that the cortical layers believed to be most closely associated with mentation are still developing as late as the age of sixty-three. Bacon produced the first two books of the *Novum Organum* at 59; Kant's *Critique of Pure Reason* was produced when he was 57; Harvey's great work on the circulation, when he was 72, etc. It is certain that long after memory of names and physical vigor have begun to abate, the power of comparison, inference, and above all a moral sense, which is perhaps the finest and latest of all our powers, comes to full maturity.

The ideal of a greater old age is not an idle dream and Browne insists that physicians should strive themselves to live to be 100 and to make their patients do so. The best antiseptic against senile decay is, he thinks, active interest in human affairs. This, at any rate, should be our working hypothesis. A man of 80 should realize that he has one-fifth of his life before him. He tells us of a man of 84 who attempted suicide because he could no longer support his parents, and of another of 102 who had undergone a successful operation for cancer of the lip without anæsthetics. Of course, senile involution, when cell growth is more than counterbalanced by cell decay, is the natural pathway to death, and a man ultimately dies of it when there is no question of disease. But the brain, like the lens of the eye, may become flatter and more longsighted, focusing better on objects far than those that are near. There is no short cut to longevity. Its achievement must be the work of a lifetime. Sympathy, which goes far deeper than courteous manners, is fundamental for the successful treatment of old age.

SENESCENCE

H. M. Friedman[4] begins his comprehensive treatise with biological and embryological considerations, and here perhaps he makes his most original suggestions. The higher the plane of the animal, the more marked is cell differentiation or specialization and this affects most cells. Once a degree of differentiation is observed, no backward step to a previous state of generalization, regeneration, or rejuvenation is possible. The higher the ascent of the cell in the plane of differentiation, the lower is its power of rejuvenation. Connective tissue, muscle fiber, and cylindrical cells are the least differentiated and therefore have the greatest power of regeneration. Nerve cells have the least because their work is of a high order and they are most specialized. Nerve fibers are mere conductors and they and epithelial cells have probably the greatest power of regeneration.

Again, the more differentiated the cell, the more rapid is its development, early decline, and death. Precocity even of the separate cell purports early maturity. "So senescence is an increased differentiation of the protoplasm, while rejuvenation is an increase of the nuclear elements at the expense of the protoplasm." The increase of nuclear material allows fission and the formation of new cells. Thus the degree of differentiation is greatest as fission or mytosis is least. The power of regeneration is in direct proportion to the power of cell fission. Thus "the greater the cell differentiation, the smaller the mytotic index." With maturity the decrease of the mytotic index, or the number of tissues into the composition of which the cell can enter, becomes restricted. The cells in the original germinal layer have before them the possibility of entering into the structure of any tissue, but as cells differentiate the germinal layers take on a more structural character and leave the

---

[4] "Senility, Premature Senility, and Longevity," *Med. Jour.*, New York, July 10, 1915.

field to the entrance of cells into different tissue formations more restricted, since during development the number of tissues yet unformed or undifferentiated becomes
less and less and once a cell has assumed a personality
it must continue to follow it up and cannot diverge from
it. This is the law of genetic restriction. The younger
the cells, the greater their multiplying power and the
greater the tissue possibilities they can choose. Hence
morbid tumors are formed from young cells of higher
mytotic index whose genetic restriction has not pro-
gressed far enough to inhibit range and rapidity of
growth. Before genetic restriction young cells may become one tissue or another. Injuries causing cell degeneration of the young cells are often, therefore, the
seats of morbid growths. The young or undifferentiated
cells forming malignant amorphous tumors and growing
in tissues alien to them develop rapidly, probably because
they are deprived of the "social" restriction to over-
growth that they would have in their own cell society.
Thus the presence of young cells in out-of-the-way
places or where older and more differentiated cells would
be expected should excite suspicion. "Young cells, like
young children, are safest among their own."

Generally a cell in an organism lives long enough to
reproduce its kind; else the species would die and death
does occur in many lower organisms immediately after
ovulation. The young thus grow rapidly, while old age
is the period of slowest growth; and indeed the rate of
growth depends upon the degree of senescence. The
tendency to senescence is at its maximum in the very
young and the rate of senescence diminishes with age.

As to the cause of senility, physiologically it is desiccation. At birth there is most fluid and gaseous material, but organization demands solidarity. Lactic acid
may retard the growth of intestinal flora and the up-keep
of the intestinal toilet by larvage. Intoxication of some

kind is a factor in many of the changes accompanying senility. Lorand thought age was chiefly due to atrophy and degenerative tissue by failure of the function of the ductless glands, especially the thyroid. The myxedematous look and are old. Thus the limit of life is a matter of excretion. The special organs of elimination cannot act to their full capacity or to that of vital necessity because of the replacement in senility of parenchyma by fibrous or fatty tissue. The retained waste products increase the sclerotic changes and produce a vicious circle—irritation, intoxication, and atheroma. The degeneration of the first stage produces insufficiency of the organs of elimination and the degeneration of all organs.

As to physical manifestations, there is atrophy of the higher and more specialized cells and they are replaced by hypertrophied connective tissue. The heart is enlarged but this is compensatory for the stiffening and narrowing of the lumen of the great vessels near it and so the blood pressure is increased. The changes in bone, ligament, and tendons are extreme, with increased enervation throughout the body and perhaps senile marasmus, which may bring extreme emaciation or osteomalacia and even bone deformity. This may affect nervous and mental elements, like senile asystole and changes in the blood. The temperature, however, is not affected.

As to mental manifestations, this author says they are extremely variable, insidious, and have a very wide latitude. The vitality of the mind should be far greater than that of the body. Old age dulls conscience, may bring vanity and new ambitions, petulance, irritability, misanthropy, and slows down activity. But the best average barometer of mental failure is memory, the loss of which comes as an advance guard of many symptoms. The old have no faith in the young, for example, Virchow and Agassiz would not accept evolution. There is a universal tendency to overeat, although we should "descend out of life as we ascended into it, even as to the child's diet." The first sign that food must be reduced is increased blood pressure. If only lower ideals were exercised in early life, the reversion is ominous. Age is never chronological except in the legal sense. It is often called a vascular problem. The old have immunity from certain diseases such as eruptive fevers, typhoid, phthisis, and old tissues do not seem to be good media for these disease agencies, but age is very prone to pneumonic infections and erysipelas.

As to premature senility, in general its symptoms are identical with those of mature senility. The old are particularly prone to flush under very slight emotional strain and cannot throw off care or control patience. As to the causes of premature senility, abuse rather than use is the key. There is an unhealthy tendency to force decline by overtaxing the body and the nerves. It is those who do this who take the pace that kills, taxing themselves beyond their capacities. Alcohol and syphilis are specific forerunners of arteriosclerosis but overeating is worse than alcohol, especially of meat. "Most people eat about twice as much as they need, and the high cost of living is the high cost of overeating." The dietitian's table of food values should always be consulted but there has to be wide latitude for individual adjustments. Modern efficiency ideals bring high pressure. Change is the greatest regulator. We now relegate older men to innocuous desuetude to give the younger a chance to forge ahead.

As to the proper sphere of the aged, there have been opposite views. Perhaps there are no more than five hundred really great men in history who were clearly above mediocrity. Galton thinks 70 per cent of their work was completed before 45, and 80 per cent before 50. Dorland analyzed four hundred celebrities and concluded the average age of the commencement of their activities was 24 years—in musicians perhaps as early as 17 and scientists at 32. Science is hard and requires a large fund of experience and knowledge. The greatest average for activity in all endeavors together is about 40. To enjoy life after 40 one must have attained some degree of success, for the saddest thing is to reflect on many years of effort and no accomplishment.

As to medico-legal aspects, eccentricities may prevent the aged testator from being allowed the right of testament, but in general the mental symptoms of advanced senility differ from senile dementia only in degree.

As to the future of old age, those who are not senile have a distinct place as counsellors. They should excel in strength of reason, cool judgment, and breadth of view. One may be past the age of discretion before one is old in years. The conservative tendencies of this period are valuable as checks to the exuberant impulses of youth. The dependent aged are a burden and their support is often a handicap. With modern progress the number who fail to keep pace increases with the speed of advance and this has to be complemented by the fact that the old are increasing in numbers. With few exceptions man lives longest of any animal. Everything does grow old except vanity and the more perfect the organization the earlier the aging and the sooner the end, for it is the perfect more surely than the good that die young. Every stage of life is marked by a limit, but this limit varies greatly. "Every man past forty is a fool, physician, or a divine, and most people practically throw away their lives." The lower the scale of education, the greater the hazard of life. Longevity among pure muscle workers is rare. We know little of the influence of race, but we know that women, lean people, the married, the religious, on the whole, live longest. Haeckel believed in "medical selection" and pointed to the fact that some have greater power to resist disease. Is this desirable for the integrity of the race? "Death is a process, not an event." Man does begin to die early in life. The bicycle rider has to keep going to keep erect, and so the old must keep working. The first vacation is often fatal.

Hastings Gilford [5] regards the development of the human body as a whole, or of any portion of the body, as describing a curve that ascends from the time of the union of the two genetic elements to a maximum at which there is the greatest development of specialization in function and the least in the general characters, such as those of multiplication. The curve then begins to descend, with a gradual and progressive loss of differentiation in form and function and an increasing tendency of certain cells to multiply. Decay of certain cells during advancing age leads to their becoming bodies foreign to their host, and this, in turn, calls forth the phagocytes which, walling off the foreign body, become themselves transformed into fibrotic tissue. The three characters of old age are decay, fibrosis, and proliferation of nonspecialized cells. As the more specialized cells retrogress, with the loss of specialization they take on an increased tendency to multiplication. "Reversion . . . is the keynote of the proliferation in old age wherever it occurs."

Granting the foregoing statements regarding the anatomy and biology of old age to be true, Gilford even believes that we can explain cancer in terms of senility. He says: "Thus the typical cancer is made up of a collection of cells native to the part, but of more embryonic type, and these cells are surrounded by collections of round indifferent cells derived from fibrous tissue and from other low class structures, such as

---

[5] "Nature of Old Age and of Cancer," *Brit. Med. J.*, Dec. 27, 1913.

endothelium and leucocytes." The fibrous tissue, moreover, is often increased, as it is in the senile organ.
These changes may be interpreted as follows. Certain
somatic cells become aged while the tissues around them
are still in a state of comparative youth. They express
their senility by returning to a more embryonic form,
and as they do so they increase in number, the faculty
of multiplication being one of the manifestations of
regression. But as this qualitative change takes place
they become alien to their surroundings and, as foreigners or rebels, stimulate into action the mechanism of
phagocytosis. Not only is there an incursion of lympho-
cytes into the parts but the connective tissue and endo-
thelial cells in their vicinity revert to their embryonic
state and begin the work of phagocytosis. But as a
fact they have to deal with neither the effete products
of molecular degeneration nor with an inert foreign
body, for though virtually strangers cancer cells are by
no means inactive. Hence the attack is abortive, except
in so far as the phagocytes, by forming new fibrous
tissue, tend mechanically to limit the proliferation of
the cancer cells. For in the meantime the fixed connective tissue cells are themselves rapidly proliferating,
with the result that when they cease their activity and
return to their resting stage, groups of cancer cells are
cut off by intersecting bundles of fibrous tissue, while
the whole mass is surrounded by an incomplete capsule
of the same structure. This tends to limit the encroach-
ment of the growing cancer, and were it not for the
lymph spaces or capillaries, which are the gaps through
which the growing cells escape, no doubt the limitation
and strangulation of cancers would occur far more often
than they do.

It will be noticed that the more nearly the cells of a
cancer approach the embryonic state the more rapid
will be the growth, and the less opportunity for fibrosis

the more malignant the cancer. Gilford maintains for this unique theory that it is satisfactory, based as it is, upon facts reasonably interpreted, and that it covers all of the ground.

Horst Oertel [6] holds that the origin of cancer in the liver is a transformation of multiple groups of its cells and that there was a direct change of atrophic, degenerative, existing liver cells into cancer cells while they were still in perfect continuity with each other. In this degeneration of normal to cancer cells the former lose their typical protoplasm, the nucleus grows small and its chromatin structure faint, till little of it remains, with only a faint rim of surrounding protoplasm. At this point some of these cells show a very striking change in rapid, irregular production of rich chromatin arranged in a less structural definition and leading to marked enlargement of them. There is a first destructive stage with extensive loss and granular degeneration of protoplasm. In the second, incipient regeneration shows and the nucleus is markedly enlarged, with irregular production of small chromatin granules; while in the third stage, the carcinomatous, we have a new type of cell following new laws and breaking with the former physiological arrangement and structure. The new functional type involves rapid independent growth with a distinct disregard of original source and surroundings and with progressive loss of continuity and power to secrete bile.

Thus he, too, holds that cancer seems an embryonic reversal and involves no specific changes but is a phenomenon of senescence, a degeneration of cells with an unequal decline in cell functions. Thus races of cells develop that lack the differentiation of undegenerated cells but are still endowed with vegetative and repro-

---

[6] "Degeneration, Senescence, and New Growth," *J. Med. Research*, vol. 33, 1918, p. 485.

ductive properties. His idea that the degeneration and injury to cells could be responsible for growth, was severely criticised. It was said that any change that meant injury could never be progressive but would lead to diminution of functions. But the author still holds that injury may produce growth of all kinds of tumors, for example, in the pancreas, growth and cell division is dependent upon the release of certain inhibitory influences that exist in the normal well-balanced cells. This upset may be caused by certain liquid solvents but the idea of formative stimuli on the whole seems to hold; namely, cancer cells arise out of degenerative and atrophic changes, so that injury, degeneration, and growth do not exclude each other but stand in genetic relation.

That organs that have reached full maturity and differentiation are stable and fixed in cell type and organization is false. Our organs are constantly in active regression, degeneration, and progression, and it is difficult to separate pathological from physiological changes. The pancreas is particularly in constant regression and progression. Thus it is peculiarly unstable and the limit of normality in its variations cannot be determined. Senescence is accompanied by multiple degenerative changes in many other organs and tissues, and associated with these are various benign and malignant tumors that seem to result from degenerative changes. Thus Oertel's idea of endless proliferation as a result of differentiation is not an idle speculation but rests upon an anatomical and experimental basis.

A. S. Warthin [7] says that syphilitic cases are generally regarded as cured if the Wassermann reaction is negative but there are very many cases that this escapes. It is commoner than is supposed, the usual estimates

---

[7] *The New Pathology of Syphilis*, Harvey Lectures 1917-19, p. 67.

being that from 5 per cent to 15 per cent of deaths are due to it, but this writer for America and Osler for Great Britain, place it at 30 per cent. "Syphilis is the leading infection and the chief cause of death, particularly in males between 40 and 60, and in the great majority of cases its symptoms are myocardial, vascular, renal, or hepatic, and this is often not recognized as a remote result." The author has never seen a marked case of syphilis cured. Most die as a result of mild inflammatory processes of the viscera and blood vessels rather than from paresis or tabes. It is progressive and marks the individual as damaged goods. Even immunity is bought at a price. All the organs must be examined before it is pronounced certainly absent. It is a spirochete-carrier. It tends to become mild but at any time the partnership between the spirochete and the body may be disturbed and the tissues susceptible to the violence of the spirochete may be increased so that the disease again appears above the clinical horizon. Chronic myocarditis is the most common form of death.

W. Spielmeyer [8] says that in the last decade the clinicians and pathological anatomists have discussed old age more than in preceding decades. We know that organs are used up and that their substance is not fully replaced. The functionally exciting parenchyma is injured by its own function and in this metabolism the quality and sometimes the volume of the organ is reduced. Thus old age is a function of the work of the organism and it seems to be an intrinsic quality of cells to use themselves up. Many do not regard age as a normal physiological process but with Metchnikoff think it is due to injurious substances, that is, endogenous toxins that are more important than the exogenous factors, so that blood vessels, glands, and muscle and

[8] "Die Psychosen des Rückbildungs- und Greisenalters," *Handbuch der Psychiatrie*, Spezieller Teil, 5 Abteilung, Leipzig, 1912.

ganglia cells degenerate. But the cortical cells, as the most sensitive of the organism, are more often injured. Metchnikoff thinks that the higher elements of the tissues are in conflict with the lower and are overcome by them, the phagocytes being left masters of the field.

Few, however, hold this view. Ribbert, Naunyn, Hansemann, and Nothnagel think that outer and inner injuries should have precedence in accounting for old age. But without these coöperative factors there is a physiological determinant of the organism and its parts to be used up and they become senile and lapse by physiological processes, while Naunyn thinks that it is perhaps a general law that every organ fulfills its functional task only by impairment of its complete organic integrity. This using up of an organism by its own work occurs first in the brain and the central nervous system. There is a general decline in weight, even in the fourth or third decennium, which is accelerated in the seventies and may reach one hundred grams (Naunyn) and, in pathological states, still more. It is, therefore, of great interest for the relation of function and the use-up of organs that brain atrophy is not usually uniform or diffuse but that there is often a difference between the right and left hemispheres in the diminution of their volume. The left hemisphere is more used and usually more atrophied than the right. The left convolutions, therefore, suffer most reduction.

Among the earliest and most uniform changes due to age is the regressive transformation of the blood vessels as in sclerosis. As the central tissues suffer from a using up of their nervous substance, the central vessels are soon involved. Till lately we have assumed that these disease processes in senium were a result and expression of the primary affections of the blood vessels in these organs. But it now appears that as in other organs, for example, the kidneys, grave age changes can occur while blood vessels are intact. So in the central organ grave independent age changes can occur without being caused by the blood vessels. To be sure, they often concur for the simple reason that the nervous system, like that of the vessels, is found affected oftenest and earliest in old age. But the assumption of a dependence of central nervous degeneration was an erroneous conclusion from the observation that by these frequent degenerative processes in the walls of the vessels there were, at the same time, phenomena of using up of nerve substance. "The changes of both organs can, despite their frequent combination, be the independent expression of age and quite independent one from the other."

Every study of the psychosis of regression and age must start from this fact and we must seek to distinguish the forms of weakness of old age due to central tissues from those that have their cause in the primary weakness of the blood vessels. For sclerotic senile dementia anatomy has already more or less basis. For the various forms of brain sclerosis it is now possible to propose an anatomical diagnosis, although it is impossible to have a very definite clinical picture of what takes place.

Outside these two chief groups of organically conditioned psychosis and degeneration there are many processes not yet certainly determined anatomically. These belong neither to sclerotic brain disease nor to proper senile dementia. They differ also in their general aspects from the average case of the imbecility of old age, and if they are classified with it, this rests only on superficial grounds and it is the problem of pathological anatomy to help clear up this clinical-psychological question. It is a little here as with innate and childish mental weakness, which we anatomically distinguish as idiocy and imbecility with partial success, just as we are trying to distinguish the psychosis of old age to make it conform to anatomical principles.

With the great recent progress of anatomy we are just at the beginning here, the chief result so far being the possibility of distinguishing senile involution and its morbid traits with a view to eventually being able to make an anatomical differential diagnosis, such as we must do to really get at the root of the problem of senile dementia. From this point of view other processes can readily be derived, and some of them histologically, like regression. The anatomical investigation stands in temporal relations with the idea of senile dementia and it must be defined or widened enough to do this. Perhaps we shall be able to have a good anatomical picture of senile dementia beginning with the fifth and sixth decennium and even to explain atypical forms and show their relation with the central system.

Here, then, the author, starting from an anatomical basis, begins with a study of forms that are atypical in localization, intensity, or temporal onset. Then he can discuss the mental diseases that are based on sclerosis. So he first discusses briefly those psychoses that rest upon clearly recognizable but not yet very distinctly determined brain troubles that deviate from the ordinary senile processes and those, which so far as we can now see, are really sclerotic. Then the long series of psychoses, the anatomical substratum of which we do not yet know, and the functional processes of this age can be discussed. In doing this, more than in the case of many organic processes, we shall find a great difficulty in proving for such diseases their specific senile or climacteric character. We shall constantly face the objection that we have here to do only with mental diseases that usually come in other ages and only have peculiar traits on account of the age of the patient, as is the case with many depressive and paranoiac symptom-complexes of regression that resemble those of age.

Thus the distinction of regressive psychoses from senile changes, this author thinks, cannot be carried through by grouping them in the decennia in which they arise. It would be better to distinguish them as progressive and incurable, or otherwise, but this could be done only with further distinction of our anatomical and clinical data and we shall perhaps still lack that for a long time.

When, therefore, in these regressions we start from anatomy and the psychoses connected with it at this age of life, we may seem to overestimate the achievements of histology. We at any rate do not underestimate our ignorance here. But with the great confusion of opinions based on clinical observations we believe we are justified in this point of departure. Ultimately anatomy will very likely be our guide in all clinical work as well as in the field of psychiatry, physiology, and psychology. We shall doubtless also learn very much more about the localization in which the degenerative processes of age begin.

Senile Dementia.—Textbooks and articles on old age generally state that the changes in psychic personality that occur are identical with normal ones, only in intensified degree. The traits most commonly specified are: limitation of the circle of ideas, qualitative and quantitative loss of elasticity, pauperization of interests, dwelling on *gemütlicher* activity, lapses in attention, Ziehen's "egocentric narrowing of the life of feeling," perhaps hypochondriacal symptoms, mistrust, inflexibility, lowered power of activity, and resistance against everything that is new. Works in general pathology, like Hübner, Ranschenburg, Balint, and Lieske deal with these in more detail.

In general, there is a sinking of psychic activity and change of character which suggest physiological involution, and these occur—in some, earlier, and in some later. If we compare these psychic traits it would seem that there is only a quantitative difference between normal old age and senile dementia, the latter having only gone farther or faster. The decision of this question is for pathological anatomy and here Spielmeyer's studies coincide with those of Simchowicz. The older an individual is, the less sharply either clinically or anatomically can it be decided whether it is normal or senile dementia. There are the same changes in the nerve cells, neuroglia, the myelin sheaths, and the mesoderm tissues; also in the blood vessels the changes are identical, the difference being only in degree. Fatty degenerations of the ganglion cells also occur in both. Sclerotic changes of elements are general. The neuroglia cells with normal seniles have lipoidal material in abundance, and the gliafibers, especially in their upper surfaces in the cortex, are increased. The walls of the blood vessels have undergone the same regressive changes and acquired the same fatty material by infiltration, and even the so-called senile plaques are found. Thus in general there is the same using up of the central organs. We are, thus, not yet in a position to determine from the brain alone, if we know nothing of the individual, whether he was a senile dement or a very old man. The older a man is, the more we find the Redlich-Fischer plaques. Thus the senile dement shows neither anatomically nor clinically any essential differences from those found in the normal senium.

I. L. Nascher [9] thinks that too little study has been given to the physical changes in involution and still less to the mental. Occasionally the approach of senile dementia gives rise to forensic questions. There is a general neglect of the subject of geriatrics. This author thinks

---

[9] "Senile Mentality," *Inter. Clin.*, vol. 4, 1916, p. 48.

the brain reaches its limit of physical development at about 30, but Bunsen and Mommsen both did much of their best work after their brain had grown quite atrophied, so that quality comes in. The integrity of these cells depends upon nutrition. We have few blood examinations of the aged and these do not show any marked clinical or microscopic differences between maturity and senility, while the process of senile involution rests apparently on defective nutrition of cell tissues. Those who do good work in age generally focus into one channel and their degeneration is shown in other fields. We usually do not think of our somatic state until some discomfort compels us to do so. One may have lessened interest in former hobbies or events of the day; but if impairment of reason keeps pace with that of memory, he will not know that his powers are failing. He then begins to think of his body and its preservation as more important than wealth or fame, wants to live, and gives more attention to prolonging life.

There is often a change of temperament into egoism, perverseness, peevishness, loss of ambition, religiosity, inability to bear slight discomforts and depression. The child thinks little of the future, while in maturity hope tends to paint a future haloed by happiness and in senility the future is death, notwithstanding what all philosophers, poets, and preachers say. Our mental attitude is simply a resignation to the inevitable. One patient had a daughter devoted to him whose absence for a moment he could not bear, and once this so angered him that his total attitude toward her changed to one of dislike and suspicion. In another case a woman of seventy-six underwent a complete change of character. Arrogance gave way to humility; in contrast to her former independence, she now craved sympathy. Then later she changed again and made extraordinary demands upon her children, wanted the latest styles in everything, etc. In another case memory, reason, and will grew weak in an old manufacturer. He lost his way on the street, a child could divert him from his purpose, and he clung to a notebook by day and night till complete dementia came. Another man who was noted for carrying through everything he planned, even breaking up partnerships, when old became not only susceptible to advice but could be easily turned from his purpose.

Thus senile mentality shows temperamental changes. There is introspection, with natural fears and unnatural phobias, hope for strength and vitality or even for beauty, and often overweening biophilism. Action is slow; fatigue, quick. The mind may be often trivial on all other matters but yet sound in the center of interest. Personal attainments and achievements are often magnified, and complaints are exaggerated as calls for sympathy. Moral deterioration may be first. Lapses are condoned that were once condemned. The old man may slowly come to take interest in what is low and vulgar. This moral decadence is entirely apart from the pathological condition in which the *cœundi potentia* is lost while the desire remains, and the recrudescence of desire may occur in the senile climacteric but is a forerunner of senile dementia.

The æsthetic sense causes the old often to neglect cleanliness in person and clothes, to be untidy in their room, expectorate, scratch in public, make disagreeable sounds, and disregard proprieties generally. Women show these traits, but in less degree, and depression is less pronounced. There is no sudden realizing of aging and fear of death is more often overcome by religion. Sometimes the intellectual faculties deteriorate more rapidly, but moral and æsthetic impulses change less. Sometimes old women take greater care of their appearance and seem to be vain and to fight old age. Men occasionally at a great age take a new interest in their appearance, dyeing their hair and becoming dandified, which may show recrudescence of sex.

After the climacteric depression may pass to apathy. Death is less fearful as the mind weakens; there is less concern for the future and life is more in the present. Even early recollections grow dim, although such cases may be roused momentarily. There may be marked preference for association with children. There may also be childish acts and garrulity. The family history given the physician by an elderly patient is often unreliable. Insignificant symptoms are magnified; so are former attainments. Old patients often claim they possessed wonderful constitutions, perhaps that they were never ill, despite indubitable marks of disease.

In homes for the aged there is much suggestion. If one scratches, the rest do, without pruritus, so that to isolate the author of this contagion cures it. The same is true of groaning and grunts and even tremor may be acquired by association. In one case, cutting off food stimulated to overcome tremor. Pain, cough, and stiffness are magnified for sympathy. The fear of pain of an operation may cause the denial or hiding of symptoms, although weakened mentality makes sense impression less acute, either from peripheral or central causes, so that it is hard to tell whether this is due to local anæsthesia or weakened mentality. Tests used for malingerers may be necessary to determine sensitiveness and other symptoms or even harshness and threats may bring out the truth. Though cruel, these are sometimes necessary for correct diagnosis.

Friends often observe changes sooner than the immediate family but the latter must corroborate the statements. The physician should determine if an oikiomania exists and so must be alone with the patient, as he will not encourage such an attitude in the presence of the object of his hatred. If the physician tries to reason him out of his delusion, he thinks he is in league with the hated person and therefore hates him more. If the physician has incurred the patient's dislike, he should leave him for a few days so that he may forget. Sometimes the dislike of seeing the doctor grows from day to day. One had a suspicion that the doctor was in league with a daughter, and so put him out. A few days later the doctor was called for, and only when the wife told the patient why he would not come did he remember his suspicions and thereafter refuse to see him. In one case, having incurred an old woman's displeasure by excusing her son, whom she feared, the doctor left and was soon called again, all being forgotten. The person hated should stay away and the dislike may pass, especially in the case of a physician who has been necessary to the patient.

The great factor is the senile's sense of dependence on others. The old man does not realize that one more mouth means less food for the children or that his carelessness makes work or his peculiarities alienate sympathy and affection. Perhaps he feels he is a burden and his death would be a relief to those for whom he provided in earlier years. So delusions of persecution may arise.

What can we do? Symptoms are often bettered at an asylum. Phobias vanish and so do fears for the immediate future. All energies may be guided to one channel and the person may be made useful and his fear of being useless thus cured. The old are thus often anxious to do little services to show they are not worthless and little tasks can occupy them without strain. A patient pensioned after sixty-five years of work could get no other employment, felt useless, instead of being cheery became depressed, and was cured by being reemployed. The influence of young people keeps up interest in life—especially marriage with a young person, the development of a hobby, collecting anything, such as stamps, coins, books; witnessing new sights, but not fairs, where numbers confuse.

Drugs give temporary relief. Small doses of morphine give exhilaration and arouse the imagination, but its effects soon wear off. "Phosphorus in solution is the most effective drug for prolonged use." It is a mental and nervous stimulant and aphrodisiac, increasing mental power and producing a sense of well-being. One-fiftieth-grain doses several times a day, stopping just as soon as the intellect begins to brighten, are often beneficent. This can be kept up for years. Perhaps amorphous phosphorus may be used.

Sir Dyce Duckworth[10] asks: Why are some remarkably young for their age and others old? It cannot all be explained by anything in the individual life or habits. Perhaps it is in part because the ancestors lived a hard life. We want the degree of inherent vitality proper to each individual patient. This would be as important for prognosis in pneumonia as are the hæmic leucocytes. Arterial hardening may be local only, for example, radial. There are two kinds of arterial degeneration, namely, the brittle and the tough, the former more liable to cause hemorrhages and fatty degeneration.

Very important is the discovery that the rigidity of calcified arteries is greatly increased immediately after death. The lime is present before, as disclosed by the X-rays, but it is like wet or unset mortar and only sets after death under the influence of carbon dioxide and the rapidly diminishing alkalinity of the blood. The so-called air in the arteries after death is chiefly carbon dioxide and this explains why such arteries do not rupture so frequently as we might expect. Premature death

---

[10] "Some Clinical Indications of Senility," *Inter. Clin.*, vol. 2, 1914, p. 93.

of parts of the body is constantly occurring, for example, baldness, teeth. One may be vulnerable to one and another to another type of injury or bacilli. Syphilis is mainly a conjoined trait or infection and greatly predisposes to tubercle. Indeed, a syphilitic patient may be regarded as a prematurely aged one in spite of a good constitution, because there is always the possibility of sequels or parasyphilis, general paralysis, etc.

Among the early mental signs of interstitial nephritis is an explosive temper. Fits of hilarity and weeping may alternate (first pointed out by Clifford Allbutt). The costal cartilages ossify generally before the sixth decade and this is often premature. A hobby may no longer avail to preserve mental activity, and "the golf ball to-day is not seldom one of the beneficent agencies for this purpose." Cirrhosis of the liver is longer averted in the patrician than in the plebeian because the laborer becomes senile sooner than others owing to his life of strain in all weathers. In arthritis, the nodosity of joints, especially in the fingers, in the form of *Heberden's* nodes, is thought by some an indication of longevity. They are often found in those who have few classical symptoms of gout and few reach eighty or ninety without these trophic changes. Dupuytren's contractures and the camptodactylia of Landouzy, or incurved little finger, are among indications of a gouty habit and are not truly rheumatic lesions. Indolence of the bladder does not imply prostatic symptoms. Very common are widespread catarrhal disturbances, as for example, tussis senilis, with much flux of mucus, often rich in sodium chloride. Fits of sneezing, also of hiccough and even gaping, are frequent.

The main treatment for early senility is physiological righteousness (Sir A. Clark). We must especially know the degree of vigor, of vitality, and specific habit of body. We must pay attention to the degree of blood pressure and early indications of renal inadequacy, orthostatic albuminuria, the tendency to epistaxis, and maintain as our keynote moderation in all things. The best idea is that of universal service which would bring all the world together on a high plane. The author refers with a good deal of skepticism to Metchnikoff's Bulgarian bacillus but mentions Saundby's book with great praise.

Robert Saundby, M.D.,[11] has given us what is, to date, the best handbook, both for practitioners and for old people who are intelligently interested in conserving their life and strength, on the common infirmities and care of the aged, exclusive, for the most part, of nervous and psychic symptoms. He first describes normal old age, then its diseases in successive chapters—diathetic infections, and those of the circulatory, respiratory, digestive, and genito-urinal systems. Perhaps most practical are the dietaries he gives for different stages of old age and different diatheses. He commands a wide knowledge of Continental literature on the subjects he treats. He has a just sense of the dangers of stressing specifics from, for example, Pythagoras, who thought there was a special virtue for longevity in honey; Bacon, in sweating; Harvey, in avoiding acids; down to Blanchard, in sal volatile; blood drinking cures, olive oil, licorice, etc. He believes that Metchnikoff's panacea and the undue stress laid by Lorand on thyroid therapy have not escaped the dangers of undue focalization. He allows a very wide latitude not only in regimen and exercise but food, condiments, and even stimulants, for the aged.

No one can read his account of the changes that take place in each part and organ of the body as they are successively described and the very different treatments that each needs as it goes wrong, without a sense of

[11] *Old Age: Its Care and Treatment in Health and Disease,* London, 1913, 312 pp.

the fatality with which these vast cohorts of life-quelling
symptoms advance and, in view of the many strategies
the lethal processes make use of to undermine the
fortress of life, without experiencing a profound sense
of the hopelessness of watching out in so many directions and realizing that, as differentiation proceeds in
the different organs, any regimen helpful to one would
almost certainly be harmful to others.

Arnold Lorand, an Australian physician,[12] bases his
work on the principle that man does not die but kills
himself. He does not philosophize but tells us that while
it is impossible to create a young man out of an old one,
it is quite within the bounds of possibility to prolong our
youthfulness by ten or twenty years. In other words,
we need no longer grow old at forty or fifty. We may
live on to the age of 90 or 100 years instead of dying
at 60 or 70. Old age is just as amenable to treatment
as chronic diseases. He has great faith in the present
possibilities and still larger hopes for the future of
serum therapy, for to him life is most of all connected
with the glands. He discourses upon the hygiene of
throat, lungs, heart, kidney, liver, stomach, bowels, reproductive organs, and the rest with a bewildering
volume of details but good perspective, and the reader
is again disheartened to find that the treatment prescribed for one organ is deleterious to another. Indeed,
Lorand's somewhat encyclopedic and undigested data,
despite the common sense and practical spirit in which
they are presented, bear, on the whole, less upon
old age itself than upon general hygiene at all stages of
life, so that his title is to that extent a misnomer.

He sums up his practical conclusions in the form of
twelve commandments, which are, briefly, to keep in
the open and take plenty of exercise; eat according to

[12] *Old Age Deferred: The Causes of Old Age and Its Postponement by Hygienic and Therapeutic Measures,* Philadelphia, 1911, 572 pp.

rule; bathe and move the bowels daily; wear porous underclothes; early to bed and rise; sleep where it is dark and quiet; rest one day each week; avoid emotional strain; get married; be temperate in the use of alcohol, tobacco, tea, and coffee; and avoid over-eating and -heating.

T. D. Crothers, M.D.,[13] thinks we have not sufficiently considered the abilities of old age from a medico-legal standpoint. He also thinks that if we do not live to be 100 something is wrong with us or our ancestors. We all carry a large reserve that many die without drawing upon, and this reserve is especially available in old age (he develops this point psychologically). Many old people with melancholia, hallucinations, and the characteristic physical defects of old age have, nevertheless, a higher kind of sanity to which their juniors do an injustice by the tests they propose. They are quite capable of making wills and otherwise deciding the large questions that come before them and often do so from a broader point of view than younger men. It is possible, then, to rise to a higher level, to a kind of graduate school of life, to use the unused, etc. Again, the varied experiences of long life give mobility of mood up and down what Adler calls the life line, so that the old have a larger assortment of viewpoints and even moods, to say nothing of greater ups and downs in horizon and standpoint generally.

C. G. Stockton, M.D.,[14] suggests family records and pride to avoid mixing good stock with that which decays early. He recognizes the great contributions of the den-

---

[13] "The Medical Significance of Old Age," *Med. Press and Circ.*, London, May 20, 1914.
[14] "The Delay of Old Age and the Alleviation of Senility," *Jour. Amer. Med. Assn.*, July 15, 1905.

tist and oculist, deplores the neglect of old age, and
insists that the aged do respond to treatment very readily. He also deplores the attitude of many physicians
who discourage resolute methods of curing defects and
warding off evils because the patient is old. He stresses
the value of emunctory procedures both within and
without.

Dr. W. G. Thompson[15] deplores the fact that physicians have given so little attention to old age and that
the medical literature upon the subject is so meager.
The very old have survived all corroborative evidence
as to their age, their failing memories confuse tradition
and fact, and they come very often to take pride in their
age and so add to it. The author's study is based on
the census statistics of 1910, which record, from 90-94
years, 6,175 deaths; from 95-99, 1,427; 100 years and
over, 372. The respiratory diseases as a group took
first rank as the cause of death; organic heart disease,
apoplexy, and Bright's disease occurring in frequency
in the order mentioned. Among diseases of the digestive
system enteritis outranked all others.

As age advances and its activities and diversions become less and less, locomotion is reduced, along with
acuteness of sight and hearing, and the pleasures of the
table remain the only gratification of a monotonous
existence. Very many accustom themselves to the
habitual use of laxatives to counteract the effects of
overeating, and often we have obstructions, especially
of the rectum or colon, that may become fatal. This,
however, is more often seen in those who eat too little
and become perhaps atrophic and marasmic. These
people become careless of matters of the toilet and obstructions often cause death. Apoplexy is relatively rare

---

[15] "Centenarians and Nonagenarians," *Med. Rec.*, Feb. 15, 1913.

among centenarians and carcinoma also declines as a cause of death after the ninetieth year. Indeed, the disease that does not develop until after the ninetieth year can scarcely be due to hereditary factors and the infrequency of cancer in the later stages of life emphasizes the constitutional resistance to extraneous influences that the majority of centenarians possess in a high degree. Acute and very quick or fatal pneumonia is not infrequent.

One very peculiar difficulty in treating old patients is their prejudice and obstinacy in matters of diet and hygiene; because they have lived so long they naturally think they know better than anyone else what is good for them and, with a certain irritability, resist interference. As a rule, they are relatively very susceptible to the action of drugs and two-thirds of the ordinary dosage for adults generally suffices. Very often the very aged suffer from the neglect of personal cleanliness. There are many diseases common from the sixth to the ninth decades of life that are very rare later, for example, tuberculosis. Suicide is very rare, the census of 1910 recording only one of a centenarian and nine among nonagenarians. The latter generally have a long-lived ancestry and many families are remarkable for this trait. But this is by no means essential. The aged often exhibit no predominant symptom of any one disease to which their death is attributable, and hence "senility" is so often given as the cause of death. Tranquillity, moderation, and regularity seem to be the chief factors in securing a long life and a peaceful death.

M. L. Price, M.D.,[16] attacks Metchnikoff's theory of old age by assuming that in addition to all toxins and inflammations there is always an old-age exhaustion of

---

[16] "Ancient and Modern Theories of Age," *Maryland Med. Jour.*, vol. 49, Feb., 1906.

a vital principle that he calls bioplasmine, that may, to be sure, be mainly caused by Metchnikoff's agencies but is equally affected by effort, exposure, growth, and reproduction. He sagely predicts that the solution of the problem of old age, which he thinks is the central theme of all medicine in the sense in which he conceives it, because every disease brings senile phenomena to some part of the organism or to the whole of it, will be solved by biochemistry, although he admits that it may take many generations of investigation to achieve this final solution.

George S. Keith, M.D.,[17] after a long life of practice, has grown suspicious of current methods. "I purge, I puke, I sweat 'em; and if they die I let 'em." As to foods, he believes that the old should only eat when they are far hungrier than they usually are and leave off eating when they now habitually begin a meal. Appetite, which seems to give momentum to all the assimilative processes, is never utilized to its full extent. Sick animals often go off alone and succeed in recovering and he believes humans have the same instinct. He is, therefore, bitterly opposed to forced feeding, even for the insane, save under very exceptional conditions. The sick should generally be allowed to eat whatever they wish, perhaps in moderation, or to go entirely without food. Probably primitive man and all animals had to undergo occasional long fasts and this serves to tone up not only the nerves but the entire digestive system. Instinct is a far truer guide than doctors who interfere with it think. Once the fevered patient who reveled in dreams of cold was kept warm; now we know better. This author has, thus, an almost implicit trust in the cravings and dislikes of the sick and would indulge them

[17] *Fads of an Old Physician* (Sequel to *Plea for a Simpler Life*), London, 1897.

almost to the limit, as the German hygienist, Sternberg, would do to a perhaps even greater degree. He is also a great believer in rubbing and massage. Hot water plays an important rôle, too, while he attaches very special value to licorice. Doctors are often too anxious to save patients from all pain, perhaps by the use of means that entail worse consequences. Pain has its place in nature and the doctor should also try to have the patient apply the cure of patience. Pain is nature's cry for help, to which she often responds as she does not to other stimuli; and benign as is the rôle of anæsthesia, it should not blind us to the tonic effects pain often exercises. So sleeplessness may not be an unmixed evil in certain cases and sleep artificially induced is usually of poorer and less restorative quality. He has found fixating, spontaneous retinal phosphenes a good soporific method. He believes that very many diseases would cure themselves if the patient could be induced to simply rest and starve. Although he is not a homeopathist, he nevertheless believes that dosages of medicine are far too large. He insists that old and experiencd physicians ought to, and that the best do, learn a great deal from experience in keeping themselves well, and that every physician should accumulate thus a store of knowledge based on self-observation, and may well, with profit, always be mildly experimenting upon himself. As age advances he would regulate diet and treatment largely to the avoidance of accumulation of uric acid in the system. He found great reinforcement for himself in making a breakfast of coffee only, etc.

J. Madison Taylor[18] notes the paucity of literature on this subject that he found in trying to read up on it and thinks it warrants far more attention. The founda-

---

[18] "The Conservation of Energy in Those of Advancing Years," *Pop. Sci. Mo.*, 1903.

tions for longevity are laid in the first few months of life and bottle-fed babies are shorter-lived and much less likely to reach old age. Those who spend their infancy and childhood, too, in large centers are less long-lived than those brought up in the country. A serene mental view and capacity for deliberate enjoyment of whatever betides he places first of all and advises self-education in serenity. The less we eat and the less variety, the longer we live, and on this the author lays great stress. We must put aside, as we advance, some articles of diet of which we are fond.

He believes dentists have greatly interfered with longevity because man was meant to be more or less toothless and thus to be reduced in old age to childish diet and fluids, while the dentists enable us to eat anything we ever did, which is against Nature. He speaks of fads and their dangers, for example, one old lady thought she prolonged her life by eating a great deal of salt. The indolence and indifference of age is a great difficulty. If one persists in trying to keep up indefinitely, the results are often amazing. Medical aid should be sought more constantly for lesser ills. Man is like an old horse—if he once gets thoroughly out of condition it is hard to bring him back. G. M. Gould has believed that unfit glasses have shortened the lives of many eminent men. But open air is a *sine qua non* always.

Tessier gives a clinical picture of approaching death —(1) heart and blood vessels, (2) lungs, (3) kidneys, (4) digestive organs, (5) the brain. Most agree that the heart plays the chief rôle in ending life and many used to think that nearly all old-age diseases were from arterial hardening. But this was doubtless much exaggerated. Old age is a progressive diminution of all functional activities. All clinicians recognize diatheses or a tendency toward disease and we can detect them in their incipiency now far more than formerly. Age diathesis means a lessened coefficient of resistance, quick exhaustion, and weak repair. The author devotes great attention to obesity, which shortens life, and he advocates various exercises of the extensor muscles, deep breathing, and thinks much can be done to tone up and increase the activity of the heart.

He thinks the effects of the menopause have been rather overestimated. Exhaustion, especially induced by emotions, fatigue, anger, grief, and fear, weaken the protective powers of the mysterious agents of immunity. The mind is very liable to become fixed upon some ailment and hyper-conscious, particularly near the menopause, and this is due to failure of the organism to offer the same degree of resistance to toxins and to a general lessening of functional activity.

He thinks we can postpone old age by the following agencies. We should develop, not discourage, bodily exercise for without it there is a slow retrogressive change. The more nearly the diet is reduced to bread, milk and fruit, the longer the person will live and enjoy good health. Some can go for long intervals without feeding though more thrive on small quantities taken frequently. He condemns all purgatives and would regulate by salads, nuts, fruit, and thinks the best drink is buttermilk, which has salutary effects on both bowels and kidneys. Next comes koumyss. Fluids are best taken in abundance, but if the heart is weak they should be avoided before exercise, for this increases the cardiac strain. If the skin is dry, he advocates dry rubs rather than cold baths and olive oil occasionally, of which he says it is amazing how much the skin will absorb. He speaks emphatically of the dangers of chills and of the trend of all tissues to harden, stiffen, or lose their elasticity. Tissues about the neck are particularly prone to lose vigor. Regulated movements of the neck and upper truncal muscles often improve hearing, vision, cerebration, and sleep, and the same is true of friction. Most digestive disturbances, even those of early middle life, are due to relaxation of the supporting tissues of the great organs in the abdomen. This dilation is found in at least 60 per cent of adults, and it produces a long train of alterations. The kidneys are supported mainly by their blood vessels, so that if they sag their circulation is impaired, and this kind of ptosis is very common. Hence faulty attitudes are very important for all visceral ptoses, while he finds much to commend in the use of abdominal corsets, even for fleshy men. Elasticity of the ribs should receive attention and the author prides himself on exercises that increase the elasticity of the basal tissues which sclerosis is prone to assail. The capacities of individuals for exercise in the open air can generally lessen the need of medical supervision. With old people, the extensors should receive more, and the flexors, less attention and there should be sufficient stretching, torsion, etc.

As to the senile heart, it is generally assumed that the old should do no more than they are inclined to do and perhaps even lead a vegetable existence. But he believes that disinclination to movement means and makes underoxidization and causes decay and he is severe on what he calls senile laziness. The healthier and happier old people are, the more active they become. The life of a hothouse plant is bad. Humphry found in most old people he examined little or no change in the arterial system. Allbutt says there are many old people in whom there is no arteriosclerosis. One common phenomenon of old age is the loss of vascular tone and defective lymph circulation. The bones lose weight and size and the walls of the shaft grow thin from within, especially toward the end of the bones and most near the head of the femur. Trunecek of Prague emitted the thesis that certain salts can be introduced into the blood current that aid in dissolving the calcium phosphate found in the structure of sclerosed arteries. So he injected hypodermically a strong solution of sodium phosphate and magnesium phosphate, which are normally found in the blood serum but only in minute quantities. Others have introduced this by both bowel and mouth. Anything that aids oxidation of tissues helps.

In another article[19] Taylor says almost nothing that is new although there is much that would be practical to aging people. The machinery has become a little worn and weaker in spots but the bare surfaces have been abraded to meet each other so that there is less friction and racking of the joints. The body cells are less irritable. Degenerative diseases are very insidious. They increase in the following order —liver, digestion, apoplexy, nerves, heart, kidneys. One's enjoyment of food is greater perhaps than discriminative. Many reminders of age are overcome by warming up. Skin emanations may be offensive. Traits of a mature mind are poise, deliberation, economy and the largest output of judgment, like the Roman senators or seniors. Irritability is common. Youth wants to know; age wants to be.

C. A. Ewald,[20] one of the most eminent of German professors of biology, gives us one of the most condensed statements on the subject of old age. He begins by contrasting the intense life of Berlin, where the lecture was given, with the fact that all paths lead to the door of death, which is nearest in war. The antique conception of death was youth with a reversed torch; the medieval, a skeletal mower taking pleasure in his

---

[19] "Evidences of Full Maturity and Early Decline," *Pop. Sci. Mo.*, 1917, p. 411.

[20] *Über Altern und Sterben*, Wien, 1913, 33 pp.

work. The martyr's love of death and even the passion
for Nirvana are probably more or less pathological. If
we assume 15,000 million people on the earth and a death
rate of 30 million per year, we should have 81,192 deaths
daily; 3,425, hourly; and 57 every minute. The baobab
tree of Cape Verde shows a life of 5,000 years. Some
have ascribed 500 to the swan. But nearly all data of
great age are discredited. Even that of Parr (152),
who married with potence at 120, and all the rest, are
doubted. But the length of life is increasing. In Sweden,
of every 100 children of five at the beginning of the
last century, 27 reached 70; at the end of the century,
48 did so. In Bavaria the number increased from 25
to 40; in Germany, in the last twenty years, it increased
from 30 to 39, so that we all have a better chance of
living long than we would have had if we had been
born a hundred years earlier. The average length of
life in 1870 in Germany was 37 years and has now
increased to 42½. In France and England it is 46 and
in Norway and Sweden, 52. Cures of tuberculosis in
the last twenty years have reduced the percentage of its
victims from 31 to 17 per 10,000, and vaccination has
reduced the death per million from smallpox to 5; while
in Russia, where it is not compulsory, it is 520. *A priori,*
death does not seem necessary and yet for even protozoa
division often involves something like a very rudimentary corpse so that investigators like Götte, Hertwig,
and Verworn accept the tenet of Weismann, with some
slight reservation, if the corpse is to be taken as the
criterion of death.

Bees and the stork and other birds of passage kill
or neglect their old, while in ancient German myth old
men often slew themselves for the good of the community. Certain species eat their young rather than
die themselves and even this is for the interest of the
species. A certain wasp lays its eggs in the female plant

and its young, when covered with its pollen, fly to a male plant to fertilize it, although this means their death. Thus death is a normative factor of development and to this extent Weismann is correct. Life has three periods. In the first there is an excess of energy and growth; then comes middle age with an equilibrium, while in old age the relation of these energies is reversed, so that the first and third stages contradict each other. But everywhere life is dependent on nutrition and all death, in whatever form, is due to its lack. So we have a kind of biological circulation and a kilogram of body substance evolves a different sum of total energy in each of these periods of life. The author gives us an interesting cut of the contraction of the vertebrae and their padding, which often in the old means ankylosis in the lower part of the spinal column.

He dissents from the Conklin theory of the abatement of metabolism as a cause of old age because he thinks this activity has a wide range of play at all stages of life, monthly and even daily. Nor does he accept without modification the *Schilddrüse* (thyroid) theory, although admitting that the endocrine glands play a very important function. Nor does he accept Von Hansemann's view of altruistic nutritive disturbance, namely, that single cell groups are more or less reciprocally dependent upon others for their activity so that they in a sense work for each other. The physiological (that is, without outer stimulation) collapse of groups of cells is especially connected with the generative cells and their departure reacts upon the nutrition of the whole body and in a sense weakens it (the atrophy of age). The loss of the generative cells is physiological because they, in departing from the body, represent the growth of a new organism. Hansemann gives countless examples but they affect only the fact and not the kind or method of growing old, which is a progressive process, and we

237

still are unable to answer the question why the generative cells in the ordinary process of life are so soon destroyed or why so few of them are devoted to this purpose.

The author sees much truth in Minot's differentiation or cytomorphosis of cells, according to which differentiation, which causes growth, is also the cause of death. Minot himself says that the biologist can no more grasp the essence of death than he can that of life. Science does not know the difference between these two despite the impulsions of our causal instinct. Horsley thinks the condition for a green old age is the conservation of a sound thyroid. With its activity is, of course, connected that of other glands.

He says it might be assumed in a period during which a whole generation dies that the whole mass of putrefaction would cause infection. But in a half-dozen German cities very carefully investigated along this line it was found that those who lived in or near cemeteries were as long-lived as others and even those who drink water that is fed by drainage from well appointed graveyards are not infected; on the contrary, in several places this water is purer than elsewhere. There is only one exhumation in Germany for criminal purposes out of 600,-000 corpses, but poison that might be detected by exhumation cannot, of course, be traced after cremation.

Instead of the remorse, anxiety for friends, dread and pain, the author, who says he has seen "many, many hundreds of deaths," never saw one that was not unconscious. There are often, perhaps even for days, physical signs of great suffering but this is never felt; and the author advocates special death rooms in hospitals because it is so hard for onlookers that it is inhuman to allow patients to die in a ward with only a screen in front of the bed. The review of life by drowning people is a myth. It is the duty of the doctor to mitigate closing pains by morphia and other means, provided these do not shorten but rather tend, as they should, to somewhat prolong life. Even in death by fire and torture the last stages are painless.

The Kamerlengo strikes the Pope on the forehead three times with a silver hammer and calls his name and, if he does not answer, says, "The Pope is really dead." This is because hearing is supposed to be the last sense to die. But often after death the muscles contract spontaneously, even enough to move the body and this has made survivors believe their friends were alive. The muscles respond to electrical stimuli for hours. The pupil of beheaded people contracts to light. In Charlotte Corday's head the eyes opened. Dr. Rousseau saw a case in which the heart occasionally beat twenty-nine hours after decapitation. Generally death proceeds from the heart and its last beat marks the entrance of death. Respiration, too, or the last breath is often the mark of death because the carbon dioxide is not removed; hence we say life is in the blood. Everyone at times wonders not only when he will die but how. And it is hard to live so as to avoid pathological death.

A French nobleman, François de Civille, in the time of Karl IX, appended to his monument the inscription: "Thrice dead, thrice buried, and by the grace of God, thrice revived." The riddle meant that he woke first from his mother's body at birth and twice in war was thought dead and placed among the dead. But the absence of personal consciousness is very unreliable because after long periods of lethargy many have rather suddenly revived. There never was a doctor present at an exhumation of a living man. Being buried alive is really a ghost that has no justification in civilized lands. This has nothing to do, of course, with simulation. Karl V simulated death in order to enjoy the spectacle of his funeral, as Juliet allowed herself to be buried. By contraction of the muscles of the neck and deep respiration the heart can be checked and the physiologist, Weber, nearly lost his life thus. Dr. Gosch tells of a Colonel Townsend who in the presence of Prof. Cheyne stopped his heart and breathing, the latter tested by a mirror, for half an hour until they were all convinced he was dead. But then he gradually came to, though he died eight hours later.

Herter and Rovighi tested lactic acid and its effects on fermentation of the large intestine and found negative results, so that we do not have an arcanum against death or old age in this sense, although insufficient excretion of toxins has much to do with it.

In his illuminating articles Professor Raymond Pearl, after showing the novelty of natural death and how even somatic cells now seem possibly immortal if separated from the metazoan body and that heredity is a prime determinant of the length of the span of life, says we must know more of the vagaries of germ plasm before society should assume to control it, although such control sooner or later will be necessary. The death rates for the four diseases that public health and sanitary activities have been most successful in treating, namely, (1) tuberculosis of the lungs, (2) typhoid fever, (3) diphtheria and croup, (4) dysentery, have been materially reduced in the last nineteen years. But if we compare four other causes of death, (1) bronchitis, (2) paralysis, (3) purulent infection and septicemia, (4) softening of the brain, on which health and sanitation have had little effect, it is found that the rate of mortality from these troubles has declined just as much, and probably a little more, in the same period of time, although the numbers in the latter group are far less. "Hence the declining death rate in and of itself does not mark the successful result of human effort."

Recognizing the fact that the essential cells in our

body are inherently capable under proper conditions of living indefinitely, the problem that confronts us is whether environment or heredity has most to do in determining the actual length of life. Pearl [21] concludes that the death rate of the earliest period of life is selective, eliminating the weak and leaving the strong, and that inheritance is "one of the strongest elements, if not indeed the dominating factor, in determining the duration of life of human beings."

The duration of life in animals also depends on the total amount of metabolic activity or work and it has been proven that rats, at least, live longer under conditions so controlled that their activity is lessened, so that the greater the total work done or total energy output, the shorter is the duration of life and *vice versa,* work accelerating the aging process somewhat as rise of temperature does. Pearl says: "The manner in which the environmental forces (of sublethal intensity of course) chiefly act in determining the duration of life appears to be chiefly by changing the rate of metabolism in the individual. Furthermore, one would suggest, on this view, that what heredity does in relation to duration of life is chiefly to determine within fairly narrow limits the total energy output which the individual exhibits in its lifetime." The duration of life of an animal stands in inverse relation to the total amount of its metabolic activity or, put in other words, to the work in the sense of theoretical mechanics that it as a machine does during its life. Or, to put it in another way, if the total activity of a unit of time is increased by some means other than increased temperature, the same result appears as if the increased activity is caused by increased temperature. Pearl thinks that Steinach's experiments on the sexual glands, whatever their results for rejuvenation, do not

---

[21] See his articles in *Sci. Mo.,* March-Sept., 1921.

prove "any really significant lengthening of the life span." Nor does he think that Robertson's experiments with tethelin from the pituitary gland, whatever its effects upon growth, show that it materially increases the length of life to a degree that has much significance statistically, so that inheritance remains a prime determinant of longevity.

We are all born in one way but die in many. By international agreement a mortality code has been developed with fourteen general classes comprising 180 distinct units. Pearl would supplement this very unsatisfactory classification by the following: (1) circulatory system and blood-forming organs, (2) respiratory system, (3) primary and secondary sex organs, (4) kidney and related excretory organs, (5) skeletal and muscular system, (6) alimentary tract and associate organs concerned with metabolism, (7) nervous system and sense organs, (8) skin, (9) endocrinal system, (10) all other causes. This would show organological breakdown rather than pathological causation. The breakdown of the respiratory system is the chief cause of death, and next comes that of the alimentary tract; these together constitute half the deaths biologically classifiable. Next come troubles with the blood and circulation. We may conceive these as three successive defense lines, and it is against the first two of these that better health and hygiene have been chiefly directed, having been most successful with the respiratory system. Child-welfare, both pre- and post-natal, is by all odds the most hopeful direction of public-health activities. Pearl's very important studies here confirm the conclusions others have reached, that early pubertal years show the lowest mortality rate, and he traces in detail for each age of life the mortality curves for each of the chief groups of disease.

Very interesting are his conclusions touching the embryological basis of mortality in which he attempts to trace the causes of death back to the three primitive tissue elements, concluding that about 57 per cent of biologically classifiable deaths result from the breakdown or failure to function of organs arising from the endoderm, 8 to 13 per cent from those that spring from the ectoderm, while the remaining 30 to 35 per cent are of mesodermic origin. The ectoderm has been most widely differentiated from its primitive condition, as best illustrated by the central nervous system, the endoderm least differentiated, while the mesoderm is intermediate in this respect. Now, degrees of differentiation imply adaptation to the environment and the endoderm, which is least differentiated, is least able to meet vicissitudes. "Evolutionally speaking, it is a very old-fashioned and out-of-date ancestral relic which causes man an infinity of troubles. Practically all public-health activities have been directed toward overcoming the difficulties which arise because man carries about this antediluvian sort of endoderm." Prior to the age of sixty the breakdown of organs of endodermic origin causes most deaths; next come breakdowns with organs of mesodermic origin, and lastly those of ectodermic origin. The rate for all these germ layers is relatively high in infancy, dropping to a low point in early youth. In infancy the chief mortality is due to endodermic defect; from about the age of 12 on, to faults of ectodermic, and after about 22 to those of mesodermic origin. The death-rate curve rises at a practically constant rate to extreme old age. From about 60 to the end of life deaths from the breakdown of organs of mesodermic origin lead. The heart generally outwears the lungs and the brain outwears both because evolution is a purely mechanical process instead of being an intelligent one. "It is conceivable that an omnipotent person could have made a much better machine as a whole than the human body which evolution has produced. He would presumably have made an endoderm

with as good resisting and wearing qualities as a mesoderm or ectoderm. Evolution by the haphazard process
of trial and error which we call natural selection makes
each part only just good enough to get by." All this, the
author believes, only strengthens the evidence that the
most important part in longevity is played by innate constitutional biological factors.

This view so commonly held, that heredity is the chief
factor in longevity is doubtless correct in general. But
it is fatalistic and directly tends to lessen the confidence
of hygienists and physicians in the efficacy of all their
methods of prolonging life in the aged. There is, we
think, good reason to believe that there is a great and
now rapidly growing number of exceptions to this so-
called law, cases in which by conformity to right rules
of living, age has been increased many years beyond that
which our forbears attained. Indeed, the very fact of the
gradual prolongation of life shows that the hereditary
predisposition to die at a certain age can be, to a great
extent, overcome. The psychological effect of this
dogma of the prepotence of heredity in determining the
length of life is itself not only depressing but may
readily become, as psychologists can best understand, a
dangerous lethal agent with the old and cause those who
have reached the span of years at which their forbears
died to succumb to their troubles with less resistance.
Indeed, it is one of the chief purposes of this volume to
show that the old-age problem is not merely economic,
philanthropic, social, or even medical, but also, when all
is said and done, perhaps chiefly psychological and that
the future welfare of the race depends upon the development of an old age due not chiefly to heredity but to
better knowledge and control of the conditions of this
state of life.

Senescence is, in no small degree, a state of mind as

well as a state of body, and the study of it as such has been so far strangely neglected but is now in order. Even doctors who have told us most about it have made few intensive investigations of its nature and there are very few gerontologists; while the alienists who have described the senile psyche have done so only in general terms that add but little to what is obvious to common experience and observation. None have sought to ascertain empirically from intelligent old people capable of telling how they think and feel about their stage in life, or to determine how far their attitude toward it was indigenous and how far it was really due to the acceptance of current traditions that have come down to us from a remote past and that no longer fit present conditions. How this old tradition still influences even physicians may best be shown by a few instances that have come under my own observation. A friend of 73 fell sick of pneumonia which soon involved both lungs. The excellent family doctor had him removed to a hospital where expert care could be added to his own. Soon all hope of his recovery was abandoned and for a week friends who called or telephoned were told that nothing more could be done and the end was certain and might be expected any time. "He is 73, you know," the doctor said. To-day he is well and daily active in the very large concern he created. The father of an intimate friend at the age of 69 fell ill from a complication of disorders the family doctor diagnosed as old age and telegraphed his son to hasten home from a distant city if he would see him alive. Upon his arrival, on the morning of the 70th birthday, he found him half comatose and convinced that this day would be his last; but he was cheered up, diverted, partook of a stimulated eggnog, his first food for two days; and when he awoke just past midnight and realized that he had entered upon another decade,

245

revived, made a slow but surprising recovery, and enjoyed not only a comfortable but a very active life for nine years. He could not, however, quite bring his mind to enter the ninth decennium. Strangely enough, my friend's mother, whom I had also known all my life, two years later passed through almost the same experience. He was called to her deathbed, reaching her three days after all hope had been abandoned. But she recovered and was nearly as well as before, and lived seven years. A friend of mine retired from a college chair at 74 and was told that he was worn out, had several grave symptoms, and must drop work and go South. "You should be satisfied," his physician told him, "with four years beyond the allotted three score and ten." But he had unfinished tasks, believed them to be life-preservers, and now at 82 is still engaged upon them. A vigorous old lady of 87 has thrice been given up by her physician within the decade. Are doctors a little falsetto in their treatment of the aged?

Seventy is, on the whole, the most dangerous milestone and the morning of that birthday is probably the saddest of all that those who attain it have known or will ever know. It brings a new consciousness that now indeed we are old; and if we still carry on as before, we are at least under the suspicion of affecting a vigor that we really lack and are liable to lapse to an apologetic state of mind because we do not step aside and give our place to our juniors who often feel that they have a right to it, even though they try not to show or even confess it to themselves. If we make partial withdrawal we find insistencies, conscious and unconscious, in those who supersede us that we might as well make it complete and the sense of being superfluous and no longer needed is bitter. Complete retirement from all our life work, whatever it is, may make us feel that we are already dead so far as our further usefulness is concerned. Yet at no stage of life do we want more to be of service than when we are deprived of our most wonted opportunities to be so. We do not take with entire kindness and resignation to being set off as a class apart.

CHAPTER VI

THE CONTRIBUTIONS OF BIOLOGY AND PHYSIOLOGY

Weismann's immortality of the germ plasm and his denial of the inheritance of acquired qualities—The truth and limitations of his views—
The theories of Hering and Simon—Metchnikoff's conception of the
disharmonies in man, of the rôle of intestinal flora and their products,
of euthanasia, and of the means and effects of prolonging life—C. S.
Minot's conception of the progressive arrest of life from birth on as
measured by declining rate of growth and his neglect to consider the
dynamic elements—C. M. Child's studies of rejuvenation in lower and
higher forms of life in the light of the problems of senescence—
J. Loeb's studies of the effects of lower temperatures, of toxins, and
ferments—The preservation of cells of somatic tissues potentially immortal under artificial conditions—Account of the studies of Carrel,
Pozzi, and others—Investigations upon the effects on sex qualities and
age of the extracts and transplantations of glands, from Claude Bernard
—Investigations of Eugene Steinach on the interchange of sex qualities
and rejuvenation by glandular operations in animals and man—G. F.
Lydston's work—Serge Voronoff's experiments and his exposition of
the achievements and hopes of glandular therapy—Some general considerations in view of work in this field.

NEXT to Darwin, though by a wide interval, August
Weismann (d. 1914, *a.e.* 80) has most influenced general
biological thought. His failing eyesight at middle age
caused him to abandon the microscope for biological
thinking, a field where there was a great need of synthesis and expert theory and in which he developed great
power and influence. His hierarchy of metamicroscopic
vital units, his dogma of the non-inheritance of acquired
qualities in confutation of the prevailing Lamarckian-
ism, and his demonstration of the continuity of the germ
plasm have been theses of great interest and centers of
very active discussion, even outside the special field of
zoölogy, although in the latter doctrine, which chiefly

248

concerns this discussion, he was in a sense anticipated by
Owen, Jäger, Nussbaum, and especially by Sir Francis
Galton, as he later found.[1] He first set forth the now
generally accepted view that most of the primitive unicellular organisms do not die and also sought to explain
how death first entered the world.[2] He says:

> We cannot speak of natural death among unicellular animals,
> for their growth has no termination which is comparable with
> death. The origin of new individuals is not connected with the
> death of the old; but increase by division takes place in such
> a way that the two parts into which an organism separates are
> exactly equivalent, one to the other, and neither of them is older
> nor younger than the other. In this way countless numbers of
> individuals arise, each of which is as old as the species itself,
> while each possesses the capability of living on indefinitely by
> means of division.

Each of these one-celled individuals thus lives on and
grows, till its surface, through which all nutritive substance is absorbed and which increases at a less rapid
rate than its cubic content, becomes relatively too small,
so that the creature can no longer be nourished through
it and the mature cell faces the alternative either to die or
divide into two halves; and, accepting the latter, becomes, by division, two smaller daughter cells that, as the
food-absorbing surface becomes now relatively greater,
are rejuvenated, although their combined substance is
exactly the same as that of the mother cell of which they
are simply bifurcations. As, thus, the substance of the
parent cells all goes over into the offspring resulting
from the fission, nothing is lost in the process, not even
an envelope or membrane, as Götte, Weismann's chief
earlier critic, thought was the case in encystment. Thus

[1] *The Germ Plasm,* 1893, p. 198 *et seq.*
[2] See his *Essays Upon Heredity and Other Biological Problems,* vol. i,
1889, especially Chaps. I, "The Duration of Life," and III, "Life and
Death."

there is no vestige or rudiment of a corpse. Nothing is sloughed off. It is in this sense that such creatures are immortal. They have gone on growing and dividing thus ever since life began and will continue to do so until it ceases. Thus there is a direct continuity from first to last that is unbroken by anything that can be called death. If once and so long as these single-celled creatures were the only or highest forms of life, death or anything like it was unknown. In all this process, of course, nothing like conjugation, mating, or fertilization occurs.

That this is not mere theory the experiments and observations of many subsequent investigators, especially Woodruff and his pupils, have shown. In thirteen and a half years he found paramecia had divided some 8,500 times, and the process is still going on as actively as at first. Of these results Raymond Pearl [3] says, "If in 8,500 generations—a duration of healthy reproductive existence which, if the generations were of the same length as in man, would represent roughly a quarter of a million years in absolute time—natural death has not occurred, we may, with reasonable assurance, conclude that the animal is immortal." Thus it is that larger, older cells are constantly being regenerated by spontaneous division and natural death does not occur among most protozoa.

They simply grow and divide in an ever alternating rhythm and this was the fundamental cadence in the song of life. If the large or mature stage is, in any sense, a prelude of old age, division in the same way represents rejuvenation. The latter is thus almost, although perhaps not quite, as primordial as the phase of growth itself, and among the most ancient and persistent of all the heritages that higher forms of life received

[3] In his able and brilliant discussion on "The Biology of Death," *Scientific Monthly*, March, 1921, p. 202.

from the lower is this power to grow young. Thus the systole and diastole of the heart of the *Zoölogos* began. The monad becomes a duad; the individual, a dividual, almost as inevitably as the former grows; and the processional through this tiny life cycle contains in it the promise and potency of countless other processes that developed from it later. Thus even a colony of the far more complex coral polyps may develop perhaps for thousands of years from a single individual.

Now, while protozoa may occasionally conjugate and thus prelude a higher form of reproduction and while the simpler metazoa may propagate by fission or budding, reminiscent of the older way, the general mode of propagation among many-celled organisms follows what seems at first a very different law. In these forms a sperm cell or spermatozoön must penetrate a germ cell or an ovum and then the zygote, or fertilized egg, immediately begins to reorganize itself from within and to divide into two, four, eight cells, etc.; and these divisions produce cells not all exactly like the mother cell but differentiation begins. In some species, as early as the first few divisions certain cells are set apart as germ cells, devoted exclusively to the purpose of reproduction. From these ova and spermatozoa arise. While others, far more in number and aggregate bulk and increasingly so as we ascend the scale of life, become more and more specialized for the production of different organs, structures, and tissues. These gradually lose the power to produce entire individuals. It is these that produce, and their descendants that constitute, all the rest of the body, or soma, and so are called the somatic cells. It is these and their progeny only that die while the germ cells, a very minute portion of the entire body in the higher forms of life, still continue, like the protozoa, to divide and grow *in sæcula sæculorum,* and it is they that, in a mundane sense, are immortal. Of course very few of the *circa* four hundred ova produced during the sex life of an average human female and vastly less of the three hundred and forty billions of spermatozoa, according to Lote's estimate, produced by the average male [4] become mature individuals. Most of them perish by the way and all those in the body at its death perish, of course, with it. But sex cells, or rather the germ plasm, even in the highest animals, including man, which attain their goal and produce mature individuals of a new generation, continuing to follow the old formula of eternal growth and division though vastly slower, remain still deathless.

Thus life is a really unbroken continuum from its beginning to its end and we are all connected, as it were, by direct physical participation with the life of our progenitors. Each individual produces a few germ cells that reach the goal of maturity and many somatic cells doomed to death; and in the next generation each repeats the same process. Some flagellate spores, for example, when they divide, lose only the flagellum, which each new individual has to reproduce for itself and this is the rudiment of the corpse that in the higher forms of life becomes indefinitely more bulky and complex; while underneath all this increasing punctuation by death, as it developed, the old plasmal immortality still persists. On the other hand, all forms of fission and agamic budding, so common a method of reproduction in plants and often found in simpler forms of multicellular animal life, such as sponges and coelenterates, are reminiscent of the protozoan fashion.

Thus we see that death came into the world not by reason of sin, as theology teaches, but because of differentiation. As cells acquired the power to produce more and more specialized organs and functions they lost the power to reproduce the entire body and they lost it pro-

---

[4] *American Handbook of Physiology,* 1897, p. 883.

gressively—almost in exact proportion as their power of multiplication became specific. Thus, as we should expect, we find in the early stages of this differentiation cells that can be influenced toward the old general or the new and more specific powers of reproduction. Yet back of all the fact remains that life itself is essentially perdurable and that we can explain death better than we can explain life. Death is thus not necessary or universal but is derived and is, in a sense, a product of slow development; and we can conceive a stage of evolution in which natural death did not occur at all but was always due to external accidents. Indeed, Weismann goes so far as to say that the difference between the germ and the soma is so great that the latter, with all its fortunes, has little or no influence upon the former; and by his doctrine that acquired traits and qualities are not inheritable he seems to draw a hard and fast line separating the mortal from the immortal parts or organisms. He also devoted the greatest ingenuity in evolving an intricate scheme of biophores, ids, idants, determinants, etc., inherent in germ cells, in order to explain the phenomena of heredity. His studies have had great influence in directing the attention of investigators to the most elementary structures and functions of germ plasm and the remarkable changes within cells that occur in the very earliest stages of embryonic development; while, as we shall see, many of the most recent researches have been directed, since his work was done, to the conditions under which somatic cells in different tissues of the animal body can be made to proliferate and grow, under carefully controlled conditions, more than it was possible for them to do under conditions afforded them while they remained parts of the body in which they were developed.

Here I deem it in point to observe that the adoption in its extreme form of the theory of preformation versus epigenesis, or the assumption that no qualities due to the experiences of the soma can have any influence upon germ plasm or affect heredity, would be to revert to views very like those of the old creationists. From Weismann we may well lay to heart that this influence is very slow and slight in any one or even a large number of generations, suggesting a very long prehistory for the germ plasm of higher organisms. But to hold that nothing in the recent past or the near future of the environment within or without the individual can ever in the least affect innate qualities is to throw ourselves into the arms of a fatalism that more or less blights all the motives of reform and amelioration of conditions or of educational influences in their widest scope. On the contrary, we hold that the ultimate goal of all the improvements of life or mores is to better heredity, that most precious and ancient of all the many forms of values and worths, and that the degree in which they do this is the final criterion of all really worthy endeavor in the world. If the good life of a long series of generations of our ancestors does not in the least tend to make their offspring a little better born and give them some slightly better chance for a worthy, long, and happy life, quite apart from all postnatal, parental, and other influences, the taproot of all motivations for reforming human conditions is cut, and all efforts in this direction become a little falsetto and every generation must start again at the beginning.

Just now we are told that the whole domain of consciousness since civilization began has had little influence upon the deeper and older unconscious elements of human nature but no one among these psychoanalysts has for a moment insisted that it had none. The moral in both cases is simply that we must now make far larger drafts upon the inexhaustible bank of Time and realize that in the one case, body, and in the other, mind, is immeasurably older than we had deemed them to be, that is, that both germ plasm and the unconscious have been very long in the making and come to us charged with potencies innate in the individual but very slowly acquired—in the one case by the ascending orders of animal life from the first and, in the other, by man and his ancestors. We certainly have not yet heard the last word from zoölogy which, while stressing the hereditary factors, for example, and individual longevity, must admit that old age in general is a more or less acquired character. Before we do so, an important correlation, to which I shall advert later, between these investigations and those in the new field of the endocrine glands and the hormones that have such new and marvelous power of speedy and profound influences upon so many parts of and processes that go on in the body, must be made.[5]

One of the chief traits of old age is the loss of germ plasm with its power of perennially regenerating life and this loss leaves the soma to slow degeneration. As germ substance decreases individuality generally increases, sometimes in the form of gross selfishness. As the body becomes cadaverous or corpse-like and the springs of love begin to dry up at their source, secondary sex qualities fade and the sexes again become more alike, as in childhood, and the extremely senile are but the husk or shadow of their former selves. Tenaciously as life is clung to, it is at the same time felt to be less worth saving either here or hereafter, for whoever heard of senile decrepitude wanting to be continued beyond the grave. All ideals of a future life assume a restoration of maturity if not of youth. Doddering, desiccating senility has always been abhorrent to gods and men and I know of no either imaginative or scientific writer who

---

[5] Mildly challenging Weismann's non-inherited ability of acquired qualities is Irving Fisher's "Impending Problems of Eugenics," *Sci. Mo.*, Sept., 1921.

has even attempted to describe the senium as it would be if prolonged to its extremest conceivable term, when each organ and function slowly ceased "altogether and nothing first"—ever shorter in stature, more shriveled and emaciated in form, hairless, the voice shrunk to a whisper, tottering, tremors, and then inability to work, move, or even eat; abatement of all natural functions, the senses slowly becoming extinct, teeth and the power of mastication gone, everything in a stage of progressive involution, increasing paralysis of all receptive or effector processes, offensive perhaps to the very senses of those about, seemingly forgotten for the time by death itself, which the poor victim perhaps longs for but is unable to command the means of attaining, feeling himself useless and a grievous burden, a just living mummy, torpid, neither really sleeping nor waking; and in the end with every natural function sinking synchronously but so gradually that observers could not be sure whether each slow breath or heart beat was really the last or just when the Great Divide had really been crossed where Sleep embraces its brother, Death. Something like this would be the fate of the soma, after it had been abandoned by the germ plasm, if a really natural death occurred, that is, if, by some of the many disharmonies that pervade the body, some organ or part did not break down before the others were worn out and drag them to its own doom, which is what always really occurs in fact.

If we look at the matter from the more psychological and Lamarckian viewpoint, suggested, for example, by the thesis of Hering, that memory is the most fundamental trait of organized matter, a view elaborated by Simon's theory of mnemes and engrams, all experience is more or less permanently registered on the most vital of living substances, which is "wax to receive and granite to retain," nerve and brain being the next best organs of registration only acting more specifically; while the most generic resultants of experience attain their ultimate goal of being recorded in the structure or functions of the germ plasm and thus becoming permanent acquisitions of the species or race. On this view the apex of life is reached at that stage of it when the influence of the soma upon the germ plasm is greatest. This, of course, ceases when the latter takes its departure with loss of the power to propagate. Thus of all the stages of life, old age and its fortunes alone can never affect heredity. Individuals who live on do so only by the momentum given by germinal energies transmitted from their parents, and only the old are completely isolated from the main currents of the life of the race. They have already died racially or to the phylum and only await a second or individual death. Thus if any large number of such individuals lived on for many decades, they would be an encumbrance; and so Nature, always intent on the interests of the species and so indifferent to the individual, has to leave them to their fate. They may still alleviate individual conditions but can contribute nothing to racial memories in the above sense. The species has "forgotten them and they are of it forgot."

Elie Metchnikoff (d. 1916, *a.e.* 71), a bacteriologist and the successor of Pasteur, who approached the problem of old age from a very different angle and collected many interesting data, was led by his experiments and observations to a unique theory.[6] He first sets forth the disharmonies in the life of animals and especially of man in a way that seems pessimistic; but both his volumes are subtitled "optimistic studies" because he finds hope at the bottom of the Pandora casket.

Old age, he thinks, is not due to loss of the power of somatic cells to divide or reproduce themselves but is

---

[6] *The Nature of Man,* 1904, 309 pp. and *The Prolongation of Life,* 1907, 343 pp.

"an infectious chronic disease, whether manifested by degeneration or an enfeebling of the nobler elements and by the excessive activity of macrophags," the latter being large wandering cells represented by the white blood corpuscles and which he holds to be true phagocytes or scavengers, which, instead of protecting as they were meant to do, are very liable to turn on and destroy the higher elements of the body. They are thus like an army raised and sent out to destroy menacing savages that may turn and attack its own city. Old age and death, then, according to Metchnikoff, are not due, as Blütschli thought, to the exhaustion of some kind of vital ferment that protozoa and germ plasm have pre-eminent power to make; nor to the mere accumulation of waste, which the more always tend to dump upon the less vital elements of the body; nor, as Delboeuf conjectured, to the precipitation of the substance of organs, which always tend to revert to their inorganic bases; nor to Roux's hypothesis that organs are always competing with each other for the available nutritive material, and that as and when there is not enough to satisfy all, those that have to starve drag down the rest; nor to the failure of the initial momentum given at impregnation; nor to the fact that at the senium the body has passed beyond the reach of the influences of sex and its products; but it is due to a very rank and variegated flora or fauna of noxious microbes, and especially to the toxic products they make, which tend to accumulate in the large intestine, making it thus a very cesspool or latrine of the most manifold infections.

Darwinists have stressed the advantages of the large intestine for convenience and the avoidance of the necessity of leaving frequent spoors by which animals might be tracked by their enemies. But many species are without it or have it only in rudimentary form and in man its removal by surgery results in no very serious impair-

ment. We may add, too, that more recently psychoanalysts have described the anus and rectum and their
functions as centers of various erotic activities, especially but by no means exclusively in children. Here
the waste products of the digestive processes are
dumped, awaiting removal, and it has long been known
that their undue accumulation caused not only local
troubles but general malaise, anxieties, and nervous and
mental tensions. Metchnikoff and his pupils showed
that very soon after birth noxious bacteria find their
way to the large intestine and flourish thereafter in
great profusion, especially in constipation, and that no
cathartics can be relied on for permanent relief, salutary
as medicine has always and everywhere found them for
mitigation of many diverse ailments. It is the microbes
that find their chief nidus here that are the principal
cause of old age and if an antidote to their lethal action
could be found Metchnikoff believes life could be very
greatly prolonged. He attempts to show that among
not only mammals but also birds, the species that have
developed the large intestine are less long-lived than
those in which it is rudimentary, so that in animals
generally its relative size and individual longevity are
inversely as each other. Most of the digestive processes
are completed before food reaches this terminal part of
the long alimentary canal and very little save water can
be absorbed through its walls, so that rectal feeding
contributes very little, indeed, to the total nutritive needs
of the body. But it is here that death finds its chief
armamentaria and establishes a receptacle, factory, or
laboratory of poisons. Not only are there many microbes
that here feed on food residues and occasionally pierce
the intestinal walls themselves, but they produce putre-
factive products that are still more lethal. The chief
of these are phenol and indol, both very complex and due
to the breaking down of albuminoids, the chief element

in meat, peas, eggs, etc. Young people may for a long time show no trace of the deleterious effects due to the absorption of these toxins, but the slight wear and tear of the tissues they cause is cumulative. They produce in animals old-age effects in kidneys, arteries, liver, lungs, muscles, testes, ovaries, and even in the brain, for senility is due to the action of these bacterial invaders and not to time or to wearing out.

So vital and rapidly growing are these bacteria that they would soon, under favorable conditions, outbulk the entire body. But while their numbers are kept down by lack of nutriment and other conditions, nature provides no adequate antidote to their activity. This was found by Woolman and was called glycobacterium, or the sugar-maker. It was found first in the dog, and it can be cultivated in the laboratory and introduced into the body. It transforms starch into sugar without affecting the albuminoids and it is not, like sugar, absorbed before it reaches the large intestine. Thus it is not sugar that is the antidote but the lactic acid of its product and this is found in nature in the bacillus of sour milk, a common article of diet among Bulgarians, who seem to be the longest-lived people in Europe. The results of experiments with this product, first upon rats and other animals, Metchnikoff thought remarkably rejuvenating; and as all know, many substances containing lactic acid were for a long time in great favor, although expectations of its effectiveness have by no means been fulfilled. The death of Metchnikoff himself, too, at the age of seventy-one, who had long and diligently used his own panacea, did not help the confidence of his disciples, for we can never forget the old slogan, "Physician, heal thyself."

In Sanger's returns to his questionnaire,[7] as well as

---

[7] See a valuable but unprinted thesis of W. T. Sanger, a pupil of mine, "The Study of Senescence," Clark University, 1915.

to my own, one often finds people who use some form of this preparation and with what they deem good results and Metchnikoff's volumes show such a unique combination of humanistic and scientific interests that they have had wide popularity.

The problems, however, with which he deals are so extremely complicated that his work may really be said to have propounded more problems than he solved. He believed he had found and even named specific phagocytes attacking most, but not all, of the main tissues and organs of the body. Cohorts of them encamp about cells, very slowly absorbing their substance and depleting their energies—some attacking muscles; others, heart and arteries, etc.; others consuming the pigment cells of the hair which, however, as Pohl showed, continues to grow as rapidly in old age as in youth, as do the finger nails; others making the bones porous and brittle by removing the lime from them and transferring some of it to the walls of the arteries; some even specializing to attack brain and nerve cells. We must fight fire with fire, and to do this we must not only introduce the sugar-making bacteria but provide them with food *in situ* in order that they may do their great work of purifying the cradle or breeding ground of noxious bacilli. Some of his disciples are still enthusiastic enough to believe that just as we purified the Panama Zone; as vaccination has almost annihilated smallpox, which once caused about one-tenth of all deaths; as Behring's antitoxin has greatly abated the scourge of diphtheria; as Wright's vaccine has lessened death from typhoid; as Ehrlich's salvarsan treatment has done so much for syphilis, and as he and Wassermann hope may be done for cancer—so we may yet find and learn how to use a specific that, although it will not realize the dreams of those who once sought an elixir of life, will nevertheless contribute to its perhaps indefinitely great prolongation. This Metchnikoff does not hesitate to call "the most important problem of humanity." His ideal is what he calls orthobiosis, which is "the development of human life so that it passes through a long period of old age in active and vigorous health leading to the final period in which there shall be present a sense of satiety of life and a wish for death." Mere prolongation of life in the sense of Herbert Spencer is not in itself desirable. When the wish for death comes, he thinks that under certain circumstances suicide would be quite justifiable. Old age, he believes, will not only be greatly prolonged but will become optimistic. Pessimism he finds commonest among young men, while many avowed pessimists have become optimistic in their old age. Young men will not so precipitately attempt to displace the old, as he finds to be too much the case now, but the latter will attain greater power and influence.

The constitution man has inherited from his anthropoid ancestors is far from fitting his present environment. The greatest disharmony of all is the morbid nature and brevity of the period of old age. Man does not round out his prescribed cycle and develop in its final stage an instinct for and love of death, as he should. He is expelled from the school of life at all stages of its curriculum but always before the final or senior year, until the fact that there was such a final grade has been almost forgotten. It was because man felt himself prematurely cut off that he developed all dreams of resurrection and of another life. Had he completed his life here he would never have wanted or dreamed of another. Had the involution that begins usually in the fifth decade or earlier gone on normally, it would have made each stage of the recessional no whit less delightful than those of the processional of youth till, having withdrawn more and more from life and being in the end quite satiated with it, the individual would have rejoiced to see the limitations that separate him from ultimate reality fall away until he merges, body and soul, into the cosmos from which he came. Only the simplest organisms are immortal and as we ascend the scale and develop a more complex soma, the more impossible does any kind of immortality become. Metchnikoff seeks nothing of this sort but would simply increase the number of years and enrich them in the last phase of our existence so that, instead of being the pitiful remnant it now is and instead of having to console itself so pathetically by the puerile and unsubstantial figments that religions and philosophies have given us, man would enter upon the full heritage that nature intended for him. Thus the highest goal of all endeavor is to overcome the present degeneration of senescence, to cultivate physiological old age; and when this ideal is realized, more and more of the complex and intricate affairs of social, industrial, political, and other forms of life will be left to the old men, for these things require not only technical training but, perhaps even more, the wide view, insight, and common sense for which experience with life is the best school.

Metchnikoff was able to discover only two ideal cases of old people in whom his "instinct for death" was well developed. But he believes that as gerontology advances this instinct will not be the exception but the rule and that the very nature of old age as we know it will be radically transformed. At present we know little more of it than the prepubescent child knows of sex or the embryo of its mother's milk. When the instinct for death is well developed, we shall long for it as we do for sleep when we are fatigued, for old age is The Great Fatigue. Many instincts of the young are reversed and pass over into their ambivalent opposite at a later stage of life; and so the love of life will, in the end, be transformed into the love of death. Both animal and human parents devote their lives to the service of their offspring during the period in which this is necessary; but when the latter are mature, we often find a reversal of this instinct. Perhaps the intense sensitiveness of ova and spermotozoa displayed in the phenomena of chemotaxis and in the marvelous power of regeneration of lost parts among many lower forms of metazoa, and the many phenomena that led Haeckel to call the soul of cells immortal, are lost later as higher, conscious psychic powers develop; and if so, this shows the marvelous transformability of the primitive impulses that dominate simpler forms of life.

Thus Metchnikoff is a humanist as well as a scientist. He sets down faithfully what he saw through the microscope, but not content with that ventures to indulge his speculative instincts and tell the world what he thinks his discoveries mean for the practical conduct of life and of mind—and that, too, in more or less untechnical terms that make his ideas accessible to intelligent laymen. For him, as for Plato, "philosophy is the art of preparing for death." He even urged that "the instinct for death seems to lie in some potential form deep in the constitution of man," and it was this he sought to develop. The only basis for all modern forms of belief in immortality roots in a platonic reminiscence of the processes of the deathless germ plasm, and from this the old soma and the, no whit less, old psyche have departed as far as possible. Psychic life, too, has its proximate beginnings in the intense vitality of germ plasm and cells and from these rudiments the adult human consciousness has so far developed that our conscious psyche knows no more of it than it does of the migrations or depredations of the phagocytes within the body. Man is the most pathetic of beings because of the two tides whose ebb and flow constitute his life—evolution and de- or in-volution, anabasis and catabasis. He has failed, on account of the action of the intestinal fauna within him, to achieve any adequate sense of appreciation, still less enjoyment of the refluent currents. Man is thus deprived of the nascent period in which this wooing of death is due to arise and does not reach his true end or final goal. Dreamy illusions about it have always haunted his soul as unsubstantial surrogates. When man now in the making is finished, what we at present call old age will be a sort of superhumanity, a new and higher story, and its completion will spontaneously bring with it new and deeper insights; and he will approach and finally enter Nirvana with the same zest and buoyancy with which he now takes possession of life.

Crude and amateurish as often is Metchnikoff's philosophy, his courage, candor, and the strength of his convictions are commendable, and the faith he adds to his knowledge is full of hope. From his ideal thinker, Schopenhauer, he caught the flavor of the Vedanta and Upanishads but he did not see how these very ideals also underlay the mystic hermetic philosophy of the medieval alchemists and their royal art, as modern symbolists like Hitchcock and Silberer interpret them; and to this I shall revert later. If he overestimated the value of his panacea and ventured into fields of other experts in which he was ignorant and where he was often mistaken, he has at least made a very valuable addition to the yet all too meager literature on senectitude, which all thoughtful and intelligent aging people can read not only with profit but with pleasure, if only they have escaped from the narrow limits of orthodox Philistia. To have really edified this now ever growing section of all civilized countries is a real culture service. His work is uniquely inspired by a spirit psychologically very akin to that which impelled Buddha when he set out on his mission of finding The Way, stimulated to do so by the sight of an aging man and a putrefying corpse.[8]

Charles Sedgwick Minot, an embryologist, (d. 1914, *a.e.* 62) devoted most of his maturer years to a study of the phenomena of growth, keeping and daily weighing many young animals, especially guinea pigs, and he has left us a good compendium of his life work.[9] Stated in the most general terms, he held that old age and death were progressive phenomena that began in the individual with life itself, that the best method of measuring vitality was the rate of growth, and that this constantly diminishes and finally ceases. As soon as, for example, guinea pigs recover from the disturbances caused by their birth, which are great and last two or three days because they are born at a very advanced stage of development, they add from 5 per cent to 6 per cent to their weight during a single day. But this percentage diminishes, so that by the end of the first month they add only 2 per cent; at ninety days, only 1 per cent; and the diminution continues, rapidly at first and then more slowly. Calculating the time to make successive additions of 10 per cent, there are twenty-five of these addi-

---

[8] In her fascinating life of her husband, "Life of Elie Metchnikoff," (1920) the widow of Metchnikoff describes him in his last days as anxious "that his end, which seemed premature at first sight, did not contradict his theories but had deep causes, such as heredity, and the belated introduction of a rational diet, which he began to follow only at fifty-three." He was very anxious that his example of serenity in the face of death should be encouraging and comforting. He had no illusions and knew for a long time that he was living only from day to day. He speculated whether the end would come to-day or to-morrow and had several specific "death sensations," pledging his wife to hold his hand when the end came. He was interested in the completion of her biography of him, begged for enough pantopon to bring an eternal sleep, directed his friend how to perform his autopsy and what to look for in the different organs, provided for his cremation and the final disposition of his ashes, etc. All was done as he wished, with no funeral and no speeches, flowers, or invocations, and his ashes now lie in an urn, as he directed, in the library of the Pasteur Institute.

[9] *The Problem of Age, Growth, and Death; A study of Cytomorphosis,* 1908, 280 pp.

tions; and not until we reach the seventeenth addition do we find nine days or more necessary. The twenty-second addition takes four days, the later ones being somewhat irregular. The first ten per cent increment often comes in two days.

Chicks, too, are born highly developed, and so lose during the first day. Then the daily percentage of increase is greater than in the guinea pig. From the sixth to the tenth day inclusive the average is nearly but not quite 9 per cent; at the end of the third month, only 2 per cent. Rabbits are born very immature and, being less developed, grow more rapidly. The average for males of the first five days of growth is over 17 per cent. The rabbit thirty days old has about the same daily percentage of increase as the new-born guinea pig. The human child takes 180 days to double its weight; a horse, 60; a cow, 47; goat, 19; pig, 18; sheep, 10; cat, 9½; dog, 8; rabbit, 6-7, these rates depending, in part, on the quality of the mother's milk.

In embryos the rate of growth is still more rapid. The increase in the guinea pig in the first five days is 3,520 per cent, or an average of 704 per cent daily. From the fifteenth to the twentieth day it is 1,058 per cent, or an average of 212 per cent per day. Thus the rate of growth during the foetal period is far more rapid and it is more so in the earlier than in the later stages of embryonic development. The farther back we go, the more rapid is this rate. Thus his curves show a very steep decline in the rate of growth, even in its earlier stages, and this decline continues, although at an ever decreasing rate, to the end. Thus from this point of view the younger creatures are, the more rapidly they are dying. The weight of a fertilized germ he estimate at 0.6 milligram (and he tells us that 50,000 of these could go by mail for a two-cent stamp). Thus the human embryo at birth has increased 5,000,000 per

cent of its initial weight. Old age is merely the later
result of changes that have gone on at a diminishing
rate ever since the ovum from which we originated was
fertilized.

Life is growth; the retardation of growth is old age;
and its cessation is death. "Senescence is at its maximum in the very young stages, and the rate of senescence
diminishes with age" (p. 250). The embryo in its
earliest stages rushes toward old age at an almost inconceivable velocity, the new-born infant runs, the child
walks rapidly, youth saunters, the adult mopes, and old
age only crawls on toward death. In other words, the
momentum of life given by impregnation at the age of
zero is retarded—most at first and with a diminishing
rate at every stage.

Something like this same paradoxical law holds, Minot
believed, for the human brain and mind. In one of his
Harvey lectures he tells us that the brain of a child
at birth is but little differentiated. During the first year
it learns all the great adaptations in the physical and
human world: time, space, ego, etc. "It learns more
during the first year than in all the subsequent years of
life" and from birth on the power of learning is rapidly
diminished. It declines very fast during infancy, more
slowly in childhood, etc.

Accepting Metchnikoff's dictum that senility is
atrophy and that toxins of intestinal origin poison and
debilitate tissues so that they succumb to, if they do
not actually attract, the predaceous phagocytes (though
not proposing his substitute of sour milk for religion
and philosophy), Minot points out that we are always
throwing off dead cells. Blood corpuscles collapse and
are utilized by the liver; the skin is incessantly shedding
dead cells, as is the whole intestinal tract and each organ;
stature declines some 13 cm.; the brain loses some 19
gms. in weight; the rate and depth of respiration sink;

the heart, although growing larger and from the age of prime to senility beating some eight times per minute faster, is nevertheless obstructed in its action by rigidifying arteries; the bones grow spongy and their hard outer part becomes a thin shell; the muscle fibers decline both in size and number, exercise being able to increase only the former and not the latter; both structure and function go on to rigidity and inflexibility after sufficient firmness and size have been attained, till the part becomes too hard and inflexible to function and then is shed as the ripened leaf falls in autumn. But none of these processes are abnormal and hence death is in no sense a disease. Indeed, the power of repair and even recuperation persists far more in the old than has been generally recognized.

The more specific cause of what is generally called old age he finds in the increase of the quantity and the hyperdifferentiation of the structure of the protoplasmic envelope of the nucleus. This protoplasm constitutes the body of the cell. In the earliest stages of cytomorphosis, which follow impregnation, the total amount of nuclear material increases fastest, while later and especially in the senescent cells it is the protoplasm that does so. In the early stages of their embryonic development, too, the cells differ relatively little; but those that constitute the adult body differ so greatly that any skilled observer can tell from which organ they came, whether from the brain, muscle, skin, stomach, liver, etc.; that is, they differentiate more and more as these organs mature. This differentiation is, however, all on the way to death and is never reversible; that is, old body cells never grow young. Nuclei change but it is the protoplasm that changes the most and acquires a new structure, while the composition of the nucleus not only changes less but always retains certain fundamental traits. "The increase of the protoplasm, together with its differentiation, is to be regarded as the explanation (or should we say cause?) of senescence" (p. 134). This is necrobiosis. All old cells, from whatever organ, are thus as recognizable as old faces. "Growth and differentiation of protoplasm are the cause of the loss of the power of growth" (p. 161). He even holds that the first stages of the segmentation of the ovum must be called rejuvenation. On page 167 he says:

The life of the cell has two phases—an early brief one during which the young material is produced and the later and prolonged one in which the process of differentiation goes on; and that which was young, through a prolonged senescence becomes old. I believe these are the alternating phases of life, and that as we define senescence as an increase and differentiation of the protoplasm, so we must define rejuvenation as an increase of the nuclear material. The alternation of phases is due to the alternation in the proportions of nucleus and protoplasm.

In adults, and even in the old, there are always young cells in reserve, often grouped in certain foci, for example, the marrow of the bones, which can in emergencies come forward, take up the function of growth, regenerate lost tissues or, in lower animals, even lost organs. At and even after the death of the aged there are always cells and even parts that are relatively young and growing. There are also, of course, the cells and their matrix, which are very early set apart for the purpose of reproduction, and these, of course, are least of all differentiated. Most cells of the body, however, follow the law of genetic restriction. This means that as differentiation proceeds, the possible directions in which cells can develop become more and more limited till finally they cannot divide at all and lose even the power of nourishing themselves, and so die. The cell and all of it represents life, and Minot has no use for any of the smaller metamicroscopic vital units, gemules, plastidules, plasomes, ideosomes, granules, etc., but thinks that if we wish to accept any kind of ultimate elements of this sort, Weismann's scheme of them is perhaps, on the whole, the best.

As to the practical questions, how we can help rejuvenation and delay senescence, he states that he has nothing to suggest, although he believes it possible that some time in the future a means may be found of increasing the activities and volume of the nucleus and restricting the growth and differentiation of the protoplasm, which would mean a prolongation of youth.

Minot concludes his volume with a glance at paidology in order to stress the great relative importance for both the bodily and mental development of the early stages of life. The baby develops faster than the child; the child, than the youth, etc., and the rate of psychic unfoldment declines very rapidly from the first, as does that of the body. Week by week, from birth, there is a remarkable expansion of life. Each one of the senses learns how to function effectively and most of them learn to attract the attention, the power of correlating movements and making voluntary ones, and the rudiments of memory and association are laid down, as are the bases of disposition. The infant from the earliest months of its life knows much of the persons and objects in its environment and perhaps has even discovered its own ego. It touches, handles, tastes everything; is an inveterate investigator in an ever widening field of research; has at least a sense of intercourse and companionship; is already at home with time, space, cause, and relation; its feelings, will, and even intellect are developed, and in this order; and the foundations for knowledge and achievement are laid. Thus the child of school age is already senile so far as its infancy is concerned and the boy's psychic processes are retarded, hard, and unspontaneous. Learning begins to be difficult. Nature no longer shoots the mind up the phyletic ladder but it must climb and grow henceforth by work as well as playwise. Thus man's mental powers show the same law of progressive retardation as does his physical growth. Instead of drawing the dead line at forty, as Osler did, Minot draws it at twenty-five. Had he been versed in paidology or even known the Freudian conceptions of infancy, he might have greatly amplified his treatment of this stage of the psychic life with which his volume closes. But as it is, there are certain definite criticisms of his conclusions concerning gerontology.

First, as I have said, he only attempts to show the cause and has nothing to say as to the cure of senescence. But he was not in quest of a panacea and was too true to the limitations of his science to pretend to have found one. This will be a disappointment only to those laymen who read him in furtherance of this pragmatic quest.

More serious is the objection that, according to his criterion and curves of declining growth rate, we are really old when we stop growing, for the mature young man and the very old one both are living but a very little above the deadline. On this view, the extinct saurians that grew all their lives were far more vital than creatures that attain a relatively fixed and constant size early and then stop growing. Growth is one measure of vitality, but surely function is another. The dynamic curve of energy and the power of work rises rapidly as that of growth declines and the curve of brain work reaches its apex somewhat later. Determining the increment of pounds or even of foot pounds of energy is not the sole measure of vitality.

Again, if all differentiation is progress toward death, evolution itself, instead of being progressive, is really retrogressive and the ascending orders of life are only a funeral march to the grave. Minot admits this in principle but says that although the advance it brings is bought at the price of death, it is worth all it costs. So it is, but it will not be if the organization and its increase in heterogeneity of structure are only mor- phological. It pays because of the quest for the good, the beautiful, and the true; because of science, law, love, the control of nature, the organizatiou of society; be- cause of the supreme joy of just being alive and the exhilarating sense of progress. The more evolved all creatures are, including man, the more the pleasure field overlaps the field of pain.

As the hypercivilized mind often longs back, like Rousseau, to an idyllic state of nature; or the world- weary pietist longs back to God; and, we may now add, as the psychoanalyst finds what he deems a psychody- namic equivalent for this trend, in a perhaps yet more exaggerated form, in the flight from reality, seen in dementia præcox and in longing for the mother's lap and, as Ferenczi says, even for her womb; so Minot's view of life might almost justify a kind of homesickness for the state of the ovum or the immortal germ plasm, for in this state of incipiency a single-celled organism performs all the functions of life, not only nutritive and reproductive but sensient and motor. It is at this stage, when all cells do all things, that the spirit of life cele- brates its highest triumph. The sigh for lost youth is here deepest. Life itself as we know it from this view- point seems a little falsetto and pathetic, for it is throughout, in a sense, a fall.

The analyst is also tempted to venture a little farther and to raise the question whether the life of the author of this view itself did not subconsciously contribute a little to reinforce his theory. With a none too rich and full childhood and youth, waiting for years for adequate recognition, passionately if not precociously devoted to the study of embryology, in which field he became one of the ablest and most accomplished of all leaders,[10] it would not be surprising if he found certain compensations in devoting his life to a study of that stage in which is manifestations are most active, and ably developed in this field apperception centers he somewhat overworked, while his self-affirmation and the instinctive impulse we all have for due recognition give a subtle self-satisfaction in reiterating the paradox that death is most active near the beginning rather than the end of the life cycle. Whether this suggestion has any validity or not, no one has ever more challengingly presented the problem of why the rate of growth declines from first to last, and whether it be due to an inevitable loss of the initial momentum or biological *élan vital* or to checks, arrests, and inhibitions of it, some of which may be removed. The very intensity of its early manifestations, if it gives us a haunting sense of loss also reinforces the hope that the high potential with which we all started somehow, sometime, may be better conserved, so that perhaps here, again, as with Metchnikoff's views, the morale of Minot's conclusions is, on the whole, optimistic.

Charles Manning Child, professor of biology in the University of Chicago, has given the most comprehensive statement of his problem to date from the standpoint of his science, although, as we shall see, much has been done since.[11] His most interesting and important contribution for our purpose is his refutation of the older view that life is always a progressive process and that true rejuvenescence does not occur. Of course, in higher animals the progressive features are predominant and development ends in death. But the above general-

---

[10] See his monumental textbook, *A Laboratory Textbook of Embryology*, 1903, 380 pp.

[11] *Senescence and Rejuvenescence*, 1915, 481 pp.

ization does not take due account of what occurs in lower organisms, while even in man and other mammals the different tissues do not undergo senescence either alike or synchronously. Some, for example, cells of the epidermis remain relatively young till and after the death of the individual. In other tissues such replacement of old, differentiated, or dead cells by younger ones occurs more or less extensively and tissue regeneration following injury occurs more or less in all tissues save only the nervous system. Such regeneration retards the aging of the tissue or organ as a whole. Minot thought that in such cases regeneration arises from cells or parts of cells that have never undergone differentiation, so that even in such cases development is progressive and not regressive. Even if he is right in maintaining that fibrillar substance cannot regenerate, it must be noted that new fibrillar substance does arise in continuity with the old, while isolated cells apparently do not produce it. Child maintains that there is differentiation in such cases and that these regenerating cells have returned to a kind of activity characteristic of the early stages of embryonic development; that is, that cells *can* assume an activity characteristic of an earlier stage. "Even in the outgrowth of new nerve fibers from the central stump of a cut nerve there is return to a process of growth and development which is normally characteristic of an earlier stage of development." Thus regression and differentiation do occur in most tissues of man and higher animals, although cells of one tissue can never produce those of another.

Again, after hibernation regeneration is often extensive. The large proportion of young cells in the body in such cases renders the animal as a whole appreciably younger than at the beginning of hibernation, so that the periodic cycle of activity and hibernation is much like an age cycle. This rejuvenescence may begin during the hibernation, when the animal is living on its own substance. Again, we see periodic changes that resemble the age cycle in glands. In the pancreas cell, for example, the loading of the cell is both morphologically and physiologically similar to senescence, and the discharge, to rejuvenescence. In this case the change occurs in individual cells without cell reproduction. Even the cells of the nervous system throughout mature life possess no appreciable capacity for differentiation and regeneration beyond the power to regenerate fibers arising from them. Child believes that the effect of a change in mental occupation or of a vacation may afford "some slight degree of rejuvenescence of the nerve cells." Verworn, he tells us, distinguishes between fatigue due to accumulations that check metabolism and exhaustion due to lack of oxygen, both of which may cause senility in nerve cells. "Thus exhaustion resembles senility as death from asphyxiation resembles death from old age." Recovery from exhaustion is not the same sort of change as rejuvenescence except as it involves increase in the rate of oxidization. But fatigue and recovery constitute a cycle resembling closely the age cycle.

Studies of starvation suggest the same thing. Various experiments have shown that in the later but premortal stage of starvation there is a certain activation of vital processes, including heat production, and it is possible that this has some significance for regeneration. Higher animals are apparently unable to use their own tissues as a source of nutrition to any such extent as the lower forms can do, and this is probably connected with a higher physiological stability of the tissue components. The body weight often does, however, increase and become greater after starvation than it was before, so that a fasting period is followed by an increase in vigor and body weight and hence the wide belief in its therapeutic value. On the other hand, the injurious effects of overnutrition in man are supposed to be due to the accumulation of food or to intoxication, but it is possible that overnutrition actually increases the rate of senescence by augmenting in the cellular substratum not only the decomposition of food but other substances that decrease the rate of metabolism. There are certainly many instances of longevity in man on a low diet. Again, after certain bacterial diseases, for example, typhoid, the body weight often becomes greater and vigor increases. While low diet often does good, it may, on the other hand, aggravate many diseases. Frogs and salamanders may live a long time without food and undergo great reduction, and starvation sometimes has a directly rejuvenating effect. The animals grow much more rapidly afterward and use a larger percentage of nutrition in growth and attain a larger size than those continuously fed.

Death of cells apparently from old age occurs at every stage of development and many cells do not die when the individual does, for he does so only because some tissue or organ that is essential reaches the point of death. Some have thought glands are primarily responsible for it; but others, whose view Child adopts, hold that it is the nervous system, especially its cephalic part, that dies first in man. In various insects and, for example, the salamander, death occurs almost at once after the exclusion of the sexual products, but this is exhaustion. In most, the length of life of the individual is determined by that of the shortest-lived essential organ or of the tissue that is least capable of regression and rejuvenation and the development of which, therefore, remains most continuously progressive. In cold-blooded animals where the rate of metabolism is dependent on external temperature, senescence can be reduced by cold, and in certain lower invertebrates by the simple method of underfeeding. When cells lose the capacity to divide, they differentiate, grow old, and sooner or later die, although death everywhere is the result of final progressive development if this process goes far enough and is not interrupted by regression caused by the need of repair, reproduction, or lack of food. Death is due, thus, to increased physiological stability of the substratum of the organism or to an increasing degree of differentiation that this general stability makes possible. And as individuation increases, death becomes more and more inevitable. Rubner calculated the total energy requirements in calories for doubling the body weight after birth and the requirements per kilogram in body weight for the whole period of life, for a number of domestic animals. His totals for all, except man, showed close agreement, and hence he concludes that the amounts of energy required are the same in all species except for man, who has a far greater amount of energy, that is, a smaller percentage of the energy of food is consumed in growth and maintenance of body weight and more in activity than in other animals. Very likely domestic animals expend less energy than their wild congeners but it is certainly difficult to correlate these results with Minot's criteria of age as measured by the decrease of growth.

Child concludes that senescence is more continuous in man than in the lower forms. His long evolution has given a physiological stability to the protoplasmic substratum and a high degree of individuation results from this. But the central nervous system, being least capable of progressive change, always dies first, so that the length of man's life is that of his nervous system and physiological death and senescence inhere in its fortunes. In the lower forms the death point may never be attained under normal conditions because of the low stability of the substratum and the consequent decrease of individuation that permits the frequent occurrence of a high degree of rejuvenation. But in the higher forms of life the capacity for the latter is limited by greater stability; and this, again, has been acquired through a process of evolution lasting through so many millennia that we must certainly "admit that this task [man's rejuvenation] may prove to be one of considerable difficulty."

Thus, according to Child, whose views are the most philosophical and insightful in the field of biology up to date for our purposes, senescence and rejuvenescence are both going on all the time in all cells and organs and are not special processes. In most cells and in most lower organisms dedifferentiation and despecialization of structure and function, which we may term in general regressive tendencies, are always less pronounced than progressive impulsions, while the latter predominate still more in the higher forms of life. It is "quite impossible to account for the course of evolution and particularly for many so-called adaptations in organisms without the inheritance of such acquired characters, but since thousands or ten thousands of generations may be necessary in many cases for inheritance of this kind to become appreciable, it is not strange that experimental evidence upon this point is still conflicting" (p. 463). Germ plasm is not something apart from or uninfluenced by all that goes on in its immediate environment within the body. Regression and dedifferentiation involve reconstitution and always approximate reproduction. To state the matter roughly, all processes involved both in growing old and in growing young might conceivably be arranged on a kind of Porphery ladder with agamic forms of indefinite reproduction, as illustrated in unicellular organisms or in germ plasm at the lower or *summum gens* end, and the most differentiated cells that have progressively lost the power of reproducing the whole organism, regenerating lost parts, power to grow, divide, and nourish themselves, at the top of the ladder, representing the *infima* species. On such a ladder, development, differentiation, and individuation is progress up, and all rejuvenating activities are descent toward the most generalized function of perpetual self-reproduction. This conception is in very suggestive harmony with the analogous psychoanalytic law of restitution to mental health by reversion to a more primitive state of psychic development, for all these methods might be called rejuvenation cures.

Physiological integration, with its increasing stability of the structural substratum, makes senescence cumulative as we go up the scale of evolution, so that it is ever less balanced or offset by rejuvenation, reproduction, or other regressive changes, as is the case with simple organisms whose life cycle consists merely of brief alternating phases of progression and regression, for the large protozoan cell about to divide is old compared with the two smaller daughter cells formed from it. Senescence is retardation and rejuvenescence is the acceleration that works by transforming, readapting, and even sloughing off old and useless structures. It will take long to modify the course of evolutionary processes that are the result of millions of years of alternating progressive and regressive changes, but not only the phenomena of rejuvenescence but "sports" and saltatory mutation, to say nothing of the findings of recent experiments showing how life and even activities of somatic cells separated from the body and given a more favorable environment may be indefinitely prolonged, point toward a vast reservoir of vitality. Thus we come to a new appreciation of the incalculable energy behind all the phenomena of animate existence and the hope is irrepressible that somehow, although we have as yet no idea how or when, we may abate or inhibit the forces that check or repress it and man may emerge into a fuller and even a longer life.

Jacques Loeb, of the Rockefeller Institute, has devoted himself for many years, with a rare combination of great learning and originality, to problems directly or indirectly bearing upon old age and death.[12] As his studies of tropism show, he is prone to mechanical and chemical interpretations; and since science has more or less eliminated smallpox, typhoid, yellow fever, malaria, rabies, diphtheria, meningitis, etc., the citizens of scientific nations will sometime, he thinks, be guaranteed a pretty fair probability of a much longer duration of life than they now enjoy. If we define life as the sum of all those forces that resist death, which means disintegration, the latter is comparable to digestion, which transforms meat into soluble products by two ferments, pepsin in the stomach and trypsin in the intestine. These ferments break up the mass into molecules small enough to be absorbed by the blood, and both of them exist not merely in digestive organs but probably in all living cells. They do not destroy our body, perhaps because the co-operation of both is required to do so and this is possible only at a certain degree of acidity, which cannot be reached in the living body because respiration is constantly removing acid. Death thus really comes when respiration ceases.

Of course there is another cause of disintegration, namely, microörganisms from the air and in the intestines. During life the cells are protected by a normal membrane that is destroyed in death and then the action of the microörganisms can superpose itself upon that

---

[12] For our purpose his views are best summed up in his *The Organism as a Whole from a Physiochemical Viewpoint*, 1916, 379 pp. See more specifically his "Natural Death and Duration of Life," *Science*, 1919, p. 578 *et seq.*

of digestion. Thus in man death is stopping the breath and this may be done by poison, disease, etc. The problem is whether there is any natural death, for if not we ought to be able to prolong life indefinitely. But we cannot experiment on man because neither the intestines nor respiratory tract can be kept free from microbes. A Russian, Bogdanow, solved this problem for the fly, putting its fresh eggs into bichlorid of mercury, which a few survived, with no microörganisms on the outside. These eggs were then developed on sterilized meat in sterile flasks and Guyemot raised 80 generations of fruit flies thus. Loeb himself and Northrop raised 87 generations. Their dead bodies were transferred to culture media such as are used for the growth of bacteria and more were produced thus for years. Hence fruit flies freed from infection and well fed would not entirely escape death and probably higher organisms would thus die from internal causes were external ones excluded. Eggs, for example, those of starfish, ripen and disintegrate very rapidly if not fertilized by the process of autolysis, which acts only after the egg is ripe. The fertilized egg, however, does not degenerate in the presence of oxygen but dies in its absence, so that we might say that the fertilized egg is a strict aërobe and the unfertilized, an anaërobe. The entrance of the spermatozöon saves the life of the egg.

Is natural death due to the gradual production in the body of harmful toxins or to the gradual destruction of substances required to keep up youthful vigor? If the latter, the natural duration of life would be the time necessary to complete a series of chemical reactions that would produce enough of the toxins to kill. Now, the period necessary to complete a chemical reaction diminishes rapidly when the temperature is raised, and increases when it is lowered. This time is doubled or trebled when the temperature is lowered by 10° C. The influence of temperature on the rate of these processes seems typical. If the duration of life, then, is the time required for the completion of certain chemical reactions in the body, we should expect it to be doubled or trebled when we lower the temperature. We can test this only where, as in our flies, infection is avoided. Northrop put their fresh eggs on sterilized yeast at a temperature of 0.2° C., and the higher temperatures selected were 5°, 10°, and 25°. All the flies died at nearly the same time when kept in the same temperature. The total average duration of life was 2½ days at 30° C., when nearly all of them died. At 10° C. it was 177 days. Thus heat accelerates all chemical action, and here we have the duration of life increased from 200 to 300 per cent. In man the body temperature is constant, for example, 35.5° C. whether in the tropics or the Arctic regions. If we could reduce our temperature, we might live as long as Methuselah. If we could keep the body temperature at 7.5° C. and follow the above ratio, we should live about 27 times 70 or about 1,900 years. Thus the duration of life seems to be the time required for the completion of a chemical reaction or a series of them. The latter may be the gradual accumulation of harmful products or the destruction of substances required for sustaining youth. Not only are unicellular organisms immortal and the life of all their successive generations a continuum, but a bit of cancer tumor can be transplanted to other individuals and there grow larger, and a bit from this second individual transferred to a third, and so on indefinitely; so that the same cancer cell continues to live on in successive transplantations throughout many individual lives. It has thus outlived many times the natural life of the mouse. Indeed, it seems to be able to live on indefinitely and Carrel has shown that this is true of other normal cells. Thus death may not be at all inherent in the individual cell but only be the fate of more complicated organisms in which the different types of structure depend on each other. Certain cells are able to produce substances that slowly become harmful to some vital organ or center and its collapse brings death to the whole.

In man there is no sharp limit between youth and maturity unless it be marked by puberty, but in lower forms of life it is demarcated by a metamorphosis. The tadpole, for example, becomes a frog in the third or fourth month of its life and this process can be accelerrated by feeding the creature with thyroid, no matter from what animal. Gudernatsch was able to make frogs no larger than a fly. Allen showed that the tadpole with the thyroid removed can never become a frog, although it may live long and continue to grow larger than the usual tadpole; but if such aged tadpoles are fed with thyroid they promptly become frogs. Salamanders metamorphose by merely throwing off the gills and changing the skin and tail, and the Mexican axoloti maintains the tadpole form through life; but even it, when fed with thyroid, promptly metamorphoses. Schwingle induced metamorphosis in tadpoles by feeding them with a trace of inorganic iodine. Thus the duration of the tadpole stage seems to be the time required to secure a certain compound containing iodine. Insects hatched as maggots will become chrysalides and then flies, but if thyroid is fed to the maggot it accelerates the metamorphosis, although we do not know whether it is due to the accumulation or formation of definite compounds.

Loeb sought to determine whether the duration of the maggot in the larval stage could be due to temperature and he found that this had effects similar to those described above. The larval period lasted 5.8 days at 25° C. and 17.8 days at 15°. The total duration of life was 38.5 days at 25° and 123.96 at 15°, both ratios being

1 to 3. Thus the influence of temperature upon the larval period was like that which it exerted on adult life. The same effect he found in salamanders, all of which suggested to him the conclusion that the duration of life and of the larval period is really the time required for the completion of certain chemical reactions. The cessation of respiration, which means death, and alterations in circulation, which mean metamorphosis or the death of youth, are critical periods and perhaps both points are reached when a certain toxin is formed in sufficient quantity or when a necessary substance is destroyed or reduced. Thus a shortened youth can, in amphibians, be prolonged by modifying the temperature or offering the specific substance that causes metamorphosis, namely, iodine or thyroid. There is no end to the substances capable of hastening death; shall we ever find one that can prolong life?[13]

Pearl's experiments on the fruit fly[14] show that where long- and short-lived strains are mixed, the first generation they produce is longer-lived than either par-

---

[13] Prof. W. J. V. Osterhout, "On the Nature of Life and Death," *Science,* April 15, 1921, thinks that we can measure by quantitative methods such fundamental conceptions as vitality, injury, recovery, and death, by electrical resistance, which, he thinks, is an excellent index of what is normal condition. He believes that this holds for both plants and animals, for all agents known to be injurious change the electrical resistance at once. He also thinks this resistance proportional to a substance he believes he found and decomposed by a series of consecutive reactions and that on this basis we can write an equation that permits us to predict the course of the death process under various conditions, so that we can say that at a certain stage it is one-fourth or one-half completed. Stated chemically, the normal life process consists of a series of reactions in which a substance O is broken down into S, and this in turn breaks down into $A, M, B,$ and so on. "Under normal conditions M is formed as readily as it is decomposed and this results in a constant condition of the electrical resistance and other properties of the cell. When, however, conditions are changed so that M is decomposed more rapidly than it is formed, the electrical resistance decreases" and other properties are simultaneously altered. Thus death results from a disturbance in the relative rates of the reactions that constantly go on.

[14] *Sci. Mo.,* Aug., 1921.

ent and that for subsequent generations Mendelian laws
hold even for longevity, so that there is increased vigor
in the hybrid generation due to the mingling of germ
plasms that are different. As to bacterial invasion, the
stability and resistance of the organism is also a factor,
but by rearing insects kept free from all such invasion
it appears that "bacteria play but an essentially accidental rôle in determining the length of the span of life
in comparison with the influence of heredity." Pearl
criticizes the conclusion of statisticians like Hersch that
poverty shortens human life, despite the fact that this is
perhaps the most potent single environmental factor
affecting civilized man to-day. But we have no real
evidence that if the conditions between the rich and poor
were reversed the death rate would also be reversed.
The influence of high temperature, which is known to
accelerate all the metabolic processes, does not interfere
with the predominant influence of heredity because it
only accelerates life processes exactly in the same way
that it accelerates chemical activities and the same is
more or less true of the influence of the secretions of the
endocrine glands.

Pearl concludes[15] that it has already been demonstrated that cells from nearly every part of the metazoan
soma are potentially immortal, even in the case of
tumors by transplantation, though of course not yet for
such exceedingly specialized structures as hair and nails.
Under artificial conditions cells from nearly all organs
can be made to long outlive the body from which they
are taken, just as grafts from apple trees may be passed
on indefinitely to successive generations. Thus death is
not a necessary inherent consequent of life in even
somatic cells but "potential longevity inheres in most of
the different kinds of cells for the metazoan body except

---

[15] *Sci. Mo.*, Apr., 1921.

those which are extremely differentiated for peculiar functions." The special conditions under which this occurs are often very complex and differ greatly for different tissues and animals, and we shall probably know far more later of the chemico-physical conditions necessary to insure continuous life, for these studies are new, having begun barely twenty years ago. The reason that all these essential tissues are not actually immortal in multicellular animals is that the individual parts do not find in the body the conditions necessary for their continued existence, each part being dependent upon other parts. This view differs from Minot's that there is a specific inherent lethal process going on within the cells themselves that causes senescence. Pearl concludes "that these visible cytological changes are expressive of effects, not causes, and that they are the effects of the organization of the body as a whole as a system of mutually dependent parts and not a specific inherent and inevitable cellular process. Cells in culture *in vitro* do not grow old. We see none of the characteristic senescent changes in them." Thus it may be inferred that when cells show characteristic senescent changes it is because they are "reflecting in their morphology and physiology a consequence of their mutually dependent association in the body as a whole and not any necessary progressive process inherent in themselves. Thus senescence is an attribute of the multicellular body as a whole consequent upon its scheme of morphologic and dynamic organization." The lethal process, thus, does not originate in the cells themselves. "In short, senescence is not a primary attribute of the physiological economy of cells as such."

It has long been known, as we have seen, that unicellular organisms could go on dividing indefinitely and that germ plasm had a potential mundane immortality; but no one had suspected that highly organized and differentiated somatic cells, which had lost the power of producing the whole individual and could only produce cells of their own special tissue, had this power. Recent experiments, however, indicate that under certain highly elaborated conditions they, too, can be made to live and even grow indefinitely and that this growth can not only be observed but measured under the microscope. Many attempts had been made by many individuals to grow tissues artificially to see their development, their functions, and decay, in both health and disease. This can now be done by taking pieces of living tissue from the body, for science has never produced a single living cell, and placing it in artificial media made out of blood plasma especially prepared, for nutrition for such a bit of tissue deprived of access to the normal circulation of the blood is the prime condition for such growth.[19] Indeed, until Carrel, who had long been interested in the regenerative processes of scars, succeeded in actually causing cells of the connective tissue to grow after being deprived of the circulation of the blood, this was supposed to be impossible. Leo Loeb had already produced artificial growth within and without the body as early as 1907, and in such processes that utilized the body fluid it was found that the same course was followed as in nature, so that the processes in such culture media approximated those that followed grafting. In 1907 Harrison gave details of such a process that

---

[19] Genevieve Grandcourt, "The Immortality of Tissues: Its Bearing on the Study of Old Age," *Sci. Am.*, Oct. 20, 1912. Also "What is Old Age?: Carrel's Research on the Mechanism of Physical Growth," *Sci. Am.*, Nov. 23, 1918.

C. Pozzi, *"Vie Manifestée Permanente de La Tissue,"* *La Preusse Médicale*, p. 532.

Alexis Carrel, "Present Condition of a Strain of Connective Tissue Twenty-eight Months Old," *Jour. Exper. Med.*, July 1, 1914, and "Contributions to the Study of the Mechanism of the Growth of Connective Tissue," *Jour. Exper. Med.*, Sept., 1913. See also *Science*, vol. 36, 1912, p. 789.

seemed convincing, although he worked only on cold-blooded animals, cultivating nerve fibers from the central system of the frog. Carrel extended this method to warm-blooded creatures and mammals, studying especially the laws of regeneration of tissues after surgical wounds.

The method of these remarkable achievements, now often repeated, is to put tiny bits of living tissue in a plasma of blood serum that will coagulate. The blood must be deprived of its cells by the centrifugal process and must generally be taken from the animal for which the tissue is to be cultivated or, at any rate, generally from the same species, although this is not without exceptions, for chicken tissue has been grown in the blood of human beings, dogs, and rabbits; morbid tissue, perhaps, like cancer, being most indifferent. The tissue is taken from an etherized subject, with every possible precaution against bacteria, chilling, or drying, and so liable is it to be killed by exposure to air that it is best dissected in serum. Both plasma and tissue are kept in cold storage and the time during which it can be thus kept varies very greatly with different animals. The bit of tissue must be very small because only the outer edge can get the nourishment when deprived of the normal blood circulation, for when the piece of tissue is large, all but the periphery dies. To see these changes of form, small bits of tissue are grown on the inside of a coverglass of a microscope slide that has been overlain with a prepared plasma, sealed with paraffin and put into an electric incubator provided with a microscope. The period before growth begins varies but when it occurs, the microscope shows the direct division of the nuclei and the growth taking the form either of layers or of radiating chains, depending on whether epithelial or connective tissue is being developed. Each tissue, whether normal or morbid, develops very precisely tissue of its own kind, and sometimes as, for example, with cancerous tissue, the growth is so rapid that it can be observed with the naked eye. This, of course, opens an immense field of observation and experiment, for example, immunity, protection against antibodies, redintegration, regulation of growth of the whole or parts, and perhaps especially rejuvenation and senility, to say nothing of the character and the influence of the secretions from all the glands. The trouble at first was that the artificial growth was so short-lived; but by changing the medium often and by frequent washing away of the waste products in a salt solution, it was found that the life and growth of these isolated bits of tissue could be very greatly prolonged. It seemed that the process of decay was due to the inability of tissues to eliminate waste products. So in 1912 Carrel's problem was whether these effects could be overcome.

To solve this problem bits of the heart and blood vessels of a chick embryo were grown. These growths were immersed in salt solution for a few minutes and then placed in the new plasma and it was soon found that thus the tissue could be made to live on indefinitely. Growth is more rapid the earlier the stage of it and it soon declines; hence the advantage of using tissue from embryos. But by subjecting these artificial growths to washings it was found that they were many times greater at the end than at the commencement of the month, showing that they do not grow old at all. Thus C. Pozzi says:

The pulsations of a bit of heart which had diminished in number and intensity or ceased could be revived to a normal state by washing and passage through a new solution. In a secondary culture two fragments of heart, separated by a free space, beat strongly and regularly, the larger fragment 92, the smaller 120 times a minute. For three days the number and intensity of pulsations of the two parts varied slightly. On the fourth they diminished considerably in intensity, the large fragment beating 40, the smaller 90 times. When the culture was washed and placed in a new medium, the pulsations again became strong, the larger one 20, the smaller one 60 times a minute. At the same time, the fragments grew rapidly, and in eight hours they were united and formed a mass of which all the parts beat synchronously.

Pozzi again says:

On January 17 the fragment of a chicken heart embryo was placed in plasma. It grew readily on a thick crown of conjunctive cells. In three days the pulsations, which were regular and strong at the beginning, grew feeble and ceased completely, and this state continued for more than a month. On the 29th of February, the culture, which had been subjected to fourteen passages, was dissected and the central film placed in a new medium. After the fifteenth passage it contracted rhythmically, with pulsations as strong and frequent as on January 17, *viz.*, from 120 to 130 per minute. During March and April this fragment of a heart continued to beat from 60 to 120 times per minute. As the growth of the conjunctive tissue became more active, it was necessary, before each passage, to extirpate the new connective tissue formed around the muscle. On April 17 the fragment beat 92 times, agitating all the mass of the tissue and the neighboring parts of the middle of the culture. On May 1 the pulsations were feeble and they were given their thirty-fifth passage. In the manipulation the muscular tissue was stretched and torn so that the contractions ceased.

Thus experiment seems to establish the fact that even connective tissue, composed of not the most highly developed but of vigorous though low-level cells, is immortal. Senility and death result because in normal conditions the blood does not succeed in removing waste products. Could science only wash them away in a living organism, life might be indefinitely prolonged. It is these connective tissues that give support to the textures that compose the body and that chiefly make up bone, cartilage, ligaments, and the lymph network, the cells of which are endowed with special properties of growth and play a great rôle in rejuvenating injured tissue. All this work, in a sense, started from Claude Bernard's principle that the life of an organism is dependent on the interaction of its cells and the medium in which they grow. Thus, to understand the process by which the body develops and why it must yield to decay and death, we must inquire into the cause of the loss of character of these interactions; and this was impossible until tissue could be grown outside the body so that the processes might thus be brought within the range of the microscope and all its conditions under control. Carrel's first effort, thus, was directed toward the way in which the medium affected the life of the cell and in constituting this medium of plasma from the blood of dogs and chickens he found that the older the animal from which the blood was taken, the less rapidly and extensively the tissues grew in it. In the blood of a relatively old animal the increase became so slight as to be practically *nil.* These comparative experiments were made, Grandcourt tells us, with the blood of animals from five months to five years of age, and there was enormously greater activity on the part of the blood of growing animals. Thus it would seem that when an animal attains its size and stops growing, its blood undergoes progressive changes till it lacks, more and more, the dynamic power of youth. So the problem was whether the plasma could be given the force of youth so far as its action on growing cells was concerned and this was accomplished by mixing it with juices extracted from the embryo. Experiments, too, were made with a strain of connective tissue cells that had been kept in artificial life for more than sixteen months. It was divided into two parts, one of which was grown on adult plasma and the other in a mixture of two parts, one of plasma and the other of embryonic juice. In two days

292

the ring of tissue around the second part was three times as great as that around the first. Some of these tissues, passed through a salt solution 130 times, doubled their area in forty-eight hours. Another, washed 57 times, increased in volume fifteen times in ten days, etc. These rapid growths, however, could not be duplicated in normal plasma which was then further modified. Thus the different media have a pretty constant effect upon the rate of growth. Carrel says: "The special rapidity of the growth of the tissue depends so much on the composition of the medium that it may become possible to use as a reagent of the dynamic value of the humors of the organism a strain of cells adjusted to life *in utero.*" If human connective tissue could be preserved in the condition of permanent life as the connective tissue cells of a chicken are preserved, the value of the plasma of an individual might be approximated by the cultivation in it of a group of these cells and by the observation of the rate of their multiplication. Such observations do suggest some indication of certain values of the blood of an organism and may give us some clue to old age.

Thus in the course of development the activity of the tissue is apt to vary in the body as a whole and in its parts. It therefore became a question whether each particular condition was permanent or whether the dynamics of the cell changes through the action of the medium upon it. To determine this, several bits of tissue, each having its own dynamic power, were cultivated in media exactly alike and differences in the character of the growth were noted. Then the influence of the medium began to tell. Measurements of the changes undergone on the part, in turn of a fast- and slow-growing tissue, showed that the former had lowered its activity one-half in forty-eight hours, while the latter had multiplied its activity by six. This process continued until the level of uniformity was reached, when the conditions of growth remained equal in all cases. Thus it appears that though, in the beginning, certain substances that the tissues had accumulated had the effect of accelerating or retarding its activity in the medium, yet in time the latter overcame these conditions and growth was brought under the laws of its own special mechanism. Thus the sum of the investigations on the influence of the medium on cells is that it may not only change the dynamic possibilities of the tissue but the character of the change may be regulated by a carefully considered modification of the medium (Grandcourt).

All this work involves the theory that the cells make such demands upon the nutrition supplied by the medium that they deplete it and then become indirect means of introducing into the life process a chemically destructive activity (catabolism). The result is a gradual slowing down of cell growth, which is progressive aging and death. A very analogous course was that followed in the earlier artificial cultivations. The tissues lived a short span of days and then died. But the process of degeneration could be obviated by salt solutions and other processes so that tissues now grow *in vitro* for a year and a half and may continue to multiply faster than those of the embryo. Thus for such tissues senility does not exist and the question naturally arises whether we can ever hope to accomplish anything of this sort inside the body.

Carrel in 1914 reported a strain of connective tissue that had undergone 358 passages and had then reached the twenty-eighth month of its life *in vitro*. It was detached from the heart of a chick embryo seven days of age, which pulsated for 104 days and gave rise to a large number of connective tissue cells. These multiplied actively for the first two years, a great many cultures having been derived from this strain every week. The fragment of the tissue usually doubled in forty-eight hours, though rapidity of growth was subject to fluctuations. One striking result is seen by comparing the amount of tissue produced by a given culture in forty-eight hours this year with that produced in the same tissue by the same strain of cells a year before. This shows that the activity of the strain had increased, although this might, of course, be due to improvement of technic or possibly to a progressive adaptation to life *in vitro*. Carrel says: "Thus it is conclusively shown that the proliferating power of the strain has in no wise diminished. During the third year of independent life, the connective tissue shows greater activity than at the beginning of the period and is no longer subject to the influence of time. If we exclude accident, the connective tissue cells, like infusoria, may proliferate indefinitely." In the latest report at hand one of these cultures had been kept alive and growing thus for seven and a half years.

The original and indefatigable American-Frenchman, C. E. Brown-Séquard (1817–1894) who in 1878 succeeded Claude Bernard in the chair of experimental medicine in the *Collège de France,* was one of the first experimental physiologists to study the functions of glands and to realize the importance of their secretions. After investigating the suprarenals in animals as early as 1869 and finding that their removal always caused death, he returned to this subject twenty years later to investigate the testicular fluids which, discharged into the blood, "exalted the power of the nervous system and kept up the vital energies." He even injected the fluids extracted from the testes of animals into his own system hypodermically, with results that he thought distinctly beneficial to himself and says that he "at the age of seventy recovered the force and energy of youth, with manifestations unknown for a number of years." He thus believed that he had discovered a new therapeutic agent of great rejuvenating power. Berthelot says, "The subject required delicate manipulation, not only because of the extraordinary precautions required for this kind of investigation but of charlatanism, always ready to possess itself of new curative procedures. He did not protest against the abuses by which his name was used to cover industrial enterprises." He persisted in his idea, and he, more than anyone else, should be called the founder of opotherapy or treatment by extracts from organs. His name will always have a prominent place in the history of endocrinology or the science that deals with the glands that secrete inwardly, a subject that already has a vast and rapidly growing literature, with an essentially new body of facts and insights and, at its present stage of development, yet far more precious hopes and expectations of great discoveries just ahead.

Some of the many commercial products of testicular juices, so very difficult to prepare in a form that can be preserved, were for many years widely used and the best known of these, Pohl's spermine preparations, are still more or less in demand. But despite Brown-Séquard's enthusiastic belief in his age-deferring cure, it lapsed from general attention, partly because the initial expectations were too high, until a very few years ago when the problems it had suggested were approached in a new way by a few investigators whose results have not only a high value in themselves but give promise of yet more important and definite subsequent discoveries—and that despite the conservatism and criticism that all efforts to deal scientifically and fundamentally with human sex problems always encounter.

BIOLOGY AND PHYSIOLOGY

Professor Eugene Steinach, who founded a laboratory of comparative physiology at Prague and was later
made director of the biological institute at Vienna, continued to work there until his institute, for which Roux
and others have solicited contributions from men of
science, to have it opened again, was closed by the war.
He began to publish his epoch-making results in 1910.
In spring frogs brought to his laboratory he found 8 per
cent impotent and also that testicular injection from
normal frogs seemed to restore or intensify the em-
bracement impulse and the strength of the forelegs.[17]
The effect lasted, however, only a few days. Nevertheless he suggests that in borderline cases it might permanently restore fertility. The same process in castrated frogs showed the same effect, only in much less
degree, and the injection of substance from the cerebro-
spinal centers of these activities seemed to have a certain but very slight effect upon the sex nature.

When ovaries and testes were transferred in guinea
pigs a few days old, he found, in general, that through
the influences of the hormones from these glands the
character of each sex underwent "slow but radical transformation over toward the other." [18] In the one case
the male organ atrophied and the breasts were developed, with a disposition to nurse, the hair became finer,
the method of growth was transformed into that of the
other sex; and the converse occurred when the transplantation was in the reverse direction. The change was
thus both morphological and functional and Steinach
believes that there is a distinct antagonism of the sex
hormones due to transplantation of a heterological gland
and that this is not due to biochemical differences of

[17] Geschlechtstrieb und echt sekundäre Geschlechtsmerkmale als Folge
der Innersekretorischen Funktion der Keimdrüsen," *Zeit. f. Physiologie*,
Sept., 1910.

[18] "Pubertätsdrüsen und Zwitterbildung," *Archiv. f. Entwicklung der
Organismen*, vol. 42, 1916, pp. 307-332.

blood but to a distinct antagonism between male and female hormones, which have a sex specificity that is the main factor in directing growth. He distinguishes between the specific sex influence and the antagonism that brings about heterological sex signs, which favor the development of other pubertal glands and control growth, even to the dimensions of the skeleton, both stimulating and inhibiting it. The transplantation can be so effected that the glands of both sexes, in a sense, inhibit each other, so that something like experimental hermaphroditism can be caused. These changes last sometimes through life and occasionally there may be periodic milk secretions in males. Each element checks and may throw the other out of function.

In a later article [19] Steinach published results of experiments upon the exchange of sex glands in other animals between the different sexes and found that the female masculated by being given the testes of her brother followed more or less his development rather than her own, almost equaling him in growth, weight, and robustness. This Steinach calls hyper-masculinization and a degree of this follows the development of the glands after transplantation, which the microscope showed was attended by real intussusception. He also showed hyper-feminization, so that we have a change of the ovaries into hypertrophic but analogous pubertal glands, with corresponding change of traits, dependent upon the degree of success or completeness of the operation. Thus he thinks, too, we can explain somatic and psychic precocity by the hypertrophy of these glands. In another article [20] the author emphasizes the great variability in the development of sex, both as to size of

[19] "Erhöhte Wirkungen der inneren Sekretion bei Hypertrophie der Pubertätsdrüsen," *Archiv. f. Entwicklungsmechanik der Organismen,* vol. 42, 1916, pp. 490-507.
[20] "Klima und Mannbarkeit," *Archiv. f. Entwicklungsmechanik der Organismen,* vol. 46, 1920, p. 391.

organs and their functions in different individuals and believes that besides environment, heredity, race, etc., climate has a great deal to do with it. He finds that in warm countries the advent of sex maturity is somewhat earlier in all its aspects, although there is some suggestion that these accelerations may be connected with the development of other secondary traits. Experiments made with animals in artificial climates point to the same result and changes in this direction are observed in animals accustomed to cold that are transported to warm climates.

Interesting as these experiments on the interchange of primary and secondary sexual qualities are, they were, for Steinach, only preliminary to what chiefly concerns us here, namely, his studies of rejuvenation [21] and his problem was to see whether by his operations he could shed light upon the problem of whether age is a condition we are defenseless against, like an incurable disease, or senescence can, at least within certain modest limits, be influenced. He says his experiments have decided in favor of the latter alternative. He had first to determine whether orthoplastic, homoplastic, or a combination of both methods was the best. The former was chosen because it was quickest and easiest and independent of earlier implantation material, especially with men. And so, with his colleague, Lichtenstern, various operations were performed, of which three type cases are as follows:

Case 1. Man of 44, lean, weak, wrinkled, incapable of physical work by reason of easy fatigue. Libido failing for years and almost extinct, testicular pains, and double-sided hydrocele. With local anesthesia the typical Winkelmann operation was performed. On both sides there was ligature of the vas deferens

---

[21] "Verjüngung durch Experimentelle Neubelebung der alternden Pubertäts Drüse," *Archiv. f. Entwicklungsmechanik der Organismen*, vol. 46, 1920, Part 4.

between the testicle and the epididymis. The cure took a week and the patient was soon discharged. A few weeks witnessed a striking change. He increased in weight, the wrinkles almost vanished, and in five months he had won back muscular power and become a hard worker, carrying heavy burdens. "Libido and potence returned with great intensity." The upper part of the thigh grew hairy and both hair and beard increased so that he had to shave more often. Improvement continued during the year and a half in which he was under observation and he seemed in every way a vigorous and young man.

Case 2. Man of 71, of large business, who came to the hospital with an abscess in the left testicle with septic signs—chills, high temperature, etc.—so that it was necessary to remove the source of maturation *in toto*. At the same time the right, sound testicle was subjected to ligature of the passage from the epididymis to the vas deferens. In twenty-four hours the patient lost his fever and in three weeks left the hospital. Quite apart from the acute symptoms, this patient had for years suffered marked signs of age, especially calcification phenomena—dizziness, shortness of breath, weakness of heart, great fatigue, tremors, etc., with libido extinct for eight years. Within a few months a marked change occurred. A feeling of masculinity returned and in nine months the patient described his own condition in a letter in which he says in substance that, to his great surprise, certain nocturnal phenomena had recurred, his appetite was so great that for a long time it was difficult for him to satisfy it, instead of previous depression he found himself again full of the joy of life and considered himself very elastic for his age, while his friends often remarked the great change that had taken place and could not believe he was seventy-one. He suffers little from fatigue, calcification and dizziness have ceased, he can think clearly, had to go to the barber more often, and all his functions have greatly improved.

Case 3. This was a wholesale merchant of 66 who for some five years had shown senile symptoms, such as difficulty of respiration and in thinking, weak memory and also muscles, and libido almost gone. In this case there was rapid prostatism and catheterization, also emaciation, and occasionally more pronounced psychic disturbances. The first operation on this case was prostatomy but this did not arrest loss of weight or increasing weakness. Then there was ligature of the vas near its entrance into the epididymis on both sides, which was followed by a very rapid recovery, with improvement of nearly all symptoms.

Thus the author thinks that in fighting old age ortho-plasty is by far the best method, and to the objection that these cases are not true psychic senescence but only symptoms of intercurrent disease he replies that this only gave occasion for the operation and that the disease itself was the result of age. Thus, in general, he concludes that for advanced senescence the ligature of the vas, as above, gives the most remarkable results, and that for those before the senium also it may often work very favorably. The same is true of premature old age, the advent of which has immense individual variations.

As to checking the advance of old age in women, Steinach is not yet ready to make any positive report, but in view of what has already been done with animals he thinks a good prognosis can be made and that the best method is by implantation of young ovarian material. The difficulty of this orthoplastic process is found only in the dependence upon the material of implantation, which is very difficult to secure. The effort is directed in all such cases to the influence of the aging ovaries, whether operative by orthoplastic transplantation or by the use of Roentgen rays. The former, on account of the earlier involution of ovaries, is confined within certain limits to women. The phenomena of fatigue, etc., have been removed by this method, which has been so successful that improvement has been noticed by friends.

In Steinach's experiments with rats, which pass through the life stages so rapidly, he used the method of transplantation of testicular glands furnished by three-months-old individuals and this grafting need not necessarily be *in situ* but in various parts of the body. If intussusception took place, as it generally did if the operation was well performed, the change here was generally marked within two weeks, as his photographs show. More or less of Steinach's work has been confirmed, Ebstein tells us, by other observers who have shown that not only in rats but in guinea pigs the transfer of ovaries and testes between the sexes makes the male, to some extent, become female, and *vice versa*. Sex differences, Steinach thinks, do not result from anatomical differences in the organs transferred but are due to functions residing in certain cells, especially those of Leydig or Lutein. It is their secretions that determine sex characteristics. Indeed, they are really glands and vitality and vigor depend upon their state. Youth is the freshening up of these glands. No one has recognized more clearly than Steinach that there is a false old age that has been, in a sense, imposed by civilization upon elderly people and given them a rôle they have more or less passively accepted, just as in the same way there are spurious forms of other diseases. Some of Steinach's critics have suggested that all he has done is to throw off these artificial inhibitions and give old age the true character nature intended it to have. But even if this criticism has any weight against his conclusions respecting old age in man, it certainly cannot apply to his studies of senescent animals, for in them the traits of old age were unmistakable, as not only photographs but, far more, activities showed. They certainly do seem to be really rejuvenated and not merely to be laying aside a sham old age.

Of the half-dozen or more expert opinions upon Steinach's work nearly all have been by his own countrymen and by far the most exhaustive and, on the whole, highly favorable is that of Paul Kammerer.[22] For a very condensed account of it in English see A. Granet's résumé [23] in which he says (1) that Steinach's work is

---

[22] "Steinach's Forschungen über Entwicklung, Beherrschung, und Wandlung der Pubertät," *Ergebnisse der Inneren Medizin und Kinderheilkunde*, 1919, vol. 17, pp. 295-398.
[23] "Eugene Steinach's Work on Rejuvenation," *N. Y. Med. J.*, vol. 112, 1920, p. 612.

based on a new conception of the puberty gland as the internal secretory portion of the gonads. This consists of the interstitial cells in the male and of the lutein cells in the female. (2) Steinach began by studying animals with a protracted rutting period in alternating stages of development of the interstitial gland and the generative gland proper. He found a periodical hyperdevelopment in the evolution of every individual, the interstitial gland predominating in infancy and attaining its maximum development at puberty and adolescence, when growth and vital energy are also at their maximum. At this time the generative gland increases and both the interstitial and generative portions continue to be about equally active till the climacteric, after which there is rapid recession of the interstitial gland, and this causes senility, which is not due to the ultimate using up of all elements but to the lack of potential stimulus due to degeneration of the interstitial gland. (3) Steinach used this alternating balance of nature in the mixed gland by artificially inhibiting the generative portion and thereby causing compensatory regulation and revival of the interstitial portion with all its rejuvenating effects and the recession of the traits of senility. This he accomplished by three methods (a) simple ligation, under local anæsthesia, of the vas deferens. This causes regression of the generative gland and a compensatory regeneration of the interstitial portions. A one-sided operation is sufficient in all cases and has the advantage of preserving in addition the power of procreation. Of course ligation of the Fallopian tube in the female does not produce this result. (b) Repeated mild exposure of the gonads to the X-ray is a slower but apparently just as effective a means of obtaining the same result for both ovaries and testes. And lastly, (c) the effects of rejuvenation may be experimentally produced by transplantation in the old of the respective gonads of the young animal of the same species. For years Steinach bred and reared healthy generations of laboratory animals and studied their dispositions, habits, physical and psychic traits, until he has become unprecedentedly expert in diagnosing age, to say nothing of sex. The increased resistance to disease and the actual prolongation of life of the operated animals he estimates at about 25 per cent but after a time senescence sets in again.

For women in the climacteric the X-ray method is, by general consent, best. But Steinach contends that increased well-being and capacity thus caused are really due to regeneration of the interstitial ovarian structures. General debility and climacteric metrorrhagias are distinctly helped by this method because the interstitial portion of the ovary is not affected by the X-ray whereas the colloidal-albuminoid precipitation occurs in the cells of the Graafian follicles, which are radio-sensitive, the same as the metaplastic cells. The affected cells disappear by autolysis. Menopause sets in and the interstitial portion alone whose hormones produce the rejuvenating effect remains functioning. The effects of transplantation, too, are the same and the shrinking of the transplanted gland seems due to atrophy and should not prevent rejuvenating effects.

E. Payr [24] calls attention to the fact that Steinach's puberty glands, which correspond to the Leydig cells, are those that secrete internally and that it is these that act so powerfully upon secondary sex qualities and bring what often appears to be a renewal of youth. His operation is especially indicated in the case of subjects with healthy internal organs who are growing prematurely old and who give evidence of loss of function of secondary sexual characteristics.

---

[24] "Steinach's Rejuvenation Operation," *Central. f. Chirurgie*, Sept. 11, 1920.

BIOLOGY AND PHYSIOLOGY

G. F. Lydston [25] describes nine cases of men with atrophied testes, injured, or removed, which were replaced *in situ* surgically by those from the bodies of boys recently dead. The glands from the boys were removed within a few hours after death and generally subjected to cold storage for some hours and then ingrafted upon the older patient. The boys from whom they were taken were healthy boys who had suffered sudden or violent death and there might be an interval of many hours not only between the death and the removal but between the latter and the implantation. In all these cases Lydston reports more or less improvement by the operation, which in a few cases was marked. The transplanted glands atrophy and disappear more rapidly when the recipient has more or less well developed testes of his own. Apparently permanent local results were best obtained in those cases in which the patient had very little gland tissue. Lydston thinks that there may be a sort of parasitic action of the patient's own glands upon the transplanted ones. His own organs probably contribute the nutritive pabulum otherwise available for the implanted ones but the therapeutic results are obtained and sustained even when the implanted gland eventually disappears. He thinks that the notable result obtained by Dr. I. L. Stanley, where the glands from a Negro hanged for murder were implanted in the scrotum of a white moron, apparently with remarkable results, suggests that atrophy may take place more slowly when the donor is of the same race as the recipient. The author doubts whether there is much advantage in anastomosis as to either betterment of nutrition or preservation of the spermogenetic function. He thinks "we run more risk of failure of the implant from the greater traumatization of the tissue necessary for anastomosis." He

[25] "Further Observations on Sex-Gland Implantation," *Jour. Am. Med. Assn.,* vol. 72, 1919, p. 396.

thinks, too, that the spermogenetic epithelium of the testes degenerates in all cases rather promptly.[26]

In his book, *Impotence, Sterility and Sex Gland Implantation* (1917), which seems somewhat ill-digested, Lydston claims priority on eight points and formulates twenty-one conclusions. It seems to me that he has not sufficiently assimilated the best European work in this field or profited as much as he might have done by the far greater refinements of technique of Steinach; while such results as he claims are, as he himself admits, always wide open to criticism.

Serge Voronoff, like Metchnikoff, combines research with humanism and gives free rein to his idealism. He is professor in the medical school of the *Collège de France* and deals with old age and death from the standpoint of endocrinology or the study of the glands of internal secretion. Accepting Weismann's doctrine of the continuity of germ plasm, he says that the nameless and ever unassuaged horror that everybody really feels for death is "because an intimate memory of our immortality" survives or because we recollect creation's first intention as expressed in plasmal immortality. Man has inherited this longing from the deathless unicellular creatures from which he descended not only in the form of quests for elixirs of life here but in all his manifold beliefs of a life beyond the grave, at the same time for

---

[26] H. E. Goodale of the Massachusetts Experiment Station, Amherst, says (*Science,* Oct. 23, 1914, p. 594.) : "A brown Leghorn male was castrated completely when twenty-four days of age, and the ovaries from two brood sisters, cut in several pieces, were placed beneath the skin and also in the abdominal cavity. At the date of writing the bird is as obviously female as its brood sisters. Skilled poultrymen have called it a pullet. While it has all the female characteristics, there can be little doubt, from the scars still visible as well as other things, that it was a male." It is not likely that its peculiar individuality was feminized owing to constitutional condition. The author believes it was feminized by the implanted ovaries in similar fashion to the rats and guinea pigs of Steinach.

this life accepting the gospel of renunciation to death as something inevitable. The ghastly thought of death not only clouds all our life but predisposes even most scientists to think that research in this field cannot be successful.

The background view of the work in Voronoff's field, roughly stated, is as follows. Somatic cells, having lost the power to propagate the whole body, as they develop and multiply become more and more special, not only in form but in function, until they finally lose the power of multiplication or of regeneration. These are higher and perform the most particularized functions. Besides these most individualized cells, so characteristic of every organ that a cytologist can at once distinguish cells that form the epithelium, intestines, brain, muscle, glands, etc., there always remain other far less differentiated or more primitive cells, chiefly leucocytes or white blood corpuscles and the connective tissue cells. The former float in the blood and can pass out through the thin walls of the capillaries into other tissues. The latter constitute all the firmer supportive framework of every organ. They are very robust, fecund proletarians and are largely made up of the former. From birth they wage unceasing war upon the nobler, more professional and expert, but less independent cells which have sacrificed most of their cruder, pristine powers for service to the body corporate. These higher cells represent the extreme division of labor within our bodies. They are no longer sufficient unto themselves but each class of them depends upon the work of others. The low, banal, barbaric but vigorous cells of the conjunctive tissue, on the other hand, always strive to destroy and to themselves take the place of the higher cells and it is this process slowly going on everywhere that constitutes old age and all its processes of hardening, atrophy, disintegration, etc., for these lower cells cannot discharge the functions of the higher ones they have supplanted and hence comes anarchy within the organ or body. We die because nature tends so strongly to develop the cruder type of cell that makes up the connective tissue.

Now, secretions of the thyroid gland check this aggression of the lower upon the higher cells, as is shown in the studies of cretinism, which is in so many respects nothing but premature old age brought on because the thyroid fluid, the special function of which was to retard this process, was not supplied; and when it fails, old age comes on precipitately and even children often look and act much like prematurely old men and women. On the other hand, the Metchnikoff ferments of the large intestine weaken the higher cells and leave them with less power of resistance, so that they become more easily the prey of the lower cells of the connective tissue. The enemy, however, for the endocrinologist is not primarily a microbe entering from without but a more formidable and subtle foe that springs up within. The difficulty in meeting the situation is immensely enhanced by the fact that the cells of the conjunctive tissue are not only useful but indispensable for the work and the development of every organ at first and continue to be so as long as they do not transcend this their original function and trespass outside it. The white corpuscles, although the source of the connective tissue cells, are themselves our chief defenders. It is they who attack and devour invading microbes but they consume not only these but also higher cells that have, by the action of microbes or otherwise, become debilitated. They are, however, on the whole, so serviceable that we cannot intervene against them but only against our more dangerous and insidious enemy, the conjunctive tissue cells.

Not only the thyroid but yet more the tiny parathyroid glands secrete a fluid, the absence of which brings convulsions and death. A knowledge of the function of these glands, no larger than a pinhead, as well as that of the adrenals or of the far more complex pituitary body (hypophysis), each lobe of which plays its own particular rôle, has been nothing less than revolutionary. The effects due either to excess or deficit of the secretion of these glands, which have been studied experimentally in animals and observed in man, show that they have great power even to arrest or accelerate growth itself. It is they that do much to keep us young or make us old. In a sense they furnish the power that makes about all the organs do their work efficiently, as an electric current from a battery may start, or its absence stop, the most diverse kinds of electric machinery. Thus glands have come to play a great rôle in physiology, medicine, and even psychology, and their activities have come to be recognized in very many phenomena both of health and disease, which till recent years no one had suspected. Some of these glands contain a relatively small number of cells but do a vast amount of work and manufacture fluids that no chemist can duplicate and that seem almost magic in their effects. We owe to them growth, health, and vitality.

Most important of all, and the chief source of human energy in man, are the sex glands, which distribute energy to all the sixty trillion cells of the body, making each carry out the function assigned it. Voronoff made personal studies of eunuchs in the East and among the many traits so often mentioned he finds them not only arrested along various lines of bodily and psychic growth but short-lived and perhaps old before they are forty. They are often selfish and crafty. Sex glands stimulate not merely amorousness but all kinds of cerebral and muscular energy, pouring into the blood a species of vital fluid, and give a sense of vigor and well-being and plenitude of life, which later vanish when their source begins to run dry in age. Can this wonderful source of human energy be placed, in any sense, in man's control? It has already been proven that trituration of the sex glands does not produce its entire product and particularly lacks the active element. Moreover, all preparations of this liquid change very rapidly and may even become toxic. This method has passed beyond the stage of ingestion in the stomach or subcutaneous ingestions.

Voronoff undertook to graft young sex glands themselves into bodies older than those from which they came and if they lived and throve in the body of the host, the product they secreted would be complete and also vital. He says of the testes: "To graft this gland is to participate at first hand in the work of creation, to imitate nature in the procedures which she has elaborated in order to secure the harmonious functioning of our body" [27] (p. 65). He published his first results in 1912. He then showed a lamb born of an ewe whose ovaries he had removed, replacing them with the ovaries of her younger sister. His most important paper was read in October, 1919, on "Testicular Grafts." He had been experimenting on flocks of sheep and goats, grafting the whole gland in twenty-five, large fragments in fifty-eight, and small ones in thirty-seven individuals. Transplantation was effected subcutaneously sixty-five times, in the scrotum itself thirty-two times, and twenty-three times in the peritoneum. Anastomosis did not follow; nor was it necessary. Testicular tissue, he thinks, has remarkable aptitude for transplantation and a microscopist, M. Retterer, shows us with abundant illustrations just what takes place. The nutrition of the small fragments was more easily assured than that of the large fragments or the whole. Sometimes where sex power is restored in old animals so that they bear young,

[27] *Life: A Study of the Means of Restoring Vital Energy and Prolonging Life,* New York, 1920, 160 p.

the parental instinct seems weakened, but the rejuvenation effects of this process, as his many photographs show, are marked. The old and debilitated animals become well, lively, vigorous, and belligerent.

Voronoff is very candid in admitting that his interest and enthusiasm may cause him unconsciously to overestimate the rejuvenating effects of his grafts, and he also admits that he does not yet know how long the beneficial effects will last. That they have done so for two or even three years is beyond question. He is conscious of the incredulity of biological experts but reminds them that a society of physicists, when first shown the phonograph, insisted that it was ventriloquism. He calls attention to the great difficulties in his field, due not only to prejudice but to laws that forbid the taking of organs of healthy men killed by accident. He does not expect surgery will ever remove glands or even portions of them from the living young to revitalize the old, in human subjects, although he thinks that perhaps "the restoration of the vital energy and the productive power of Pasteur may well be worth the slight pain inflicted on the robust porter." Most men, however, would prefer to lose an eye rather than one of these glands, as the price proposed by a few who offered themselves for this purpose shows.

Voronoff sees a great future possible for glandular transplantation and grafting between men and animals but shows that this can never be very effective for man save with apes, to whom he is so much more closely related, even in the makeup and properties of his blood, than to any other species. Thus the organ of an ape transplanted to man will find there nutritive and other conditions very like those it was used to. Surgery has done much and wonderful grafting in the war, even of bones, and now man, "the talented ape," as Huxley called him, is recognizing his simian ancestry in a new way. A fibula congenitally missing in a child was successfully transplanted from an ape, and the radiogram showed complete intussusception, no absorption, and it functioned well. Voronoff transplanted the thyroid gland of an ape into the neck of a boy of fourteen, who was lapsing to cretinism, with remarkable results which he describes in detail and with photographs, although the ape from which the thyroid was taken died. The transplanted gland was not merely tolerated and then expelled as a foreign body or resorbed but the graft seemed to really take and its effects to be permanent and not temporary, like those due to the ingestion of thyroid tablets. The boy changed in his habits, his school work improved remarkably, and the last heard from him was that he was a soldier at the front. Here the beneficial effects were marked and traced for six years and seemed to promise permanence. Other grafts from apes for cretinism have been made, but because chimpanzees, which are best for this purpose, are very hard to procure in sufficient numbers, this process must always be limited. Voronoff has, however, made no grafts, even of thyroids, from parent to child save in one case; and here, although the young imbecile was nearly twenty when the operation was performed, marked improvement took place. The ape is, in a sense, however, superior to man, as represented by the quality of these organs, owing perhaps to a more robust physical constitution; or it may be due to the fact that with the first boy the graft was from a young ape and the latter from his mature mother.

For woman, for whom old age has perhaps even greater terrors than for man, such restoration has not yet been made. Indeed, ovariotomy has less effects upon young women than does castration upon man, so that here we face a new problem that cannot yet be solved. The problem now is whether we can generalize yet from these special studies, including bone grafting and the surgery of transplantation of other organs. Kidney grafting has been successful as yet only on cats and dogs but opotherapy or the administration of glandular extracts of animals when our own fail is in its infancy, although it does seem to give promise of deferring death and increasing the vigor of human life. Indeed, he thinks that the renewal of worn-out glandular mechanisms by grafting may even become a commonplace. The vital fluid supplied by these organs "restores energy in all cells and spreads happiness and a feeling of well-being and the plenitude of life throughout our organism." The idea of controlling this marvelous force and placing it at our service when the natural sources of our energy begin to dry up with the advance of age has long haunted the minds of investigators, and Paul Bert and Ollier decades ago dreamed of a day when old organs might be set aside like wornout clothes and replaced by new ones. "Several of these animals operated upon have exceeded the age limit which animals of their species generally attain and, instead of showing signs of decrepitude and senility, they give promise of astonishing vigor."

Louis Berman, M.D.,[28] tells us that infancy is the epoch of the thymus, childhood of the pineal, adolescence of whatever gland is left in control as the result of the life struggle, and senility is the epoch of gradual endocrine insufficiency. The discovery of the effects of endocrine secretions he compares with that of radium and thinks that by control of this function we may be able to modify the rigidity of Weismann's dogma and affect heredity itself. He draws a very long bow and even attempts to characterize important personages and races according to the predominance of thyroid, pituitary, or

[28] *The Glands Regulating Personality:* A study of the glands of internal secretion in relation to the types of human nature. New York, MacMillan, 1921. 300 p.

adrenal secretions and sees here the fundamental determinants of human character and conduct. Well informed and expert as he is in this field, his views, though bold and interesting, are, it must be admitted, more or less speculative in the present state of our knowledge, and he devotes little consideration to old age or to the methods of deferring it.

If we conceive life as the sum total of all the forces that resist death and death in its essence as the queller of life, it is to biology, not to theology or philosophy, that we must look for our most authoritative and normative ideas of both life and death. We must examine not only the now very copious data that this science already supplies but also the instrument that defines, delivers, and interprets them, namely, the mind, so that psychology must henceforth have a place here second only to biology in formulating conclusions. Now, psychology teaches not only that there are certain determining tendencies that always, in part at least below the threshold of consciousness, direct the course of thought, slowly build up centers of apperception and interest, and that must always be reckoned with sooner or later not only in the treatment of any subject in which their action is involved but also when almost any scientific laws of nature are formulated, but also that, quite apart from their primary significance for the field in which they arose, they have a secondary anagogic value in other fields, in which they become symbols, often of great efficacy. Only the lower alchemists sought to evolve gold from baser metals and this quest we now know was always and everywhere really subordinate to the effort to evolve the *summum bonum* in human life. So the modern sciences that deal with life and death, health and disease, are really directed far more than they know, even in those researches upon the lower forms of life and most abnormal processes, by the deeper, determining motivation to know better and to influence more the conditions of human life. Thus a truer and larger self-knowledge for man is, in this sense, their ultimate goal.

In view of this, what psychologist can for a moment doubt that the old problem which F. W. H. Myers called the most insistent that ever haunted the mind of man has contributed very much to stimulate interest in Weismann's doctrine of the immortality of the germ plasm and for a wide lay public has given a zest and interest in phenomena that can hardly be observed at all save through a microscope and by an expert. If we had an analysis of Weismann's own consciousness from his first conception of this idea to its full development we should doubtless find the same factor. True, we search his writings in vain for any intimation that he recognized any such influence, but I think there can be no doubt that had he been a psychologist interested in the sources of his own motivations and had he left us an autobiography as intimate as that of Spencer, Wundt, or even Darwin, we should have seen that he realized that he was only giving a new answer to the oldest of all culture problems. Of course, no psychoanalyst or geneticist would claim that Weismann was seeking an *elixir vitæ* or a new fountain of youth for himself or for others, but it would be equally extreme, on the other hand, to deny that in the very use of the concept and term immortal, as he applied them to germ plasm and protozoa, he was propounding a new if partial surrogate answer to the problem of a larger life for man. Indeed, we might go further and suggest that in his extreme pronouncements against the inheritance of acquired qualities he gave way to the same basal disposition or diathesis that made theologians so exiguous in formulating conceptions of the inviolability of divine decrees.

Another underlying psychic determinant is found in the intense popular interest in investigations like those of Voronoff, Steinach, and Carrel, of which the latter is perhaps least conscious while the former is almost as tinglingly so throughout as Haeckel was of these older concepts. That highly differentiated and complex somatic tissues removed from the body and given a more fit medium, and kept from all products of decomposition, etc., can keep on functioning and growing for years, better than they had done in the body in which they originated, neither has nor is ever likely to have any real practical utility for prolonging or intensifying human life. The fact may have a certain moral for cleanliness and even for nutrition but we can never wash out the tissues of the body or keep each of its cells in an optimum environment. Yet even here the mind finds a faint if, all things considered, somewhat pathetic element of hope that old age and death may sometime be deferred.

Nor can we ever hope to ward death off by keeping the tissues of the body young and growing to the end of life and breaking the law, to which nearly all species are subject, of attaining their maximum size long before age and decline set in. It has long been realized that one of the first signs of the advent of the chronic hereditary diseases in children is the arrest of growth but man can never, of course, hope to approximate immortality by attaining gigantic size. Nor can we hope to advance toward the old idea of macrobiotism by permanently lowering the temperature within the body, as experimenters show can be done with great increase of life for certain of its lower forms, especially those called cold-blooded which take the temperature of the medium in which they live. And yet here man has a very old instinct, reinforced by modern hygiene, to avoid excessive heat, an instinct that perhaps originally impelled him to leave tropic regions and haunt the edge of retreating glaciers. Nor can we ever expect to rejuvenate man by bringing about a dedifferentiation of organs or functions because just this is the price we pay for progress, evolution, and individuation. But this concept, too, has many prelusive forms in the early developmental history of human consciousness and it has its own obvious anagogic meaning. If we follow these trends they lead us, of course, straight to Pantheism and give us a painful sense of the limitations inherent in personality itself. As to the conclusion of Loeb, that life departs with breath because the absence of a fresh supply of oxygen lets loose dissolutive chemical changes its presence prevented, the pragmatic layman can only point to the recognition that in a few generations has become worldwide, of the value of ventilation, deep breathing, and the adequate oxidation of tissues. This shows that man felt that life was closely bound up with oxygen long before he could prove it. So the biological evidence that it is the brain or nervous system that dies first and determines the death of all the other parts and functions, if it has any culture correlate, finds it probably in the hazy quarter truths of the doctrines of the mental healers, that far more human ills and far more deaths and preventions and postponements of death than we know are amenable to mind cure because they are mindmade.

The only practical hope of easement from the hardships of senescence and for the postponement of death now tenable is that now arising faintly and tentatively that, some day, some mitigation of the terrors of old age and death may be found by glandular implantation or perhaps even by the injection of the secretions of certain glands. We know that the germinal glands, and especially their products, have a unique vitality of their own and also that they exert a remarkable and all-pervasive influence upon all the organs and functions of the body; and that thyroid extract retards and its absence precipitates all the processes of aging. The new studies in this field suggest that glands may be the sovereign masters of life. These studies are yet, however, in their infancy and it will be, at the best, a long time before we can know whether they are able to fulfill their promise to the human heart and to the will to live.

I deem it, however, very significant that contemporaneously with the discovery and exploitation of endocrine functions, and especially those of the sex glands, from another field and quite independently have come the discovery and exploitation of the unconscious and the recognition that its chief content is sexual. The analogies between these two lines of advance and their real relation with each other have not yet been fully recognized, much less wrought out. But already there is promise of a new and more stimulating rapport between biology and analytic and genetic psychology. If researches in the former field ever have the therapeutic value already so abundantly illustrated in the latter, we shall indeed be fortunate. Just now this seems not probable for a long time. But the physiological dominance of sex glands and their products, and the immense rôle played by sex life, especially in man, suggest that it is in this field that the cure of his most grievous ills must be sought, just as the oldest and most persistent myths and legends have so long taught that it was in this field that the so-called fall of man took place.

CHAPTER VII

REPORT ON QUESTIONNAIRE RETURNS

Their value suggestive but only for a class—(1) Effects of the first realization of the approach of old age—(2) To what do you ascribe your long life?—(3) How do you keep well?—(4) Are you troubled by regrets?—(5) What temptations do you feel—old or new? (6) What duties do you feel you still owe to others or to self?—(7) Is interest in public affairs for the far future and past, as compared with what is closer at hand, greater or less?—(8) In what do you take your greatest pleasures?—(9) Do you enjoy the society of children, youth, adults, those of your own age, more or less than formerly? —(10) Would you live your life over again?—(11) Did you experience an "Indian summer" of renewed vigor before the winter of age began? —(12) Do you rely more or less upon doctors than formerly?—(13) Do you get more or less from the clergy and the church than formerly? —(14) Do you think more or less of dying and the Hereafter?— A few individual returns from eminent people.

PERHAPS no one but a genetic psychologist can realize how very widely the successive stages of life in man differ from each other. Underneath the tenuous memory continuum that is the chief basis of all feeling of identity between our present and former selves, deeper even than every unity of life plan and persistence of disposition, are the great changes the years bring. These are, indeed, so great that although they very commonly modulate, each into the next stage of the series by almost imperceptible gradations, we all really live not one but a succession of lives. Further than this, just as in dementia præcox the normal development of the psyche is permanently arrested in a juvenile stage, so, but far more commonly, the normal progress from maturity to senectitude is arrested; and in the decades of involution, which is just as progressive and interesting as evolution, the old cling to or leave with great reluctance their mature stage and so never achieve true senectitude. Just as the precocious dement balks in adolescence at the growing complexity and arduousness of the problems of adulthood and so fails to mature because he lacks the energy or hereditary momentum to do so, so the old very often find themselves inadequate to the new tasks involved in beating the great retreat. They cannot break from the things that are behind and reach forward to those that are before and they cling with a tenacity that is purely arrestive to a stage of life that has passed. They refuse to accept old age and to make the most and best of it, to face its tasks and to improve all its opportunities. If they do not paint, dye, pad, or affect the fashions and manners of the young (for old age may show traits of narcissism), when the call comes to move on to a new phase of life, their mentality defaults. This type of mental defect has never so far been adequately characterized but it is probably far more common than what is usually called senile dementia, of which it is almost the diametrical opposite, although because of its prevalence it has a better claim to this designation.

Believing profoundly that involution is just as interesting a phase of life as evolution and not being satisfied with the poems, essays, and meditations of literary men and women who have addressed the public on the theme of senescence, which are, as we saw in a former chapter, often more or less hortatory, consolatory, or else were composed as exercises to hearten themselves against the great enemy, it seemed worth while to try to seek a new contact with the fresh spontaneous thoughts and feelings of normal old people concerning their estate.

Years ago I had visited homes for the aged, held converse with many inmates and officials, had given each

inmate a tiny blue book and asked them to answer a few
questions and add anything that occurred to them that
they thought characteristic of their stage of life. The
records thus secured, although voluminous enough, had
very little value. Most who answered were uneducated
and the data they supplied were usually trivial, tediously
and irrelevantly reminiscent, or else descriptive of surroundings in earlier life, complaints, wishes, fears, etc., so
that I realized that true old age as I had conceived it was
not to be sought in such institutions. There was pathos
and pessimism galore, while disciplined tranquillity and
serenity were very rare. There is doubtless material
enough in even the most inarticulate and insignificant
life to repay the longest and most painstaking study.
Perhaps, too, a psychotherapy may sometime be evolved
that will launch such stranded and arrested lives out
again into the current and give them full fruition of all
the fruitage of life. But the world is as yet far from
any such beneficent ministry.

Accordingly, I turned to another source and selected
a few score of names of mostly eminent and some very
distinguished old people, both acquaintances and
strangers, and addressed to each a simple questionnaire,
also inviting spontaneous impartations in addition to
responses to the points suggested. Some of those who
did me the honor of replying, and often with much
detail, are people of national and international reputation and I wish I had not promised to withhold their
names for this would have given greatly added interest
to the following report. All are cultivated Americans
and thus they represent a single class. Most are Anglo-
Saxons and I have not been able to gather much material
from Oriental or non-Christian sources, desirable and
important as this would be. My data are, however,
sufficiently copious to illustrate the chief types of attitudes within their class. To the returns from this

source I have added data from less than a score of others of the same class with whom I have personal acquaintance and I have drawn but very little from the rich field of autobiography for my inductions. Such data can, of course, only yield results that are far more suggestive than conclusive, and so I forbear from all statistics because the number of my respondents is too small. But although what follows does not represent the great majority of old people it does have a psychological value that I deem as unique as it is pertinent to my theme. It is also perhaps significant that of those who wrote expressing interest and an intention to respond, not one has done so after an interval of several months. It should perhaps also be mentioned here that the suggestion of attempting this book came from nearly two-score letters from old people, which were addressed to me through the editor of the *Atlantic Monthly* and were evoked by an anonymous article I published on "Old Age" in the January, 1921, number of that magazine. I have endeavored to keep the following report of these somewhat heterogeneous data as objective as possible, although it would be absurd to claim that by such a method on such a theme I have entirely escaped subjective bias.

How and at what age did you first realize the approach of old age?

This realization not infrequently begins in the forties and increases thereafter, often intensively with the beginning of each new decade. The first sign of baldness, the first touch of fatigue at stated tasks, lapse of memory for names, waning potency in men; and the first gray hairs, wrinkles, fading of complexion, and change of figure, etc., in women are often specified in our returns. Such and many other signs usually gave the first sad recognition that the meridian of life was being crossed and that gradual declination was just ahead. In many a man and woman this is, as has been recognized, a dangerous age and it often comes in the middle and later thirties in women. The latter, realizing that their summer is ending, sometimes break away from old restraints and give themselves more liberties, not only social but moral. The first glimpse of the specter of senility ahead puts them in a now-or-never mood. Men ask themselves if they will be content to go on as they are so far heading, so that there will be nothing new to be written in the story of their life save only the date of their death. They wonder if the future is to be as the past and perhaps make an inventory of their unrealized ideals, hopes, and wishes, and cross many of them off their ledger as bad debts they owe themselves but can never collect. This crossing the line is for some so serious a matter that it may cause an abrupt turn in their life line, which starts off in a new direction, as is illustrated in a few conspicuous examples in Chapter I. This touch of autumn in August, however, rarely brings frost or blight but leaves only a trace of a new seriousness and perhaps sadness, while otherwise all goes on as before.

In a few cases the first realization that one is getting old springs upon the soul, as if from ambush, on some trivial occasion and clings like an obsession that remits only to recur again and again. The majority, however, promptly and ruthlessly suppress all such intimations beneath the threshold of consciousness, telling not only others but themselves that they are just as young and capable as ever, thus refusing to recognize that age is upon them till perhaps the sixth or seventh decade. Thus the old are often the last to recognize in themselves infirmities that have long been patent to others. This is one of the benignities of nature, for to no disease, not even consumption, does she give a more effective opiate. A man of ninety still retains his post as head of a great concern he created in his youth, to its serious detriment, convinced that he is better than ever and that the scores of younger men under him lack the efficiency of those of his own generation. "He was on the verge of resigning twenty years ago," said one of his subordinates to me, "but now he does not know enough to do so."

On the other hand, some seem to take a new lease of life in this youth of old age. It is not so much that they have a new sense of the value of time but because they have taken in sail in other directions and, realizing the limitations of life, have focused more sharply upon the things they deem most essential.

To what do you ascribe your long life?

Good heredity is much more often specified than anything else. There is a tendency in the old to inventory the virtues of parents and ancestors and a deep-seated belief, even in these democratic days, that blood will tell. Four correspondents believed their constitution was weak and that the early realization of this called their attention to personal hygiene, so that these individuals ascribe their long life more to their own effort than to inheritance. Next in rating is the environment of early life. In our land many have been born in the country and led a laborious life in youth and later changed to urban surroundings and to more sedentary habits, which always involves a considerable strain of readjustment. Where this change has been successfully weathered there is a strong disposition to place a very high emphasis upon the beneficence of strenuous physical activity in the formative period.

Next in appreciation comes the preservative influence of good and temperate habits, reinforced by observations of acquaintances of early life who, by reason of less moderation, have preceded them to the cemetery.

When our own associates die we tend to draw the lessons of their physical and moral life. One ascribes her longevity to the very early implantation of the idea that everything must be determined by its bearing upon her power to bring healthy children into the world. Most mention, and many stress, the absence of worry and overwork, although one insists that he had been chronically anxious from the first, suffering by day for years from apprehensions of evil and lying awake nights trying to plan the reconstruction of the universe. Several ascribe their length of years to the fact that as they advanced in age they learned betimes to give up former duties and lay off burdens they could no longer carry with impunity. It is evident that this realization of the effect of years differs very widely in different individuals and seems almost lacking in some. Several take pride in the fact that although they inherited a short life from both parents and grandparents they have succeeded in greatly prolonging it, and by diet and regimen in overcoming hereditary handicaps. One determined early in life to make the mind rule the body. One old lady ascribes her vigor to progressive self-forgetfulness and devotion to the service of others.

An interesting case, which I deem typical of many in these Christian Science days, declares that he early learned that all living animals, especially man, have "a constructive, preserving, and renewing principle or energy within them fully competent to care for the body in every particular, demonstrated by the evidence of a vast number of recorded cures of so-called incurable diseases without any external remedial agency." This element can become amenable to conscious control. "We are composed of a thousand billion cells, far greater in number than that of the entire population of the globe since man arrived and each of them infinitely complex and charged with potencies." With such a force man

should place no limitations upon himself, for he has inexhaustible recuperative energy, etc. If such a faith
has little justification for science, it may, nevertheless,
give a mental attitude that is conducive to a poise and
confidence that in itself has marked hygienic and therapeutic value. It is interesting to note that cultivated
men and women seem far less prone than the ignorant to
the medical fetishism that ascribes exceptional value to
some nostrum or single item of diet or regimen and this
suggests how fast the age-long quest for a universal
panacea is vanishing from modern consciousness. As
men grow old and have a long experience and youthful
friends have passed away, it is inevitable that they
should seek the cause of their longevity and this urge
would naturally increase with years. Therefore, while
the individual answers to this question have little scientific value, they are of both psychological and practical
interest. Underneath them all there is a tendency to
identify hygiene with morals and most men who achieve
great age thus tend to look with complacency upon their
life as a whole as a triumph of virtue, even though in
fact it may have been quite irregular.

*How do you keep well, that is, what do you find
especially good or bad in diet, regimen, interests, and
personal hygiene generally?*

In the answers to this question, as was perhaps to be
expected, we find the utmost diversity. Only two report
that they eat and do anything that appeals to them, with
no special attention to regimen. Some eschew drugs,
while one would wager that he had taken nearly every
kind of medicament and said he had used laxatives daily
for thirty-eight years. One had found great reinforcement of life from moderate wine drinking and thus found
prohibition somewhat reductive of his vitality. Some entirely eschew tea, coffee, and tobacco, while most indulge

in both of the former and several in the latter in moderation. Several found marked reinforcement when they began to rest or perhaps take a nap in the middle of the day. All praise early retiring and insist that a generous portion of the twenty-four hours must be spent in bed, even if they do not sleep. Most ascribe much virtue to daily, and particularly to cold baths, shower, spray, etc., while a very few prefer a sponge- or only a rub-down. Most stress the importance of exercise, varied and out-of-doors, particularly walking, while some emphasize the value of a little all-round indoor gymnastics that call all the muscles into moderate action. Some note the avoidance of starchy foods, while others speak of the effectiveness of bran or other agencies against constipation, which is, rightly or wrongly, felt to be one of the morbific tendencies of the old, although others believe that some degree of it is normal at this stage of life. Only one felt rejuvenated by vegetarianism, while many found it advantageous to eat less and more frequently. Most had given considerable attention to diet and had drawn up a list of things good or bad for them. Some found it necessary to regulate their lives with reference to some special morbid tendency of kidneys, intestines, heart, lungs, etc. Some laid special emphasis upon confining their occupation to things that were agreeable or congenial, while things distasteful brought fatigue early. A few were so in love with their life-work, or it had such variety, that they never felt the need of a vacation, while others were very dependent upon a more or less stated remission of work or change of scene and activity, not only yearly but at every week's end.

The problem of finding a golden mean between excess and defective diet, exercise, work, and excitement, was almost always present. The fads that individuals stressed were horseback and bicycle riding, hunting, tramping, sleeping out-of-doors on an open porch, developing a programme that kept both mind and body busy all day with objective things, indulging in one or even several avocations often far removed from the main line of interest, etc. Some stressed more or less exact routine, while others found virtue in having none but always following their inner inclination and took pleasure in breaking up old habits. One old man loved skating; another, when he was seventy-three, took up automobiling with great zest. A man of ninety has a rub-down by a nurse every night and morning, with some massage. Another is so dependent upon the food to which he is accustomed that he always takes his cook with him in his private car and even if he goes out to dinner must be served with viands prepared by this particular servitor. Then, after exactly half an hour, he leaves the table, even when he is visiting, for a brief siesta. DeSaverin tells us that old people are liable to develop Epicurean appetites and, as they advance in age, can distinguish liquid and solid viands with far greater acuteness than when they were younger. Our data do not, however, confirm this but suggest that gustatory inclinations grow more amenable to reason. Appetite, we are told, is the safest guide, pointing true as the needle to the pole, to the nutritive needs of the body. It is, nevertheless, very modifiable, and the old often easily come to like the food they have learned is good for them, although they very rarely adopt dietaries suggested for their benefit by nutrition laboratories. It does seem, however, that there should be institutions where old people can go periodically for personal surveys of all their habits and receive suggestions that, based upon their idiosyncrasies, would doubtless be marked by very wide individual variations. It is certain that the diet and regimen most advantageous for the person of one diathesis would be very deleterious to another.

328

Are you troubled with regrets for things done or not done by or for you?

In these returns there is no vestige of tragic remorse of either the old classic or theological kind, although only one disclaimed every trace of regret for anything in the past. This is not because he had not made mistakes but because he believed, as nearly all did, that regrets were vain. Most admitted serious errors both of omission and commission, while many specified waste of time and energy, misdirection, bad advice, lack of method, continuity, and system. One bitterly regretted her choice of calling, which had made her daily work a "crucifixion." Several regretted that they had not been more generous and deplored the too absorbing efforts they had made for acquisition. Others deplored their training as children, the effects of which it had taken years to overcome; while still others regretted the way in which they had brought up their own children. Some thought they had done too little for or given too little attention to their families. Some had made special efforts to cultivate forgetfulness of faults and especially rankling injustices they had suffered from others. One felt that he had come into the world not by his own will but as an accident of sexual passion and therefore felt himself under no obligations to his parents and not responsible for his life or its conduct. Some had even learned to rejoice in their mistakes because of the wisdom that had thus been taught them. Not a few took occasion to reflect upon their satisfactions, which offset the dissatisfaction with what life had brought. Many reproached themselves that they had not done more, worked harder, had more to show, etc. Other old people have a dull and sometimes corroding sense of sexual errors in their past that may have impaired the quality of all their family relations and even the constitution of their children. Some are prone to turn to thoughts of specific instances of outrageous injustice, so that their most poignant regret is that they have never been able to wreak vengeance upon those who had wronged them.

Many specified the long hardships to which they had been subjected by too strict religious and moral regimen and blamed their parents for not giving them instruction betimes during the stage of pubertal ferment. A few had been through the crisis of business failure, made mistaken alliances, or been mismated, or regretted that they had not married. Not infrequent is the regret of having been a spendthrift, wasted a patrimony; and still more frequent are the mentions of injuries to health by unhygienic habits. A few chiefly deplored the fact of not being able to believe what they felt they should. Other few deplored the dullness and languor of their emotional zests and that they take less interest in things than formerly. Most who make decided breaks in middle life do not seem to regret them, although more regret a series of circumnutations among various occupations before they found the right one.

It would seem that the very fact that man has succeeded in living and conserving tolerable health till advanced years gives a feeling that he has, on the whole, succeeded despite errors and lapses, and there seems to be at least a tacit agreement on the part of all that it is idle to regret what it is too late to help. Old age does not, therefore, seem to be a time of repentance for youthful follies and if this exists at all, it is more than compensated for by a complacency that things have not been worse than they were, and even the possibilities of the latter bring no disquietude.

What temptations do you feel, old or new?
More of my respondents failed to answer this question than any other and most answers were brief. It is very interesting and significant to note that resistances to

anything like confessionalism increase with age. If the old have long walked in ways that society condemns, their secrecy about it has been too long and habitual to be readily broken. This is one reason why psychoanalysis totally fails with the old, so that most analysts refuse to take patients over forty. The German jurist, Friedrich, said that everyone was a potential murderer, because at some moment in his life he had been angry enough to kill and probably would have done so if every circumstance had favored. So the candid and conscientious man who looks back upon a long life realizes that he has done or nearly done, at least in heart, about every crime and yielded and felt promptings to about every vice. Probably everyone, too, had actually done things that if known would expose him to obloquy. Thus the old almost never go to the confessional. Moreover, there is a benign but deep instinct in us to forget things we have done that would disgrace us and perhaps especially those things at which our own moral sense and self-respect most revolt, where qualms of conscience would be so painful that we refuse to face them. And this is connected with the fact that in those churches that stress a radical change of heart, with deep conviction of sin, conversions of the old are very rare. Martial[1] says of the fortunate old Antonius viewing the years behind:

> Back on their flight he looks and feels no dread
> To think that Lethe's waters flow so near.
> There is no day of all the train that gives
> A pang; no moment that he would forget.
> A good man's span is doubled; twice he lives
> Who, viewing his past life, enjoys it yet.

All, of course, want to do just this, so that "the good

---

[1] Book X, Epigram 23 D.

men do" may live "after them," while "the bad is interred with their bones."

Edgar Lee Masters, in a little volume of clever poetic skits,[2] describes the dead in a country churchyard as sitting up, one after another, in their graves and belying their epitaphs. One says in substance, "They called me good and pure but I was a villain"; another, "They called me philanthropic and generous but I ground the faces of the poor and all my charities were to camouflage my selfishness and extortion"; and so on through a long list of rectifications, showing that while men generally follow the precept of saying nothing but good of the dead there may be, after all, at the bottom of the soul a certain impulse to have all the worst in us known. But this is not true of modern life, if it ever was so in the past.

Some of our respondents specified temptations to overeat, to under-exercise, to take life too easy or to be too tardy in throwing off responsibilities, to read or think too much, to be censorious and intolerant, irritable, to resent the cocky infallibility of the young, the excessive urge to speed up, the danger of getting cranky, of brooding; and a few speak vaguely of temptations of the flesh. Nearly all say that they are less prone to yield to temptations than in middle life.

It is perhaps from this standpoint that we see most clearly the danger to which the old are subjected in the progressive loss of self-knowledge. It is very hard for any but the strongest mentalities to realize the changes that age brings, to adjust to, feel at home in, and come to terms consciously with it, so that most would probably be surprised if they knew how clearly those closest to them understood their weaknesses, tolerated their idiosyncrasies, and made allowances for their failures. Self-control, poise, a calm, judicial state of mind even

---

[2] *Spoon River Anthology.*

with regard to things that concern us most deeply, are among the chief, if also among the rarest, virtues of senescence. Everyone carries with him to the grave many a secret that it is well for him and for the world is buried with him; and the impulse to be known even by God Himself exactly as we are, although it has so many expressions in prayers and religious formulæ, lacks in our day, we must conclude, any real depth of sincerity.

What duties do you feel that you still owe either to those about you or to the world?

Some place first the duty of providing wisely and well for their families and friends after their death. A few are oppressed by the thought that they still owe the world far more than they can pay, although one who has lived a life of very large usefulness thinks the world owes him now far more than he owes it. Some have a dread amounting almost to horror of being useless and wish, above all things, to be not a burden but serviceable. A few feel the same old duties, with no change. Others feel called to give to the world, or at least to those about them, advice and admonition based upon the rich lessons of experience. Some who have been lifelong slaves to duty resolve that they will now emancipate themselves and live henceforth according to their own pleasure. Some feel that their time and strength for doing good have so abated that it is vain to try to accomplish anything more and that they must devote themselves to being, instead of doing, good, and would thus cultivate every grace of character and let their light so shine as to be examples to others, so that self-development must henceforth be their chief effort.

In such answers as are before me two things stand out with special prominence. The first is that the men of science, who constitute about one-third of all, have unfinished studies, which they feel it is their supreme duty to complete before their powers abate. It is less often new themes to which they would consecrate their energies than old ones on which already very much work has been done and that they rightly feel no one else could properly finish and that would thus be lost to the world unless they themselves were able to complete it. These men are less intent upon public reforms or special civic duties than upon adding at least a tiny stone to the great temple of science, although only a few in their own specialty will ever appreciate or be benefited by their work. The world has certainly lost much, although probably less than those concerned think, by the death or the incapacitating senility of savants who left an unfinished window in their Aladdin tower. We all think of great novels, which the authors did not live to complete; of promising, intricate researches, which were perhaps bungled by the imperfect reports of the half-competent who undertook to present them to the world; of papers left by the old to be edited by their children or their advanced students, some of which had better have remained untouched; of belabored manuscripts, which survivors can make nothing of and which are perhaps piously preserved for years and eventually consigned to the flames. It is such fates for the children of their brain that some of our respondents seem to dread chiefly and it is this that prompts them to dreams, which are generally fatuous, of literary executors or post-mortem publications.

The most general conclusion from these data is that the old are very prone to develop, if they have not had it before, a kind of educational instinct in the larger sense of this word; they wish to admonish or exhort, if not the world at least some section of it, to better and wiser living, to the acquisition of the knowledge that is of most worth, to the cultivation of peace and amity, or to a simple and perhaps more strenuous and efficient life and to the development of good habits. The lessons they would teach often impress the young as being trite and commonplace, but if they are so, they are charged with a depth of conviction and enriched by a wealth of experience that give them a greater significance than the young can appreciate.

Is your interest in public, community, or in far future or past things, as compared with interest in persons and things right about you, greater or less than formerly?
Here we have two very distinctly opposite tendencies. On the one hand, more frequently in women than men and much more common in the uneducated classes, the horizon of interest tends to narrow to the immediate environment and to the here and now of each day and if health is impaired, the chief concern may be personal well- or ill-being, in which case we see the egoism and selfishness of old age in its extreme form. On the other hand, and as we would fain believe more normally, we have an increase of breadth of view and of interest not only in local affairs of the community but of the state, country, world, and humanity, which may be intensified as decline necessitates withdrawal from more active participation in affairs nearest in time and place. Two great events have had an incalculable influence in this direction that often appears in our data. The one is the World War, the new era of history it has opened, and the whole problem of the future fate of civilization. This has made a tremendous appeal to those of contemplative habits and has stimulated them to follow the course of world events, to study the past and peer into the future as never before, as well as to want to live on to see the next act in the great drama. Suffrage and the new enfranchisement of woman have marked a great increase in public life and opened new spheres

335

of influence for her sex in political, civic, and moral fields that are proving so absorbing that the former tendency which advanced years brought—to focus on persons at closer range and on narrower human relations—is superseded by a new and larger humanism. Not only have these tendencies greatly enriched old age but there is no reason to think they will ever be transcended or reversed. In this sense there has been no age in the world in which it was so good to be old and the last decade or two have contributed far more than any other to give old people a stronger hold on life and to bring it more of just the kind of culture needed for its legitimate development, as well as to very greatly strengthen the will to live.

In what do you now take your greatest pleasure?
While a few find it only in the same sources as before old age supervened, most have discovered new sources of satisfaction or at least find joy in more abandonment to inclinations that had to be more or less sidetracked or almost tabooed before. Reading is most often specified. A few who used to read novels voraciously have lost all interest in love stories and turned to biographies, which they now pursue with almost the same zest as they formerly felt for romance. A few turn to history in general or perhaps trace the earlier stages of the development of their own field of work. Several find a great resource in meditation or even reverie, giving more time to day-dreaming than before. A very few feel a new urge to give some message to the world before they die, and perhaps try, with or without success, to write for publication, while some do so merely for their own edification. Two old professors who have taught successfully all their lives, on ceasing to do so were impelled to address a larger public by print and were dismayed to find their efforts unsuccessful. Others con-

336

fess to a loss of ambition to do anything to better the world but would confine their efforts to making those about them wiser or happier. Many find a new charm in nature, for example, walks in the open, gardening, birds, stars, celestial phenomena, or perhaps reading the works of naturalists and out-of-door observers of animals, flowers, plants, trees; while others, like Socrates, prefer human relations and indulge more freely than before in companionships, correspondence, or perhaps things that absorb them in their immediate environment, or in a wider rapport with current events, and give more time to newspapers, etc. It is not uncommon for cultivated old people to reread the classic standard literature they perused in their youth and sometimes to abandon themselves to the study of the best things in ancient literature, which they had only known before by name and always felt inclined but never had time to indulge in, feeling perhaps that they are thus tardily making up for lost time. Only a few specify greater keenness of æsthetic enjoyment for works of art, music, drama, etc. Men very rarely, and women somewhat more frequently, confess to taking greater pleasure in dress, so that while we only seldom find dandified old men who affect the fashions and dress of youth, women not infrequently feel that as their personal charms decline they must compensate by richness of attire, jewels, and perhaps lavish ornamentation, coiffure, etc. One old lady in the eighties regretted bitterly that lavender was the only color in which she could now dress without criticism. Perhaps excess in this direction is, on the whole, more pleasing than the growing neglect of these things with years, which is so much more common.

Of the three muses, solitude, society, and nature, while all have a new if not stronger attraction it is the first that, from our returns, would seem to increase most with age. Deafness, or perhaps impatience with the

337

overactivities of the young, may weaken the social bonds and physical infirmity may limit contact with nature but nearly all our respondents seek and find solace in themselves more than before. We find few old people who, like many younger ones, have a horror of being alone. Several have daily periods of retreat or retirement when they are "at home" only to themselves, perhaps to digest what they have lately read or to adjust with more equanimity to changes within or without. Thus the old generally find resources within themselves that more or less compensate for their growing isolation, although some reproach themselves or others that they find these resources too meager. One old philosopher says in substance that, realizing that he must sometime meet death absolutely alone and reach a point where he must take final leave of all and everything about him, he feels that he must strengthen his soul by practising for the most solitary of all experiences. Thus there is a certain hermit or recluse motive, which of old sent so many aging persons into the desert, wilderness, mountains, etc., a motif that may possibly have received some psychogenetic reinforcement from the dangers of ill-treatment by their fellows to which in cruder stages of life the old were exposed. It is entirely impossible for youth to fully sympathize with age because this would mean nothing less than to anticipate it, and so the aged often feel, deep in their souls, that there is a slight falsetto or conventional note, even in the greatest consideration shown to them. This condition, in morbid cases, may amount to suspicions of insincerity or a sense that kindness masks the opposite feeling. Happily, however, most of the aged do not seem to suffer acutely from this feeling but accept what is done for them at its full face value.

Nature, on the other hand, is probably at no stage of life felt to be so motherly, so sympathetic, or so full of moral meanings. Quite apart from the nature that science teaches us, the old seem to feel a recrudescence of the old anthropomorphic feeling that once made the nature-myths and has inspired so many of the parables, similes, tropes, and what are now called anagogic interpretations, by which man has read into nature's phenomena the experiences of his own life. The old man feels in a new way that not only all bibles but humanity itself came straight out of the heart of nature, so that contemplation of her various aspects may become for him again a kind of navel-gazing. He sometimes becomes an annotator of weather and temperature, to which he has a new susceptibility, and feels a new kinship not only with the sun, storm, forest, mountain, shore and sea, but even with celestial phenomena. He welcomes the advent of spring with a trace of the old jubilance once expressed in many vernal festivals; feels and is perhaps depressed by the analogy between his period of life and winter; often indulges the hope that he may die in his favorite season and not be buried when the world is ice-bound; and is in the closest rapport with climate and often makes much sacrifice to live in one he has found most favorable. In general, he is responsive, probably far more deeply even than he realizes, to all the moods and tenses in which nature expresses herself. Perhaps his very wakefulness gives him a new rapport with the night through all its watches.

The old who have access to the country often select favorite and generally retired nooks where they can sit for hours and be alone with nature and thus entertain their souls. One old man who did this habitually every summer in a spot in what he called his coign of vantage told me that at each successive year, on revisiting this spot, he was conscious of some deep change, of a certain new sense of closeness to nature's heart, which, although he could not define it, seemed to mark a new step in

his development and which he thought somehow normative for his whole life during the year, for he often
went to sleep thinking of the charm of this place, etc.
The psychology of solitude, both chosen and enforced,
shows that it often brings an almost rapturous delight
in the contemplation of some simple object of nature—
a flower, shrub, insect or tiny animal, which causes for
a moment a kind of temporary focalization that gives
it something of a fetishistic power. All this, however,
does not lessen but perhaps rather augments, by the law
of change and alternation, the growing charm that humanity in the large sense always has for old people who
conserve their faculties. The sphinx riddle, what is man
and what is the worth and meaning of all his strivings,
never fails to come over the matured mind, despite the
fact that it is the most baffling and insoluble of all problems, for "age brings a philosophic mind" and with it
comes a new realization that the greatest study of mankind is man.

*Do you enjoy the society of children, of young people,
adults, or those near your own age more or less than
formerly?*
Responses here differed very widely but certain common traits appear. Those who grow deaf are often
condemned to a progressive solitude and this affliction
has a pathos of its own. The friends we knew in youth
and college are scattered and most of them, and perhaps
most members of our own family, are dead, so that
associates of our own age are generally very few. But
besides this the old often develop idiosyncrasies highly
distasteful to others and we find complaints of the stupidity or querulousness of other old people. Despite the
fact that we have occasional instances of intimate friendships in the latest decades of life, the herd instinct that
prompts each to flock with those of near his or her own

years is less insistent, while with happily married pairs even love seems to take on the character of friendship. There is, indeed, no doubt that the gregarious instinct tends to wane, and as men advance in years they tend to withdraw from clubs and associations, not only because of infirmities but because increased individuation is itself isolative. On the other hand, I think we detect, not only in these returns but in life, a tendency to prefer associates of the next generation, that is, those of such an age that they might have been our own children. Some old men especially state that they prefer the society of men of middle life and it has often been thought that young teachers are best for young and older teachers for older children and that the young have a certain attraction for those near the age limits of their parents. A few of the very old like children, but often with reservations or best at a distance, and are prone to be annoyed by their noise or too great familiarity. It is pretty clear that age does incline to youth and perhaps becomes dependent on it for a kind of vicarious rejuvenation. Old professors often feel in a peculiarly close rapport with those of student years but this is partly due to habit. The old sometimes take, with peculiar interest, to pets and not infrequently have strong likes and dislikes, which they can only explain on the basis of congeniality or antipathy.

There can be no question that old people to-day are just as fond of acting as mentors for the young as they were in ancient Greece, although now it takes the very different form of a propensity to give advice and warnings. But our civilization has not yet found effective ways of making even god-fathers and -mothers really sponsors or assistant parents, although the teaching instinct is closely allied to the parental and is more or less developed in all. It is the testimony of those familiar with old people's homes that their inmates do not tend to fraternize and although crony friendships are not infrequent, there is no analogy to "mashes" or "crushes." Indeed, pessimists have often intimated that no one could really love very old people and so far as this is true we could hardly expect them to love even each other in return.

The above applies more to men than women and the case seems quite different with the latter, who are much more prone to be interested in the young, even in the very young, than are old men. The grandmother may lavish too much, while the grandfather gives too little, attention to the grandchildren. On the other hand, both are often very critical of the larger liberties allowed to and taken by children and find it hard to adjust to new notions and social customs and especially to the now rapidly increasing license given to both their conversation and conduct, which can hardly be said, in its turn, to involve greater respect for age than formerly.

Would you live your life over again?

All answered this question, but three could not decide. One had found it all so enjoyable that he would gladly start over again and repeat all identically. One recoiled "with horror" at the thought and rejoiced every week that it was ended forever. Even the pleasant experiences had such an alloy or aftermath of pain that one subject could not bear the thought of repeating a moment of it.

"What is the use?" said another. "I would probably do the same thing over again." Some would live parts of their lives again or begin at a certain stage. Most would repeat it if they could start with some of their present knowledge or experience and thus improve upon what they had been or done. Most, too, had such a sense of progress that it would seem painful to them to go back to more primitive conditions. Two felt so assured of progress beyond the grave that the future drew them more than the past. One did not see how his life could be materially improved for he had fallen victim to no temptations, made very few mistakes, etc.; while many specified often radical changes they would make, errors or mistakes they would avoid, etc. There were no expressions of remorse; no bitter imprecations of fate, heredity, or nature; no vain longings for rejuvenation; and these data suggest that the vivid pleasures of childhood, the joys of youth, and the intoxication with life that characterizes its immature stages had vanished and left no trace in the memory of these respondents, or perhaps that life had palled and brought a certain satiety. One said:

I have lived three more or less independent lives, as naturalist and explorer for the love of it, as science teacher for the love of it, and as administrator because I knew men and the value of money; and finally, as a matter of duty, as a minor prophet of democracy. If I had the chance I would take them all again. There is pleasure in it and the world badly needs men willing to be counted in the minority.

In the attitude of these old people to this problem the psychologist can glimpse a little of the *tedium vitæ* that perhaps first produced and then discarded the Oriental doctrine of eternal recurrence of life and death, a psychic trend that gave birth to and vitalized metempsychosis and that impelled the Buddha to break away and find a goal beyond it. It needs little psychology to see that such attitudes of mind imply a deep dissatisfaction with any form of future existence that would be in essence a repetition of life here, even with moderate improvements on our present state of existence. A postmortem form of survival or revival that is, in any large sense, a reduplication of this could never bring a deep satisfaction. All ancient creeds and all modern philosophies of recurrence, for example, that of Nietzsche, have always been strongholds of pessimism and are really anti-evolutionary, although they are sometimes said to presage modern theories of development.

To the genetic philosopher it would seem, from such data, that senescents tend to lose the sense that infancy and childhood are more generic than adulthood, that the latter brings the "shades of the prisonhouse," and that every stage of individual development brings added limitations, so that our matured consciousness is only a very partial expression of the vaster life of the race, most of which is more and more repressed and incapable of coming to consciousness as life proceeds. If each of us might have lived very different lives from what we have done, and if many and varied lives are required to express all the possibilities with which we all start, it would seem as if each individual would have chosen, when he had played one part, to assume another in the *comédie humaine* and then another, and so on; that the slave would want to complement his defects of opportunity by becoming king—if not, indeed, *vice versa.* When the psychic life of the race was young and rank, great minds did dream even of living out every phase and stage of life: of being animals, of experiencing every lot and station of humanity. But now that the world is older and the hyperindividuation that comes with age has supervened, this passion to taste everything possible to our estate is lost. Instead of sampling every dish we make a full meal of one and other viands are refused for we are sated. Biology teaches, as we have seen, that specialization is death and a hypertrophied personal consciousness is psychic specialization.

For myself, I confess I even retain in old age some vestige of my strong childish desire to be a horse, lion, ape, dog, fish, and even insect; or, in a word, to know how the world looks from under the skull of our older brothers, the beasts. Still stronger is the wish to have

344

lived as a troglodyte, Indian, to have been a fire-wor-
shiper, totemist, a woman, millionaire, tramp, or even
a moron or a genius—if not, in some moods, to have
experienced various insanities and even diseases. But
strangest of all is the wish that I could be set back to
happy childhood, even if it had to be with the smallest
modicum of the experience I have acquired, and try the
game of life again. It has been, on the whole, so fortunate that I would even repeat it identically, if I had
to, rather than to face the future I do. But the chief
charm would be not so much to improve it and avoid
errors but to vary it and give my more generic self a
less one-sided expression so as to bring out latencies
that are suppressed or slumber and to invest the same
old self with a new set of attributes. I have only seen
one very small aspect of life and know but a single
corner of my own soul and my knowledge of the world
is too limited to my own narrow specialty. The future
not only of my department but of all lines of human
activity is so full of possibilities yet unrealized but which
have aroused such eagerness of interest, that I would
accept another life here under almost any terms in order
to see the swelling drama unfold; while I revolt unspeakably at the realization that I must be cut off when
so many things in which I have the keenest zest are in
the most critical or interesting phase of their development.

Of course I am answering my question in a different
sense than that understood by most of my correspondents. In fact, in a way it was an idle and perhaps
foolish question, because to exactly relive a present life
is so impossible that it is hardly conceivable. But let us
oldsters realize that if we are sated, it is because our
appetite has flagged and not because viands are scantier
or less toothsome. Perhaps we all wish we had been
born later so that we should be now in our prime. Most

of us would probably have sacrificed a few of the earlier, if by so doing we could add a few more to the later, years of our life. Perhaps the very restlessness of old people, their retirement from activity, their propensity to a change of scene or mode of life, or their not infrequent *Wanderlust,* is the result of a blind instinct to exploit unused and submerged faculties and thus to complement or vicariate for the loss of certain possibilities always involved in realizing other careers. Certain it is that even those who do not make a clean break with their past develop views, interests, habits, modes of life, personal associations, or perhaps take pleasure in becoming novices, apprentices, or amateurs, in new fields and find thus a certain rejuvenation, the strong instinct for which has found so many unworthy forms of expression that the term "second childhood" as applied to age is commonly one of reproach and the affectations of youth by the old are ridiculous. We all tend to live our lives over again in our children and grandchildren and this impulse is another expression of the deep instinct for renewal and living other lives again. How shall we explain, too, the so common inclination of the old to plant trees they will never see mature or build houses they can hope to live in only a short time; or to get into and keep in such sympathetic rapport with the young; to engage in works of charity; or to grow tolerant of errors, of persons, and of opinions they once bitterly opposed. What can all these phenomena mean save that the barriers of egoism are falling down and that we tend to live more and more not only for but in others by a kind of sympathetic identification with them. Three of my correspondents had a period of reorienting themselves to new interests as if to find themselves again, which is suggestive of the period in youth when one vocation after another is taken up and abandoned before a fit life purpose has been found.

Whether these tentatives in the old were a recrudescence of a series of earlier circummutations, like those of a climbing vine seeking a fit support, our data do not show.

Did you experience an "Indian summer" of revived energy before the winter of age began to set in?

Only five responses were affirmative to this question. One of the most eminent men of science with a world-wide reputation reported, at seventy-two, that he had never worked so effectively and was now engaged on a program that would require from ten to twenty years of strenuous activity for its completion, besides answering several scores of letters daily. Another scarcely less eminent, at the age of seventy-three, had lately undertaken an arduous line of investigation that would "require many years to complete" but was confident that he could finish it, for "a task is a life-preserver." My returns suggest that men engaged in scientific research have more power to "carry on" than any other class and that those engaged in the professions are perhaps least likely to do so when they cease active practice. Several specify greater mental clarity in seeing through delusions, shams, and vanities. Others feel a certain exaltation at times, dependent perhaps upon digestion or the weather. Others specify new and deeper self-knowledge. Others find much satisfaction in the settling of a few fixed and cardinal ideas or convictions. A few feel new ambitions to begin new enterprises. Several found in the war and its results a mental stimulus that they felt to be rejuvenating and longed and believed that they must live on to see the settlement of some of the great questions now so wide open. Four had observed such awakenings in others. Most, however, felt themselves going on about as before, with no change save gradual abatement of energy. Some felt as strong physically and mentally as ever until they set themselves to some serious task and then realized that this feeling was illusory. Others were sure they would have felt a revival of springtide but for some infirmity or disaster. It is, however, hard for others to judge on this matter and harder perhaps for the individual to answer the question for himself.

The remission of responsibilities and the dropping of burdens would of itself give a certain sense of exaltation, because all such changes involve a new balance between ambitions and accomplishments. Retired clergymen often feel a great relief from being no longer accountable to others for their opinions and some often find a joyful sense of emancipation from old doctrines surprising, not only to others but most of all to themselves. One writes, "I found, on sober second thought, I no longer really believed certain dogmas I had preached all my life and that in my inmost heart I really believed certain things I had often condemned as heresies." He found an intense mental stimulus in thus reconstructing his own creed. A clergyman of seventy-nine once told me he had ceased to preach, even as a supply, because since his resignation his new views gave offense. Old physicians, too, sometimes, though far more rarely and to a less extent, drop as illusions certain fundamental principles by which the practice of a lifetime had been regulated.

Again, the new lines of interest to which the old, set free from the tasks of their lives, sometimes turn show that there is a half-delusive and half-real sense of psychic rejuvenation associated with the pursuit of a new topic. On the whole, however, it would seem that withdrawal from exacting duties, the freedom from the necessity of self-support and the leisure thus resulting, the abatement of the *vita sexualis* and the storm and stress this is now known to cause, the fact that one is now no longer anxious lest he do or say anything that would interfere with his own future career, and the sense that he can both live and think as he lists, would altogether constitute a loud call to revise his views, to get down to fundamentals, be more sincere and independent, to get better acquainted with his inmost self, review his past life, and draw from it its lessons. Morale, as I have elsewhere tried to show,[3] consists in keeping ourselves, body and mind, always at the tiptop of condition and this is ever harder to do as age advances. But I think we may conclude that just in proportion as this is done there is a perhaps prolonged and delightful "Indian summer" that is caused by the kind of mental housecleaning that dispenses with all non-essentials and consists in warming up the deeper emotions, quickening the intellect and reinforcing the will, and that this period combines uniquely the charm of summer and fall without excessive heat and without dangerous chill. All invites to synthesis, for the age of excessive and diverting specialization that is forced upon the young and immature in our day is past and the season for harvest has come. And it is just this that our distracted world now most lacks and needs. Sane and ripe old age has a new sense of values, relations, perspectives; and no form of culture man has ever produced is ripe until the fruitage it contributes to morals and life has been garnered. To show how all our achievements affect human conduct is the thing the world most needs to-day and needs far more than at any other period in history. This is what our age calls so loudly upon the old to supply. Just in proportion as civilization advances and life becomes more and more complex and distracting, the need of older and wiser men increases, for only from their outlook tower can things be seen in their true perspective. Wells's new

---

[3] *Morale: The Supreme Standard of Life and Conduct*, New York, D. Appleton Co., 1920. 376 pp.

349

conspectus of history represents the old man's view and one of my correspondents writes that in a long literary life he has never come upon anything quite so stimulating and absorbing. It is this sort of work that should have been done by an old man and such tasks can only be accomplished by those younger men who have the rare power of genius to anticipate the choicest gifts of age. Plato saw that the proper business of old men was to philosophize; and what is religion, to which so many senescents turn, but a condensed philosophy put in the form of symbol, myth, and rite.

Old women, perhaps even more than old men, seem to enjoy an "Indian summer" of life. The best of them grow serene, tolerant, liberal, often devote themselves with great assiduity to charity, to causes, to helpful and intelligent ministrations to others, perhaps with utter self-abnegation; while others carry on affairs, conduct enterprises of moment, and really guide all about them without their knowledge and without realizing themselves that they are doing so; still others read with an abandon that they have never experienced before and are often wise in counsel, even subordinating their own daughters, husbands, and perhaps sons in a way that suggests the possibility of a new matriarchate. They sometimes develop a therapeutic skill that is a modern analogue of the old grandmother's medicinal herb-lore and is as unexplained as the old countryman's weather wisdom. They are almost always more religious than old men but rarely dogmatic or theological and often grow indifferent or almost oblivious of the creeds they affected in their earlier years. Thus they illustrate at every stage of life what is true of all its stages, that woman lives nearer to the life of the race, is a better representative of it, and so a more generic being than man, and is thus less prone to dwarfing specialization.

Do you rely more or less on doctors or find that you must study yourself and be your own doctor?

In the answers to this question there was a general consensus to the effect that doctors were resorted to only in emergencies of illness, accident, or perhaps surgery, and several mentioned the old saw to the effect that in the fourth or fifth decade a man is either a fool, an invalid, or a physician to himself. Only a few followed the practice of having a look-over at intervals as a prophylactic. Two had special friendships for a particular doctor, except for whom they would have no use for the profession. Several expressed their gratitude to physicians who were responsible for a vacation, a tour, or other change. Several had turned away from the regulars to homeopathy, osteopathy, or Christian Science. Some allowed doctors to examine and prescribe and then used their own judgment as to how much of their medicines should be taken or prescriptions followed. Some relied much upon physicians who had known them personally for a long period or practiced in their family but had little faith in new physicians. One doctor professed loss of confidence in his profession and had "returned to nature." A few had found fasting of from twenty-four to forty-eight hours beneficial for most of their ailments. None doubted, and several expressed very special gratitude to specialists, particularly ophthalmologists and even surgeons. There is a very general aversion to drugs, although a few dosed themselves for years, tried many patent medicines, and one thought he had exhausted almost all the pharmacopœia. Aging people often regret the replacement of the old family physician by experts who in prescribing for one defective function ignore and perhaps injure others. Occasionally old people of both sexes retain or revert to old family traditions of the virtue of herbs, which played such a great rôle in the ancient days of the herbalists. We find, too, outcrops of the fear that surgeons are too ready to operate. One old man told me that in a recent illness it took him a month to get over the disease and three months to recover from the effects of the medicines the doctor had prescribed. Another followed the precept of young doctors for special and acute, and old doctors for general, troubles and for prescriptions of regimen. It is often deplored that while women's diseases, troubles of sight, throat, lungs, abdomen, and children's disorders, have each their own specialists, there are almost none who have specialized on old age and that when the old are seriously ill, there is a general tendency in the profession to give up hope too soon, to pay less attention to those who because of age and its feebleness will die soon anyway. We have frequent illustrations of remarkable recoveries of old people who had been given up by physicians.

It must not be forgotten, however, that medicine has made great strides in the last few decades and that the older generation now passing has not yet come to a full realization of the new resources that the advances of modern pathology and the other sciences that underlie the healing art have brought to it. Perhaps we might commend to the aged, when they first fully realize that they are old, the course of one of our respondents, who made a round of the specialists for the different organs to reinforce his own hygienic self-knowledge, although he found the prophylactic prescriptions of the different experts so contradictory as to be often practically impossible. Unhappily, however, we have no agencies to examine the whole ensemble of parts and functions and suggest modes of life fit for each individual, as for example, the Life Extension Institute should do. Nothing is more certain than that every senescent should, with increasing frequency, have himself looked over that he may anticipate, at as early a stage as possible, the onset of the many physiological failures that impend.

Do you get more or less from the clergy and the church than formerly?

All answered this question, with surprising unanimity and but slight reservations, negatively. A few still loved church services, had clerical friends whom they loved and respected, went to church for the music, enjoyed university preachers, reread portions of the Bible with edification, etc. Many thought the clergy insincere or ignorant, too absorbed in money-raising, preposterously antagonistic to science, or found the same uplift in reading other great literature as in the Scriptures. Over and over we find statements to the effect that the writer has become his own high-priest, minister, oracle, captain of his soul, no longer in need of ecclesiastical mediation with the divine, etc. "Why is the church still so apologetic when science does not apologize for Copernicus?" "Why has the church waged such bitter warfare against Darwinism, when evolution is only another and better name for the revelation of the divine and should have brought such enlargement and reinforcement to religious thought and feelings?" One eminent artist finds all the religion he needs in art; students of science find it in nature; students of the humanities, in the study of the deeper nature of man. The beautiful is just as religious, if not more so, than the good or the true. "There is only one great word in the world and that is *love.*" "I preached all the doctrines and found some truth in many of them but have rejected most, and perhaps the form of all, as pulp and rind." "Each of us must work out our own salvation." "My religion is the Red Cross." Several who had been brought up pietists and had attached themselves to various churches in turn had, in later years, withdrawn from all and come

353

to depend on their own reading and meditation. "The clergy are blind leaders of the blind." In one case church was discontinued because the assumptions of pulpiteers aroused "all my porcupine quills." Some had ceased to attend divine services because they seemed irreligious compared to the deeper religion they find within. The higher criticism has brought insights to some that the church knows not of and "my real conversion was from, not to, the church. It knows and can teach us nothing about the hereafter."

Thus, in general it would seem, if our meager returns are at all typical, that the clergyman makes less appeal to the old and knows less about ministering to their nature and needs than do physicians. It must not be forgotten, however, that, as one of our respondents says in substance, the views of those this questionnaire appealed to, people of intelligence and culture, are exceptional, and probably the majority of the uneducated have at least a falsetto belief in some institutions and teachings of the church. Our returns indicate, however, the same growth of skepticism with years as that found by the far more extensive conspectus of J. H. Leuba,[4] from which he gathered that the percentage of those who believed in God and immortality decreased both with age and with education.

Do you think or worry about dying or the hereafter more or less than formerly?

Here, as was to be expected in our age of transition and *éclaircissement,* there is the utmost diversity. All my respondents answered but only four of them (three women) found anything like the orthodox religious consolations afforded by the hope of a personal immortality. Most were agnostic. "I know as much about it as anyone

---

[4] *Belief in God and Immortality: A Psychological, Anthropological, and Statistical Study,* Boston, 1906.

who ever lived, which is absolutely nothing." Four were distinctly pantheistic and found pleasure in the belief of extinction, annihilation, or absorption into the cosmos like a drop of water returning to the sea. About one-half had lost confidence in sacerdotalism and had no connection with any church and a few were bitter against ecclesiastical assumptions. Most had ceased to worry about death, a few professed never to think of it, two dreaded the pain they associated with the act of dying, and one prayed that the end might be instantaneous. Men of science wished and hoped that they might go on "thinking God's thoughts after Him" with renewed facilities and incentives for getting nearer to the soul of the great *Autos*. One's life-long religion seems to have been based on the analogy of the chick in the egg who regarded hatching as its death, when it was really coming into a vaster life. Most disclaimed all terror, although two in their youth had felt that this might recur in second childhood. The attitude of most might be described by the phrases: "one world at a time and this one now;" "consider the duty of the present moment and leave the rest;" "never be anxious concerning anything beyond our control," etc. One wished to die like a pious Buddhist in thinking on his good deeds. One expressed a strong contempt for a god who would tolerate an orthodox hell and several felt that they would sooner or later become wearied to the point of ennui with a heaven according to any conception of it. Most had reckoned with the chance of death in the plans of their business, making their wills, etc., but believed that all thought concerning the hereafter was a waste of energy. Several found consolation only in influential immortality and wanted to live on in the memory of their friends and in the service they had rendered to others, although this idea was generally connected with thoughts of plasmal immortality or living on in their offspring. One good old lady I knew who had spent a life doing good works and had always attended church said, in answer to this question, that she had been so occupied in active services that she had never found time to think much about theology but in her heart doubted all doctrines, was not at all sure that she believed in either God or immortality, and was convinced only that whatever happened would be all right. Old clergymen seem particularly prone to suffer from doubts, sometimes of the most radical nature, and even wonder if after a life of zealous propaganda they may, after all, have been wrong. Several professed themselves more deeply religious, as they understand religion, than the church itself, and even insisted upon a larger, deeper faith than orthodoxy dreams of.

It would seem, from these and other data, that the fears of death are by far most intense in youth, and that in moments when the tide of life ebbs and there are great griefs or disappointments—not only in love, where it is most marked, but along other life lines—a terrible and sudden envisagement of death often arises, although this mood is generally flitting and soon passes. When in age the forces of life abate, death has already begun its work and if belief in personal immortality remains it is sustained and fed chiefly by poetic metaphors or similes that have little justification before the bar of reason and are essentially tenuous and sentimental. Certain it is that inhibitions of the life tide do not so readily prompt thoughts of suicide; though if they do so, as statistics show, the thought of it is more likely to prompt the act of self-destruction in the later decades than it is in youth, when nearly all coquette with these thoughts. The curve has two crests, one in adolescence and the other in senescence.

The chief psychological inference seems to be that the old generally refuse to face squarely and come to terms with the death-thought consciously because it is more fatal to them than to the young, but fly to every kind of relief from it by diversion to other things and themes. In age there is often a narrowing of the intellectual horizon to the immediate environment and this itself is opiative. Thus nature alleviates in the old the fear of death, which impends and which they know to be near. They sometimes wonder just how it will come but rarely dwell upon such details as their own obsequies or leaving last messages and think more often, if their thoughts stray to such subjects, of the effects their demise will entail upon the course of life of others. The fact is, the race has always found death too terrible to be faced in all its horrors and has camouflaged and disguised its grim details by tombs and avoided the direct envisagement of it by focusing attention upon the soul that survives in ways we shall see more clearly hereafter.

Some individuals' returns transcended my rubrics and have a value in themselves that merit, and I hope will find, publication in full elsewhere. One man known and loved wherever the English language is spoken, who died in 1921 in his 84th year, had the supreme good fortune for nearly thirty years to have the almost daily association and assistance of a sagacious lady physician who entered sympathetically into all his interests and became his literary executor and biographer. This venerable man, so buoyant in his writings, grew depressed as age advanced, especially toward nightfall, although this is nowhere expressed in his books but abounds in his diaries. He developed an interest that seems abnormal in everything pertaining to diet, tried scores of new foods and drinks, only to discard them one after another, and became so averse to tea, coffee, and smoking that it was hard for him to tolerate those addicted to them. But it was on the problems connected with constipation and evacuation that his interest seems to have become most exaggerated. In his converse even with the young but especially with those near his own age he constantly reverted to this subject and his favorite theme of conversation seems to have been on topics of personal and especially dietary hygiene. He studied the chemistry of nutrition and corresponded with experts upon the subject and attempted to carry out upon himself all their findings as he understood them. Eggs he thought more or less poisonous and for a time he seemed almost to think that the hens that laid them could not be suitable food. His idiosyncrasies in this field would constitute a unique theme for study that would have lessons all its own. He was always checking his appetite and experimenting upon and observing himself. There were, in this case, somewhat unique signs of an Indian summer. He wrote twelve books from the age of 30 to 64, and fifteen from 64 to near 84. At 64 he felt that he had written himself out but soon struck other veins, so that his later books cannot be called inferior to his earlier ones. In editing poems of Nature at this time he found so many aspects of it that poets had overlooked that he undertook to supply the gap and had a period of rhyming that lasted about a year.

This suggests another octogenarian I knew, a great leader in mathematics and a man of international fame, who in his latest years believed that he had poetic gifts and wooed the muses, even the goddess of love, with canticles that amazed his friends, who wondered whether he was just making his acquaintance with poetry for the first time or had known it more discriminatingly earlier in life and lost his standards. Another eminent man I knew whose name is known throughout the literary world, and who was also a physician, believed in and practiced frequent naps, in which I have seen him indulge between the courses of a long public dinner, in the intervals of which he would converse with all his old sprightliness and vigor and at the close make the best speech of the occasion. There was no record of even midday sleeps with the naturalist above described. He usually did his best work in the forenoon but occasionally, even in the last years of his life, worked till late at night and resumed early in the morning, doing this for some days as with a kind of afflatus. He also kept up an active interest in public affairs until his increasing illness compelled him to narrow down his interests more and more, so that toward the end they seemed to center entirely in himself.

A man of eighty ceased manual work at fifty and had a marked intellectual renaissance and became an author. He has come to realize the limitations of doctors and, although he employs them, is his own ultimate judge in all matters pertaining to his health. He has withdrawn from the influence of the clergy. "My science and reason say that there is no hereafter while my faith says that there is but I do not give myself any trouble about their quarrel for it will all be decided soon enough." "I am more disposed to take the far view of things and try to estimate wider relations than formerly." "I feel that my duty is to the race and to humanity rather than to any section of it." He reads science and occasionally a good story, although the latter "must have some interest besides that of love." "I formerly was fond of hunting and fishing but the killing instinct has faded with age, as it does with most people; but the forest and field, the sea and land, are beautiful beyond compare and their infinitely varied forms are more bewitching than ever." Everyone, he thinks, should have some Bohemia into which he should retreat when overtaken by age and has leisure, and his has been genealogy, mainly getting acquainted with his own ancestors and trying to visualize them as men and women, feeling that he owes to them all his qualities, mental, moral, and physical.

A liberal clergyman approaching the eighties after a life of unique eminence and service writes: "As for a future life for the soul of man, I believe it is a moral necessity to explain and justify his ethical conduct in the present sphere of existence. If, nevertheless, after death there should be no continued existence, individually and consciously, I am ready to accept this solution as also wise and right because ordained by Him who is all-wise and good—'I cannot drift beyond His loving care.'" He believes that his devotion to great causes that he has seen advance, while "conserving divine ideals below, which ever find us young and ever keep us so," has contributed to his exceptional vigor and his message to the young is to prepare for old age physically, economically, intellectually, morally, and religiously. He grows more charitable and appreciative, feels deep personal gratitude to physicians, who have more than once saved his life; blesses his long-lived parents for the rare constitution that has not only carried him through but given him a recuperative power at which he has often marveled, dreads the excess of sentiment he often notes in others of his age, who too readily become lachrymose; deplores the excessive freedom and growing self-affirmation, lack of restraint and modesty, courtesy, and thoughtfulness for others in the rising generation; thinks, with Goethe, that if as he grows older he has less keenness of sympathy for suffering, he thrills more deeply in the contemplation of every noble and disinterested act; finds satisfaction in knowing that his ashes (for he has long been an advocate of cremation) will lie near other dear ones on a beautiful hillside in sight of the Pacific; and takes satisfaction in reviewing his life from a large ethical standpoint.

QUESTIONNAIRE RETURNS

A naturalist of seventy-two of international reputation, who has done perhaps more creative work for the benefit of the human race in his field than any other living man, first realized that he was old at sixty-five, when digestion and elimination were very slightly reduced. Feeling the need of companionship he married at sixty-seven and found increased happiness and rejuvenation. Frail when young, he learned early to take better care of himself, restricting the amount of starchy foods and stressing the importance of the daily use of one ounce of agar-agar, one ounce of wheat bran, and half an ounce of liquid paraffin, which has become an absolute necessity. He writes three hours and works his head and body outdoors eight hours per day, covering rarely less than twelve miles. He is not only his own doctor but has often helped others by his experience. "I never worry about dying or think of the hereafter," he says. "I have done good work for my fellow men, have never injured, over-reached, or cheated a human being in all my life and hope to live in the hearts of others so that my works and words may be of value to those who follow." "I have no earthly or heavenly use for the clergy or church; am my own minister to my soul." "I have no regrets whatever for anything I have ever done through life but have been 'done for' several times by others." "Since about fifty I have taken more interest in public and community affairs and the future life of those who are to come after." His great temptation is physical and mental overwork, which it requires constant care to curb. "I am now in the 'Indian summer' of mental clarity, finding myself able to do very much heavier and better work than at any other time in life, and only wish I could continue to carry on these experiments throughout the ages but am limiting myself to experiments that will not last more than ten or twenty years." He receives several score letters a day and is editing a comprehensive work of eight volumes describing perhaps the most complicated creative work that has fallen to the hands of man to do.

One of America's most eminent educators and leaders in science, and the creator of a great university, who has made his mark on the world as an advocate of peace, believing, however, that when we were once in the war we should push it with the utmost vigor, regrets only that he has, on one or two occasions, been misunderstood. He has traveled and lectured very extensively and is widely known by his books outside his own specialty. He ascribes his vigor to his early life on a farm and his outdoor life as a student of nature. Although he became a doctor of medicine in 1875 he has had occasion to feel the deepest appreciation of the services a few other members of that profession have rendered him. He says: "I have good friends among the clergy and often preach to them. They have no special pull on my future. I shall probably have to go out alone; I came in that way." He writes:

> When man shall come to Manhood's destiny
> When our slow-creeping race shall be full-grown
> Deep in each human heart a chamber lone
> Of holies, holiest shall builded be;
> And each man for himself shall hold the key,
> Each one shall kindle his own altar fires,
> Each burn an offering of his own desires,
> And each at last his own high-priest must be.

A Quaker lady of seventy-four has reread Emerson, Browning, Tennyson, Shakespeare, and other masters, and found them more intelligible and charged with meaning than ever before. Hence she is convinced that she has a new mental clarity, not only in regard to these but to the fundamental questions of life. She shrinks from companionship with the very old and infirm but loves society more than ever, especially of those somewhat younger than herself. She feels no temptation except to indulge too much in day-dreaming, has less love for young children individually but found more enthusiasm than in anything else in a cause that saved the lives of many and improved the condition of yet more. She is deeply religious, reading the Bible daily and hoping to see her departed friends in another life, although "I have my doubts."

One venerable respondent wrote in substance that no words could describe the rest and peace that slowly supervened after he had ridded his mind of every vestige of the old belief in which he was trained of a future personal life and realized that he would live on only in the contribution he had made to the sum of human knowledge and welfare, in the grateful memory of his friends, in his posterity, and that his individuality, with all its limitations, would be resolved into or rendered back to the cosmos with his mouldering corpse. When he realized that death would end all forever for him and was once free from all the harassing hopes and fears about a postmortem state, the new serenity and poise made him believe that he had penetrated to a deeper psychic level than that explored and bequeathed to the Christian world by the marvelously gifted but epileptic apostle, Paul, and that he had struck the bedrock of humanity and attained a fuller and larger completeness of life as it was meant to be and will be if man ever comes to full maturity. He compares the attainment of this new attitude toward death to the change that took place in Bunyan's Christian when he turned his back upon the city of Vanity Fair and faced the Delectable Mountain.

An able respondent who has given much attention to these subjects concludes that deep in his soul every candid mind feels that all arguments for immortality are more or less falsetto and do not ring true, are factitious, and are neither born of nor have the power to bring inner conviction. Their propounders, if they are honest to the core and also if they have the power to analyze their own mental processes in constructing such so-called proofs, feel, though they may not know it, that they are really reasoning against their own profounder convictions or seeking to convince themselves against their own intuitions. They vilipend skepticism because they hope thus to drown its still small voice in themselves. In no other field of thought does it begin to be so hard to be sincere with ourselves and in no other domain of belief do men accept such specious and inconclusive evidence. Most demonstrators of immortality within the Christian pale fall back sooner or later, some more and some less, upon the myth of revelation and the postulated faculty called faith which, when we study its psychology, turns out to be only a hope-wish born of the unspent momentum of the will-to-live and this deploys in the individual in which it is thus falsely interpreted, as egoism wants it to be. Rich and rank as have been its products for the imagination, they are fancy bred and, in fact, superstitions, extra-beliefs or *Aberglauben* of the psyche and their acceptance as authentic or final is always and everywhere a craven flight from reality, for the sentence of execution is already passed upon all of us and is only suspended for a season.

One thoughtful respondent who is facing his sunset years says that he has heard some sixty-five hundred sermons and has reversed certain of his opinions so that he has felt compelled to resign as a trustee of his church since he has a new and clear idea of the kind of church he wants. He cannot longer believe in the kind of deity who likes to be flattered, thanked, entreated, and listen

364

to Te Deums. "We inherit such ideas from vain Oriental kings." "Symbolisms a thousand years old are not suited to us or to our times." "I cannot subscribe to that stock idea—'the religion I got from my mother's knee is good enough for me'—for by the same token we should now be idolaters or Druids." "Now that the church has become a man it ought to 'put away childish things' and should no longer use 'bottles' and ceremonies two or three thousand years old." "If we judge the church by its results in suppressing selfishness or even vice, it is a failure and any other agency in any other field or business not being able to show any better and faster results, that is, in reducing crime, unrest, selfishness, and hate between classes, races, and nations, especially as evidenced by the experiences of the decade 1911-1921, would have to resign." "If Christianity had not been, almost from the very start, handicapped by the church in creating irrelevant and quarrelsome issues and diverting emphasis to a future life, instead of improving the conditions of the present one, it is fair to say that our present social, moral, and spiritual condition would have been very different from and better than it is." The church atmosphere, hymns, prayers, sermons, ceremonies, "are all age-musty and dominated by and saturated with miracles and sanguinary and puzzling atonement and trinity theology, things with which I am no longer in sympathy and the emphasis of which is offensive to me." "I think all these things are man-made incrustations. I sometimes think the wonder is not why so many men stay away from church but why so many attend it. Religion must be rescued. I do not know how but it has got to be done."

CHAPTER VIII

SOME CONCLUSIONS

The early decades of age—The deadline of seventy—The patheticism of
the old—The attitude of physicians toward them—Fluctuations of youth
—Erotic decline—Alternations in the domain of sleep, food, mood,
irritability, rational self-control, and sex—The dawn of old age in
women—Dangers of the disparity when December weds May—Sexual
hygiene for the old—Mental effects of the dulling of sensations—Lack
of mental pabulum—The *tedium vitae*—Changes in the emotional life—
Age not second childhood—Women in the dangerous age—Need of a
new and higher type of old age—Aristotle's golden mean and the magnanimous man—The age of disillusion—Increased power of synthesis
—Nature's balance between old and young—The eternal war between
them—Superior powers of the old in perspective and larger views—New
love of nature and the country—Their preëminence in religion, politics,
philosophy, morals, and as judges—Looking within and without—Merging with the cosmos—The three ways of escaping the decay of civilization.

To learn that we are really old is a long, complex,
and painful experience. Each decade the circle of the
Great Fatigue narrows around us, restricting the intensity and endurance of our activities. In the thirties the
athletic power passes its prime, for muscular energy
begins to abate. There is also some loss of deftness,
subtlety, and power of making fine, complex movements
of the accessory motor system, and a loss of facility for
acquiring new skills. In the forties grayness and, in
men, baldness may begin and eyesight is a little less
acute so that we hold our book or paper farther off.
We are less fond of "roughing" it or of severe forms
of exercise. We may become so discontented with our
achievements or our environment that we change our
whole plan of life. In the fifties we feel that half a
century is a long time to have lived and compare our
vitality with that of our forbears and contemporaries

of the same age. Memory for names may occasionally slip a cog. We go to the physician for a "once over" to be sure that all our organs are functioning properly. We realize that if we are ever to accomplish anything more in the world we must be up and at it and give up many old hopes and ambitions as vain. Perhaps we indulge ourselves in certain pleasures hitherto denied before it is forever too late. At sixty we realize that there is but one more threshold to cross before we find ourselves in the great hall of discard where most lay their burdens down and that what remains yet to do must be done quickly. Hence this is a decade peculiarly prone to overwork. We refuse to compromise with failing powers but drive ourselves all the more because we are on the home stretch. We anticipate leaving but must leave things right and feel we can rest up afterwards. So we are prone to overdraw our account of energy and brave the danger of collapse if our overdraft is not honored. Thus some cross the conventional deadline of seventy in a state of exhaustion that nature can never entirely make good. Added to all this is the struggle, never so intense for men as in the sixties, to seem younger, to be and remain necessary, and perhaps to circumvent the looming possibilities of displacement by younger men. Thus it is that men often shorten their lives and, what is far more important, impair the quality of their old age, so that we yet see and know but little of what it could, should, or would be if we could order life according to its true nature and intent. Only greater easement between fifty and seventy can bring ripe, healthful, vigorous senectitude, the services of which to the race constitute, as I have elsewhere tried to show, probably the very greatest need of our civilization to-day.

In the seventies we often begin to muse on how our environment will look and what our friends will do when we are gone; and now the suspicion, hitherto nebulous, that there are quarters in which our demise would be welcome may arise to consciousness and perhaps take definite form. There are those who, also perhaps unconsciously, are waiting for our place or positions and so we grow hypersensitive to every manifestation of respect or esteem and not only resist being set aside or being superseded but seek to find new kinds of service that will be recognized as useful. The seventieth is the saddest of all birthdays and if we "linger superfluous on the stage," we feel that society regards us as, to some extent, a class apart; and so we instinctively make more effort to compensate our clumsiness by spryness and gently resist the kindly offices and tokens of respect to which the young incline or, perhaps more often, are taught to render the old. We are a trifle more prone to lose or mislay things, perhaps almost resent the family's solicitude for our glasses, slippers, cane, overcoat, diet, and quiet. We have to give ever-increasing time and attention to health and to nursing ourselves and in many exceptional experiences feel that we are seeing persons and may be doing things for the last time. All our plans and efforts and prospects directed toward the future have a new element of uncertainty and tentativeness. We can easily be spoiled by kindness or soured by neglect and our own personality requires so much attention in making the new adjustments that are necessary that we are in new danger of becoming selfish; while our nerves are liable to grow irritable and there is a new trend to depressive states as our activities abate.

It is not strange that one of our grievous dangers is patheticism. One who begins to suspect waning love on the part of those in his sphere may come to accept and even crave pity in its place and farther on in the infirmities of age a husband or wife may do the same and magnify to their partner ailments and symptoms to this end. A little farther yet in this direction lies what may be called the hysteria of senescents. We may come to love to be waited on more than is needful and thus grow into a fictive helplessness and dependence on the ministrations of others. We love to pour our troubles into sympathetic ears and may be spoiled by the too great devotion of our married partner, sons, or daughters, whom we sometimes permit to become slaves not only to our infirmities but to our very whims and notions. Who has not known old people otherwise excellent who almost seem to have lived by the precept of never doing for themselves anything they can get others to do for them. There are fathers who, with no thought that they are selfish, monopolize the love and services of their daughters, and mothers who do the same of grown sons, and these of the younger generation may lavish upon their parents the devotion that was meant for a mate or a family of their own. We know that marriage, when it comes to such people, is likely to be unhappy unless the wife is in the image of the fondled mother or the husband in that of the too much loved father. We are prone to forget that for the old, as truly as for the young, it is more blessed to give than to receive and that we must not insist on our rights and forget that each has its corresponding duties. The old are rarely oppressed by a sense of gratitude and may come to feel that because they have reared their children they have laid them under obligations of a return service that can never be fully discharged, forgetting that beyond certain limits they pay us best by rendering the same service not to us but to their own children. Most of us are or are destined to become a real burden and this we should strive to delay and lighten and not to accelerate or increase, and we should not come to make a luxury of our sense of dependence. Thus if the old have savings, however small, they should never expropriate but retain and use them wherever and when their help will be most serviceable. The fact that we have withdrawn from larger outside activities naturally inclines us to strive to be of compensatingly more account in the smaller circle left us but this must not make us arbitrary in this narrowed field for self-assertion and we should not feel that as we become less important to the world we must become more so within the family circle. We have, in fact, a new place and must exert ourselves to learn and keep it, without interference with those who are taking ours or making their own careers.

In his dealings with such cases the physician needs a special sagacity. He must realize the great satisfaction it gives his aged patients to have him listen patiently and sympathetically to all their ills and should encourage them to trust him fully and with no reservations. This not only shields others but by humoring the wise doctor can not only gain full confidence but may be able to bring such patients to see their own selfishness and thus effect a real cure even in their physical condition. I have known cases where such ministrations were a benediction to the family. Where old patients have thus built up a system of half-fancied ailments, placeboes may work wonders, the therapy being in fact chiefly mental. Such insidious dangers to which the aged are exposed cannot be reached by medicaments but rather by pithiatism in the sense of Babinski or persuasion in the sense of Dubois, Merchenowsky, Rosenbach, or Herbert Hall, who heal by prescribing activities, physical and mental, found possible after painstaking analysis. The old often feel a falsetto invalidism that may be cured by a vigorous appeal to their moral sense or, again by changes in their daily program or regimen or by exposing them to fresh streams of rich outer impressions that correct the mental stagnation to which

SOME CONCLUSIONS

they are prone or keep their attention from themselves by giving their minds a larger field and a far-off focus, as against their inveterate tendency to mental short-sightedness.

In youth erotic fetishes and pet, instinctive aversions are now known to play an important if half-unconscious rôle in love between the sexes. Eyes, hair, lips, cheek, neck, or any of her little ways of movement or speech may become a focus of special charm to the young amorist. Conversely, other or even the same features, traits, automatisms, or habits may mediate no less unconscious dislike.[1] Some of the same rapports or repulsions exist between the old and the young. The former may even have their favorite children or grandchildren and dislike others in ways they themselves could only inadequately justify. This partiality is most pronounced between fathers and daughters, mothers and sons. It is the chief factor not only in what is called love at first sight but of first impressions of strangers, which are proverbially so hard to efface. Thus what we deem trifles may loom large.

The old are particularly prone to develop peculiarities which, if they do not unconsciously alienate those nearest and perhaps dearest to them, are real handicaps to their devotion. Of this the old are rarely aware, and if attention is called to them they minimize their importance. These might be listed and weighed like their analogues in the erotic field. The roster of them on the negative side would be long. There are faults in table manners, modes of eating and drinking, using table utensils from the napkin on, etc. Mastication may be noisy or otherwise subtly disagreeable, or there is slobbering, clumsiness, or neglect of common conventionalities once observed. The toilet may be neglected, the attire soiled or spotted or imperfectly put on, and so a

[1] See my *Adolescence*, vol. ii, p. 113 *et seq.*

371

look-over needed before we go out. We do things or make noises in the presence of others that once we only permitted ourselves when alone and there is a new indifference to personal appearance. The voice is impaired in volume, richness of inflection, and articulation; our face or form are no longer æsthetic objects; we mislay things and invoke those about us to help find them; and are tediously slow in mind and body. If, in addition to all this, we become pryingly overcurious, fault-finding, exact, and forgetful, we give our friends more to put up with than we realize, and the best of them would be shocked if they became conscious of how much they repress in their psychic attitude toward, if not in their treatment of us. On all such matters we should make frequent self-surveys. On the other hand, if we cultivate not only order and control but, above all, the poise and repose of those seeking the Great Peace, striving always to do, be, and say only our best things, we may make ourselves not only respected but loved in a new way, so that we shall be turned to not only for advice but for companionship and help in emergencies and make some of even the most obtrusive signs of physical decay attractive by association with the higher qualities of soul, as the ugliness of Socrates came to be almost loved by his disciples. Art understands this and many of its masterpieces depict old age in its glory. The same is true of literature and even of the drama, despite the fact that actors who specialize in old women's and particularly old men's parts so often make age repulsive and ridiculous, for it has always been a most attractive field for caricature.

The old are subject to certain fluctuations, new in kind, degree, or both. Sleep is less regular. They have good and bad nights, one or more of each alternating, which make the next day clear or cloudy with dregs. If fatigue comes more quickly, so does recuperation by rest. They are often refreshed by a very brief nap or by recumbency, or even by a period of solitude during the day. Thus on the periodicity of day and night is superposed one of less amplitude or briefer duration, perhaps after one or each meal. Thus the distinction between the sleeping and waking state comes to be less sharp, slumber is not so deep or long, and the dreamy states of reverie invade mentation by day. The great restorer does not quite make losses good and the accumulation of these deficits explains very many of the phenomena of old age, which might be characterized as sleepiness for death, the rest that is complete and knows no waking. Capitulation to the siesta habit is marked in some by a distinct improvement of condition. They speak of a new balance between activity and repose and sleep all the better nights, while others resist such tamperings with nature's rhythm and if they acquire the midday habit find themselves nervous or less refreshed the morning after. Some retire and rise with the sun and find a certain elation of spirits in this reversion to nature and praise the morning hour or even sunrise, of which the urbanized world about them knows little and ever less; while others find a virtue in lying abed late. While we know too little of the hygiene of the aged to prescribe, it is certain that they tend to break with the old regulations and really need some of the indulgences they are often too inclined to permit themselves.

The appetites fluctuate and may readily become capricious. Some would eat more and less often than before and love to experiment with new viands. Some think some items of diet once beneficial become harmful and so eliminate them, while some like and can digest things impossible before. Sometimes they indulge for days or even weeks in a favorite dish that at intervals they cannot touch with impunity, as if there were spells of immunity broken by intervals during which the same article produces deleterious results. One says that what is at one time a food becomes for him at another time a poison. This seems particularly true of certain fruits, while the acid balance seems very liable to upsets. Most tend to overeat and are always struggling with their appetite. Yet they often have periods when foods lose their attraction, as if Nature decreed a fast. Here she is often right and a day or more of relative or even entire abstinence may prove helpful. So the former diet periods do not need to be observed; nor need the old be coaxed at such times with tempting food.

Springtime is hard on the assimilative processes of all but especially on those of the old. This is partly because the tides of life everywhere set toward genesis rather than toward individuation but still more because the calorific elements of food need to be essentially reduced and also because winter's supplies grow a little stale before summer ripens her produce. So, too, with the abated activity that years bring the need of food is reduced and hence the old can often thrive on a small percentage of what they formerly needed. Most, too, not only learn to avoid hearty meals at night but find it best to lay in most of their rations earlier in the day. Very many find in diet their chief center of interest and solicitude and the most active theme for theorization, so that in many cases more and more mentation seems to center about alimentary functions. There are very active inductions from experience and constant modifications of views hard to change in other fields. There does seem to be often a change toward either increased sensitiveness or torpidity of the alimentary tract. A few grow especially susceptible to seasoning, condiments, flavors, and even confectionery. They may become even connoisseurs in wine, tea, coffee, tobacco, while others grow indifferent and insist that they like and can eat almost anything. Nutritive ups and downs are thus more marked than before. Tendencies to decrease in weight are distinctly more favorable for prolonged life than the opposite tendency to obesity. Indeed, the former seems normal.

There are alternations of mood. Depression may be acute to-day and vanish to-morrow, depending not only upon sleep and nutrition but the weather and incidents, perhaps trivialities, in the environment. Irritability may alternate with apathy and the old may lose self-control and anon exercise a high degree of it. Some days they feel comfortable and even vigorous and on others are miserable. Now weak organs or functions, heart, stomach, bowels, rheumatism, or whatever be the besetting troubles, are much in evidence and symptoms may grow dangerous until the old have a new sense of the fragile hold they have upon life, which may end suddenly in some of these weak moments. Then these symptoms intermit and they feel well and take heart again till the next "spell." A few never allow themselves to be caught without some one or more trusted drugs kept handy for immediate use in emergencies and much, too, might be written of "warnings" and their sometimes epochal effects upon both the inner and outer life. Thus the old may sometimes give way to their feelings and become stormy, lachrymose, perhaps even violent, and they may react from this to a state of almost philosophic poise, which passes upon even their own outbreaks with objective detachment and psychological interest, phenomena that we may call the "apologetics" of old age. Thus emotivity and reason may succeed each other.

The old are very dependent upon weather, climate, and seasons. Winter is hardest on them. Not only does it mean more indoor life and less activity but cold is one of the chief enemies of the old and winter is also supercharged with subtle and profound symbolisms of their own stage of life which deploy more beneath than above the threshold of their consciousness. What old person does not shudder at the thought of being buried in snow and ice. Even the autumn is for them full of somber analogies of the stage of the sere and falling leaves, of the ripening and garnering of the fruits of the earth, of the first blighting frosts. All the old long for the rejuvenation of springtime and perhaps daydream of it when nature is snowbound. Some keep diaries of wind, temperature, and storm and become weather-wise, while those who can, seek warmer climes, especially when winter begins to break, a season statistics show is most fatal for the old. The poet who sang that he could endure anything but a series of bad days must have had the psychic barometry of old age. Thus we draw nearer to nature, our source and our home.

Even sex often does not decline and die without terminal oscillations in its course and in extreme cases apathy and aversion may alternate with abnormal erotic outbreaks dangerous alike to the health of the individual, to domestic happiness, and even to public morals. Those who have led lustful lives may resort to unnatural and illegal forms of vice and thus illustrate the various perversions of this function. While only a few indulge in orgies, very few fail to note occasional spontaneous but transient calentures here suggestive of potency long after it was deemed "closed season." Such recrudescences, though they seem to be nearly always only partial, are very prone to deceive and may lead to follies. Instead of being indulged, cultivated, or even welcomed, as by an inveterate fallacy too prevalent with the young they too often are, the old should rigorously ignore and suppress all such manifestations in this field. While the full realization of impotence brings a psychalgia all its own, it also has physiological and psychological if not conscious compensations, while belated and, especially, stimulated activity of reproductive functions not only can never result in offspring of value to the world but saps vitality and accelerates the decay of every secondary sex quality of mind and body, so that complete chastity, psychic and somatic, should be the ideal of the old. They should be not only embodiments of purity but the wisest of all counselors in this field. Only to those in whom asceticism and sublimation have done their perfect work will there come an Indian summer of calentures for the higher ideals of life and mind, while those who fail here can never know the true and consummate joy of old age.

For myself, I frankly confess that the longer I live the more I want to keep on doing so. Hence in the last two years of retired leisure I have given far more time and attention to personal hygiene, regimen, and diet than ever before and have mildly experimented with myself in many ways. I have tried eating two and four meals daily, going early and late to bed, forcing myself to lie there a fixed number of hours and at certain times again retiring and rising with no regularity as I felt like doing. I have tried systematic rub-downs, self-massage; cold and warm, frequent and infrequent baths, have equipped a modest gymnasium and taken mild but systematic exercises with various apparatus and then abandoned all this or done nothing of it without an inner prompting. I have followed prescribed diets and tried many special foods, interested myself in vitamines, beginning with Eddy's manual and trying out vegex preparations, although no one has as yet studied the effects of any of the three species of vitamines upon old age, as has been done for other stages of life. I even used olive oil, which so many of my correspondents praise both for internal and external application, stopped smoking for a week, which seemed greatly to prolong

377

each day after thirty years of mild addition to nicotine, corrected for a time and then yielded to the senescent's tendency to constipation, experimented with alcohol in several forms, even with Pohl's spermine tablets and minimal doses of phosphorus, etc. But out of all these moderate hygienic adventures I have so far found no topping specific. It would be interesting to try out the gland-grafting experiments which seem to have regenerated the famous Vienna surgeon, Lorenz, and others, and I think I would gladly offer myself as a *corpus vile* for the Steinach operation to study its psychological effects at first hand. Although I have found in the above experiences a few things that I so far believe helpful to me, I have derived from them all no advice to offer others except, if time and inclination favor, to try out all things for themselves. Plenty of moderate exercise out of doors, active intellectual interests, both just to the point of healthy fatigue but no more, are fundamental. One must have insight and considerable power of self-observation to profit therefrom. But the main thing is to develop and maintain at its highest possible morale a rigorous and unremitting hygienic conscience that will never let down but always enforce the doing of what we know to be best. Otherwise we may eat, sleep, work, and generally do or not do what seems best as we list. I am even skeptical about the almost universal counsel for tranquillity and against worrying, for more or less anxiety is not only the normal lot of man but it gives a tonic sense of responsibility which we all need.

Special forms of pleasure that have to be prepared for attract us less but we find soul-filling satisfaction in just living, contemplating nature wherever we happen to be, eating, sleeping, and in common converse. All these things acquire a charm unknown before, while "occasions," events, and sights that are rare and afar lose their charm. Thus we come to love each hour of each

378

day and the most wonted and commonplace experiences, while our work (for no one can be happy without some task) even though it seemed drudgery before becomes attractive because we can do it when and as we will and as much or little of it as our strength permits or inclination impels. Meanwhile friends grow nearer and dearer, enmities fade, and we enjoy converse with those toward whom we were formerly indifferent or even averse. Thus old age may become the most satisfying and deeply enjoyable stage of life. Hitherto the rest cures we prescribed have been more or less reversionary to youthful or even primitive scenes and activities. It may be that this is wrong and that for all such cases we should prescribe for the young or middle-aged the occupations, attitudes and regimen of the old and that this would be more therapeutic.

Sensations and movements are the basis of mind and when these are reduced, as in old age, we often have the phenomena of mental starvation because the supplies of mental pabulum are lowered. If the old have little society and do not read, their psychic powers of digesting their experience run down, not from any inherent weakness but because they are on short rations for data. The mills could often grind as fine and as much as ever, and possibly more so, but the grist is lacking. Thus there are two opposite trends in the old. On the one hand, their physical state demands attention to themselves so that they tend to have "too much ego" in their cosmos, grow subjective, and may become hypochondriacal or preoccupied with their own personal problems. The simple decree of nature is that we must give more care to our health and morale and it is excess, defect, or perversion of this deep instinct that causes so many of our pains and our ill repute. Here lies our chief need of personal study, psychoanalysis, and reëducation. The other trend is in the opposite direction, toward depersonalization. We need to look out, not in; to forget self and to be absorbed in objectives. We are impelled to escape our environment and interest ourselves in things that are remote in space and time, in nature, the stars, great causes and events, personalities, masterpieces, to escape from our miserable selves by their contemplation. We cannot see the countenance of things for their soul. It is this fugue from self that perhaps impels us to so many of our petty pastimes and diversions: solitaire, idle reveries, our predilection for amusements, fussiness about our things; as well as, on the negative side, to neglect our person, really of dwindling value in the great world and soon to be effaced. All these phenomena are outcrops of the tendency by which "the individual withers and the world is more and more," for our fate is depersonalization and resumption into nature. These symptoms are anticipations of euthanasia or, to use a phrase now current in psychology, they are extrovertive and not introvertive, just as the old were meant to be.

Thus the old need a higher kind and degree of self-knowledge than they have yet attained. They need to be individually studied and analyzed to avoid the new, peculiar, and not yet understood dementia præcox now so liable to supervene upon the youth of age. This is all the more needful now that the intensity of modern life with its industrial and managerial strain compels earlier withdrawal from its strenuosities. We live longer and also begin to retire earlier, so that senescence is lengthening at both ends. Hence, again, the need of midwives to bring us into the new world of higher sanity now possible to ever more of us. Both we and our civilization now so checked, disoriented, and misled by immaturities are in such crying need of a higher leadership that is not forthcoming! We are suffering chiefly from unripeness. The human stock is not maturing as it should. Life is so complicated that the years of apprenticeship are ever longer and harder, so that we are exhausted ere we become master workmen in our craft and the rapid age turnover this involves robs us of too many of the choicest fruits of experience.

Our retirement, even if gradual and not dated, calls attention to our age, and to our little world we grow old a decade the day it learns that we have stepped aside while to ourselves we may and ought to feel that we grow young that day by yet more. The springtide of a new stage of life stirs our pulses and we feel something of the care-free happiness of another childhood. Our intimates often remark signs of a new vitality, physical and mental. If we are normal and not too spent, we feel new hopes, ambitions, make plans to surpass our old selves and to at last be, do, say, enjoy something really worth while. As we pass our life in review, stage by stage, up to the present, it seems so incomplete, fragmentary, tentative, and altogether unsatisfying that we almost wonder whether it was we ourselves who really lived it or someone else whose career we are following with an objective detachment never felt before toward our own ego. Certain it is that a new veil falls between us and our past, gauzy and transparent though it be. Our psychic nature did not intend us for the rôle of reminiscence so persistently assigned to and so commonly accepted by us. Our juvenile memories are but the ragbag vestiges of a vaster experience that had to be forgotten to be completely incorporated in our personality and to ascribe too much significance to them is the fetishism of senility. If we write up our lives, we can make them interesting and valuable only by using our better information about and more sympathetic rapport with ourselves with the same impartiality that a close and discerning friend would do if he had all our data. It is for the things of the present and for the problems of the future that our mental vision becomes clearer than ever before. Our wish and will to achieve and make our insights known and prevail acquire new force.

How different we find old age from what we had expected or observed it to be; how little there is in common between what we feel toward it and the way we find it regarded by our juniors; and how hard it is to conform to their expectations of us! They think we have glided into a peaceful harbor and have only to cast anchor and be at rest. We feel that we have made landfall on a new continent where we must not only disembark but explore and make new departures and institutions and give a better interpretation to human life. Instead of descending toward a deep, dark valley we stand, in fact, before a delectable mountain, from the summit of which, if we can only reach it, we can view the world in a clearer light and in truer perspective than the race has yet attained. It is all only a question of strength and endurance. That is the great and only but, when we squarely face it, a staggering proviso. In all essentials we are better and more fit than ever before save only for the curse of fatigability, for age and death are nothing but fatigue advancing and finally conquering life. One single example of a hale old man dowered by nature and nurture, as immune from tire as youth is, would give the world a new idea of senectitude.

We were told that the days and years pass more quickly as we advance in age. What could be more false! Not only do the nights, of which sound sleep once made us unconscious, often drag slowly through their watches but each day is so long that we often find time hanging heavily on our hands; and when we have done all the work we can, we turn to our friends to amuse us and seek and perhaps invent pastimes or fresh occupations to kill it. Sermons, lectures, meetings of all kinds, even the drama, seem long. The winter lingers until we almost fear that spring will never come or out-of-doors attract us again. When we have to wait for things, the time stretches as if there were no limit to its elasticity, and when we turn to reveries of the past, it is a last resort from the *tedium vitae*. We really have time for anything and to spare. It is the demon fatigue that makes us so in love with diversion, for rest is more and more frequently sought and found in change.

They say our emotional life is damped. True, we are more immune from certain great passions and our affectivity is very differently distributed. But what lessons of repression we have to learn! If the fires of youth are banked and smouldering they are in no wise extinguished and perhaps burn only the more fiercely inwardly because they cannot vent themselves, as even the Lange-James theory admits for repressed feelings, inhibition of which really only makes them more intense. We get scant credit for the self-control that restrains us from so much we feel impelled to say and do and if we break out, it is ascribed not to its true cause in outer circumstance but to the irritability thought characteristic of our years. Age has the same right to emotional perturbations as youth and is no whit less exposed and disposed to them. Here, as everywhere, we are misunderstood and are in such a feeble minority that we have to incessantly renounce our impulsions. Marie Bashkirtseff has betrayed the secret of how the pubescent girl, and Karin Michaëlis, of how the woman of forty feels, but no one has ever attempted to explain the sentimental nature of aging men or women. Even Solomon and Omar Khayyam presented only the negations and not the reaffirmations of the will-to-live.

Thus it is no wonder if the old often best illustrate what Henri Bordeaux describes as "the fear of living." René Doumic thinks that there is a new disease in our old civilization and that many in their prime only make a pretense of living. "We value our peace above everything and wish to keep it at all hazards, however dearly we must pay for it. We shun responsibilities, avoid risks and chances of struggle, flee from adventure and danger, seek to escape from everything that makes for the charm and value of life. We no longer have any faith in the future because we no longer have faith in ourselves." How well this applies to those brought face to face with the last stage of life! The fact is, we must find and make new pleasures as well as new modes of escaping and mitigating the pains of body and mind and must learn anew how to love, hate, fear, be angry, pity, and sympathize aright. The serenity ascribed to us would pall and bring stagnation. It is a profound psychological truth that "out of the heart are the issues of life" and our heart is not dead; on the contrary, emotivity probably increases with years and most expressions of it, unless they become more sublimated, strongly tend to grow more crass and stormy. We were never more interested in things, persons, events, causes, in life itself. Slights rankle, neglect chills, attentions warm, affronts incense, and praise thrills us, and if we grow censorious, it is because our ideals of conduct and motive have become higher and purer and we are in a greater hurry to see them realized. We cannot help these gropings toward a new dispensation and their very persistence is the best reason for believing that they will sometime find their goal in a better stage of things and an improved race of men not in another world but here. Perhaps some of even what we now call the whimsies of the old will be seen to be the labor pains of humanity, which is striving thus to surpass itself, to improve the stock, and to really bring in a new and higher type of man.

Old age is called second childhood. This is all wrong

for there is nothing rejuvenative about it. Childhood is the most active, healthful, buoyant, and intuitive stage of life; age, the least so. What is there really common to the morning and evening of life? We even lose much of the power we once had to understand children and if we love them, we want them at a distance, while they in turn understand and like us little by nature. They inherit far less of the results of experience with grandparents than with parents, for less of us have survived to see them and the latter often resent or even criticise our relations to them. We are nearly as immune to their prevailing faults as to their diseases. They listen to our stories but do not crave our cuddling, are jealous if we usurp the offices of their parents to them and are usually a little less free in our presence. Nature has established an old and close rapport between one generation and the next. Even young teachers get on best with young, old with maturer pupils. M. L. Reymert[2] says that his general study shows him that teachers below twenty and over forty are of less influence than teachers between these ages. The most efficient man teacher is generally from 25 to 35. The best woman teacher has a little wider range—say, 20 to 40. But of course mental and physiological age are different. Helen M. Downey "Old and Young Teachers," *Ped. Sem.,* June, 1918, concludes, on the basis of questionnaire data, that the younger teacher has other interests that keep her bright and cheerful; the older teacher excels in mental and the younger in dispositional traits; the old are careless of appearance and this does not appeal to children; the older rule by discipline, not by love and kindness; the young teacher more often overtaxes her strength; the old are more set in methods, fixed in opinions, resent suggestions for improvement. Many suggest there should be an age

[2] "The Psychology of the Teacher," *Ped. Sem.,* vol. 24, p. 531 *et seq.*

limit of 60. Health and temper suffer. There are often negative psychic idiosyncrasies. Older teachers lose contact. Social traits are a very great factor in consideration of the period of rapid growth. Dispositional qualities are more impressive than any other. The favorite teacher is enthusiastic, energetic, young. Pupils' estimates do not involve age when they speak of old and young. I know an old and successful professor, interested in his work to the end, who, when he retired with powers little abated and much work yet to be completed, found that in his speech and writing he imagined himself as no longer addressing minds in the student, even graduate, stage, but wished to be at home teaching and learning from those not under forty, for at that age real wisdom begins, the effects of special training having then faded. A refocalization took place in his mind that involved not only new methods but, yet more, new topics and subject matter. What student, however mature, would care for and what curriculum in any university in the world would include, for example, the theme of this volume. And who but a *Greis* would ever have found its preparation a fascinating task! No, the old are not childish but, if they are normal, have simply reached a stage of postmaturity that involves much of what Nietzsche called the transvaluation of all values.

But if we can no longer see over the crest of the divide that separates age from youth, if the acclivity is shut off, we do see more nearly and clearly each step of the declivity and find the catabasis of life no less zestful than its anabasis was in its time, while we have the great advantage that comes from the power of being able to compare the two and this itself opens rich mines of thought. The age of the sage has bid a final adieu not only to all puerilities but to the callow ardors of the ephebic stage. He is graduated from adulthood and turns, as by an eschatological instinct, to ultimate human problems, of which younger minds, though they may be attracted to them, can have only premonitions. To hear and heed this call is the strength and glory of those who are complete "grown-ups." The trouble with mankind in general is that it has not yet grown up. Its faults, which we see on every hand, and the blunders that make so large a part of history are those of immaturity. Man has always felt the need of guardianship and because he lacked wisdom invented immortal omniscient gods—tribal, national, or cosmic—to guide him and as embodiments of what he felt lacking in himself. It is just this need of an all-wise providence that the old will come to supply if and as humanity slowly ripens.

If and so far as it is true that a woman is as old as she looks and a man as he feels, all this processional, especially its early stages, is, on the whole, probably much harder for her than for him. She feels not only that "the coming of the crow's foot means the going of the beau's foot," but the first wrinkles about the mouth, eyes, or under the chin; the loss of fullness about the neck, to which folklore attributes such significance; the first sagging of the cheeks or the bust; the first signs of fading complexion; or the first gray hair, give her bitter food for thought. Her cult of the mirror, that man progressively eschews, increases. But woman commands far more resources against all such heralds of decay than man and gives vastly more time to compensating for them. Youth is her glory and she has more comeliness to lose than man, who can, however, never quite rival the hag in ugliness. She has also great powers of compensation by affecting girlish ways and has a stronger hold on her youth than man and old women do not feel as old as old men do. Throughout married life, if she is well, woman usually assumes the rôle of the younger mate, even though she be not so in years. Though sexual involution comes to her earlier she remains in far more sympathetic touch with the young than her husband, so that there is a half truth and not mere gallantry in the saying that a woman never grows old.

The woman just beginning to feel passé has a psychology all her own of which even the devotees of that science know little and she herself yet less, but of which Michäelis in "The Dangerous Age" has given us a few glimpses. Love, wifehood, and motherhood, as the world knows, constitute the very heart of woman's life and as the chance of these supreme felicities begins to fade, something, which it is no extravagance to call desperation, begins to supervene. Its processes may and often do deploy so deep in the subconscious regions of the soul that even she is but little aware of the transformations that are taking place there. These she quite commonly ignores, camouflages, or honestly and resentfully denies. The psychopathologist sees most clearly the tragedies of aborted Eros as they are writ large in morbid symptoms. But with the same causes and conditions, the same processes are always more or less active, however repressed, and the unmated woman before the close of the third decennium has generally come to some terms with the death of the phyletic instinct within her, which is the core and mainspring of her life, and has dimly anticipated all the significance of old age.

Happily for her dawning senescence, it is one of the great achievements of our age that she has found a splendid vicarious function in culture and new social, vocational, professional, and political services, so that she can now give to mankind much that is best in her that was once confined to the narrower sphere of domestic life, and be little or none the worse but perhaps the better for it. This great emancipation is building a new and higher story to her life, so that as the amative, heyday charm of her youth begins to abate she need no longer despair. All her earlier occupational training that fits her for self-support, complete or even partial, is, thus, anticipatory of this third new stage of life that the senium now begins to reveal to her. This gives her now a certain advantage over man. Thus she has found a new call that means not only more safety but priceless service, to which all her superfluous energies can be devoted, and the world now waits with an eagerness that is almost suspense to see whether she will have the courage to grapple with the most vital problems that confront her sex and find the wisdom to solve them or, neglecting these, be content with the effort to do man's work in man's ways.

Thus, woman is older than man in the same sense that the child is older than the adult, because her qualities are more generic and she is nearer to and a better representative of the race than he and also in that she sublimates sex earlier and more completely, entering the outer shadows of senectitude in the thirties. But she is also, at the same time, younger than he in that she is less differentiated in tissues or traits, less specialized and in her early decades must learn better than he to conserve so much that is best in the physique and *esprit* of her youth. If her physiological change, when it comes, is more marked, abrupt, and datable, the psychic changes she undergoes are far more gradual and imperceptible, while her sympathy with youth and even childhood, and in general not only her moral but all her normal instincts, which are the best gift the adolescent stage of life has to offer, are keener and surer.

This critical age has its own peculiar temptations to which woman entering middle life sometimes succumbs. She, like man, is prone to ask of the future whether it is all to be like the present or past and, if so, what is to become of the unfulfilled dreams of youth. The Prince Charming never came; or perhaps her ideal has proven only a clay image; or her affection, or his, may have found another focus that seems worthier. Hence it is in no wise strange that some women, hitherto good by the old standards, now make a break with their past, impelled to do so by an augmented desire to taste all the joys of life before it is forever too late. Not only does it seem intolerable to go on to the end as they are but there is perhaps some tempter who detects and waters these seeds of discontent and helps the middle-aged woman on to feel that she has been a coward to life. Beaudelaire, who certainly thought he understood French women, said that for most of them at thirty-five who are married and perhaps for even more who are unwed, anything was possible. Even curiosity is a spur to adventure and fancy, if not conduct, may prompt to cast off all restraints. "Why not?" is a question that incessantly arises and every answer seems unsatisfactory. And how many of us can qualify, by being without sin, to cast the first stone at those who fall here. Such women are too old to enter upon a life of vice but often form secret and occasionally very happy alliances with, usually, older men, which may last for years without involving any abandonment of their stated occupation or leaving the ranks of respectability and with now, unquestionably, a growing disposition on the part of society to condone, even though it may suspect or even know.

Again, as we men grow old, we recognize that we have lost something of whatever attraction we have had for the other sex generally and often come to regard most of its members as somewhat trivial and to prefer the society of other men. Even the love of husbands and wives happily married takes on a different character; and they are fortunate, indeed, if the losses are balanced or compensated for by the gains, as they should ideally be, or if friendship waxes as erotism wanes. The old beau who devotes attention without intention to younger women can, at best, only amuse and rarely interest them, although they may feel subtly flattered Sometimes they find delectation in cajoling him and playing upon his weaknesses and they may also come to indulge in a freedom of speech and manner with him that they would never permit themselves with men of their own age; while, conversely, friendships between older women and younger men are always more sincere. The case of the doddering dotard with the flapper is rare, save in the literature of senile psychopathology and medical jurisprudence, where it is by no means uncommon. But this we shall not here discuss.

Senescent men are also too prone to attribute the other manifestations of their own abatement of philoprogenitive energy to the lessened ardor of their wives and perhaps to invoke the abnormal stimulus of some wild love to sustain, or at least to test, their vigor, not realizing that such a course accelerates rather than retards the involution that comes with age. The jealousy felt towards young, ardent wives by their older husbands lest they be made cuckold constitutes probably a far less frequent triangle and involves, on the whole, less suffering than that experienced by wives who are growing frigid with years toward their still lusty spouses. The age disparity of the climacteric may open a door for suspicions, however groundless, which may secretly sap the foundations of conjugal harmony. In this connection one must always take account of the fact that there is not seldom in man an Indian summer, of months or occasionally years, of enhanced inclination toward sex before its final extinction, as returns elsewhere reported show. From personal confessions and medical literature, studies made in old men's homes, and sporadic evidence from other sources, I am convinced that for a very large proportion of old men the progressive loss of potence, with all the complex phenomena attending it, is one of the chief, and in many cases the very most psychalgic, experience of all the changes involved in growing old. There is a very pregnant sense in which a man is as old as the glands that dominate this phase of life. Laymen, including most physicians, know very little of and find it hard to credit the devices that may be resorted to to retard this atrophy or often to conserve and even enhance the vestiges of this function, the excessive activity of which is the surest preventative of a happy old age. While there are those who late in life resort to vicious and even pathological modes of gratification, those who became debauchees in youth or middle life very rarely even attain old age and all should heed the motto to "beware the Indian summer of eroticism." Who has not observed among his personal acquaintances, to say nothing of men conspicuous in public life, the tragic consequences to health, occupation, and even life, that follow when December weds May; and what shall we say, even from the eugenic standpoint, of women who prefer to be an old man's darling to a young man's slave. We know, too, that children born of postmature parents are liable, if they mature at all, to do so precociously and to show early signs of senility, just as children born of those of premature age often fail to reach full maturity. If contraceptive methods are ever justifiable, it is to prevent offspring of both but perhaps especially the former kind.

On the other hand, we have many clinical cases in which after years of impotence from psychic causes the removal of these latter not only restored the procreative function but relieved the patient of often grave symptoms and brought marked mental rejuvenation. This has been often recorded, especially for men. In some instances, apparently, children have been born after such a period of dormancy or latency that has lasted for years. Not only is the downward slope of this curve far more gradual than its pubertal rise and, as we have seen, attended by more oscillations but there is far more individual variation in the age at which decline begins and ends, so that one man's norm would be another man's disaster and perhaps doom.

The old should be able to think most dispassionately upon such themes and should feel it incumbent upon them to transmit the wisdom born of their own experience and observation to the younger generation. In certain primitive races and modern societies and communities the old, usually of the same but sometimes even of the opposite sex are expected to initiate the members of the rising generation in the mysteries of sex. We now know the dangers and sometimes even incestuous tendencies with which such a course is sure to be beset; and if parents attempt to discharge this function for their children, or wherever it is done personally, there are perils. Indeed, none of the methods of sex education, of which so many have lately been proposed, have been entirely satisfactory. Perhaps this kind of training really ought to be one of the special functions of grandparents and they should prepare themselves for it. At any rate, while we have learned much in recent years of sex psychology, pedagogy, and hygiene for the young, we have almost no literature, and indeed know almost nothing of it for the old; and this despite the fact that they are in the greatest need of it and have practically no help in the solution of the novel and intricate problems they must now face, as best they can, alone.

One reason why treatises on the climacteric are so few and so inadequate is that the importance of the subject has only lately been recognized even by psychiatrists, gynecologists, or gerontologists; while another and more important reason is found in the extreme reluctance of the old to tell. Psychoanalysis is impossible unless it can overcome resistance, which it is often put to its wit's ends to do. Modesty and perhaps prudery have veiled the physiological and, far more, the psychological aspect of this function. This instinct of concealment is no less, and probably far greater, in the old. They balk, evade, and deceive the investigator at every step. Psychoanalysts have strangely neglected this theme and generally even refuse to take patients of over forty or fifty years of age. What can be learned in homes for old men is usually by observation, from attendants and from inmates' talk of each other, and those who answer questionnaires almost always fail to note facts even remotely related to this theme. Still, in this *terra incognita* we occasionally come upon the naked truth, only to realize that the retreat of Amor is the counterpart of its advent, as autumn is of springtide. What nature gives so prodigally in pubescent and adolescent years she garners with no less circumstance and no less attention to details, so that we are left, in the end, with no less tendencies to "polymorphic perversity" than before these were constellated into the normal sex life of maturity. Even some of the proclivities to autoerotism and homosexuality may arise. Amatory reveries may increase as dreams of this character decrease and there are often flashing recrudescences of desire.

Despite or after the long and sometimes acute perturbations of the *vita sexualis* as it draws to its close, there is very commonly a new and deep peace. We are glad that the storm and stress are passed and that we are henceforth immune to passion. This is doubtless the normal and, let us hope, increasingly common course. The sexes approximate each other in both traits and features as they grow old and thus if we can no longer love women sensually, we have a new appreciation of the eternally feminine, its intuitive qualities, and its more general and moral interests. Old women acquire a new power of sensing things from man's point of view and hence companionship between old men and women may become a noble surrogate for carnal love. Happy the old who can enjoy comradeship on this plane with a congenial member of the other sex and thrice happy is the very rare case of well-mated couples who find, when the time comes, that they have qualified for this consummation of their union with each other!

Folklore, especially in its grosser forms, but also classical and medieval,[3] and even modern literature—medical, psychiatric, and most of all the writings of psychoanalysis—abound in descriptions of the tragic results that ensue when husband and wife do not grow old together or when their age disparity is too great. Even in the purest, most loyal, and best mated pairs there is often a period of unspoken and perhaps half unconscious suspicion and jealousy, which each partner regrets and tries to banish from waking thoughts, outcrops of which often appear in dreams. Roués have always felt that the young wives of old men were their legitimate prey. The former seem more liable to fall before temptation than if they had remained single. Bitter, indeed, is often the lot of Senex who dotes on a young bride and seeks to atone by lavishing gifts and providing every kind of service and social enjoyment that infatuation can suggest for waning marital potency. While society austerely and even ostentatiously condemns such a wife who errs, it secretly judges her to be not without some excuse and has little pity, and often only covert derision, for such a husband.

Yet more pathetic is the converse case of the aging wife of a spouse yet young and lusty. The sense that she is losing her charm for the man she loves is gall

---

[3] See Burton's *Anatomy of Melancholy*, sec. 3.

and wormwood to her very soul. She, too, seeks to atone by making herself physically more attractive, not only to him but to others that he may see their admiration, by every kind of personal ministration and often by seeking literary, artistic, or other success outside the family circle. She becomes painfully conscious of the attractions of younger or otherwise more favored women whom her mate meets and easily grows suspicious, not only with but often without cause. She may feel the lure of incentives other women use to attract men which her pride will not permit her to cultivate, although she may make concessions to these more or less unconsciously. Tendencies thus repressed may find outcrops in other fields and may even take the form of symptoms, perhaps of fears for the well-being of her mate, even of physical harm, business failure, social disgrace, or perhaps religious heresy. In other cases she may be at last forced to admit infidelity on his part and then it is that she finds herself face to face with the dour problem of either trying to ignore or condone, and perhaps conceal or excuse, his fault to others and living a hollow life of sham and convention on the one hand; or of openly breaking and separating and living henceforth a more or less isolated life, on the other. She must thus very carefully weigh not only her own material interests but the future of her children and the chance of pitiless public scandal.

In the medical literature on the menopause (Kisch, who studied 96 cases; Laudet, 95; Tilt, Faye, and Mayer, 97 each; and especially the more philosophical Börner and Currier) we find very little save records of physiological and anatomical changes, so that it has remained for the Freudians to exploit the perhaps far more important psychic changes that characterize this stage of life. The love life in the new and larger sense in which this is now coming to be understood is the very heart and core of woman's nature and it plays a vaster rôle in the life of man than had till lately been suspected. Whatever thwarts or diverts the *vita sexualis* from its normal course brings all kinds of disasters in its train. About all the transformations of senescence root in the fact that by this recession of the life tide we are gradually cut loose from the more vital currents of the life of the race and individuality now has its unique innings. The debauchee, who marries perhaps late and after long experience with women of easy virtue, often finds a modest wife disappointing and misses all the arts of allurement he had found in his orgies. So, too, when the happily married man finds the earlier ardors of his wife growing cool, he is only too liable to suspect waning affection, when in fact nature is only following her inexorable course. He may even wonder if, in the inscrutable ways Eros has, his wife's fancy may have unconsciously strayed to some more engaging man or fallen a victim to some baseless suspicion of him, or at any rate grown weary of his advances and perhaps come to a new and deeper realization of some of his faults or limitations. Feeling that their present relations are not all they once were, he fails to recognize that it is the very nature of love to grow sublimated as years pass and to become more and more an affair of the soul, as it perhaps once was of the body; and that it is just at this critical point that it normally becomes richer, riper, and more truly devoted. The wife's impulse to minister disinterestedly to her husband is never so strong or pure as at the moment when the power of giving complete physical satisfaction first begins to wane and it is at this epoch that it can so easily and naturally be transmuted into the impulse to serve, help, enter into closer and more sympathetic mental relations, to know more of his inner life, struggles, ideals, ambitions and even his business and in general to enlarge the surface of personal

397

contact. This is thus the psychological moment for man to interest his mate in the affairs he has most at heart and to make her a partner, perhaps even of some of the details, of his own vocation. This golden opportunity, however, is brief, and if it passes unimproved it will soon be forever too late and each mate will, ere long, find him- or herself starting on devious ways that will lead them ever further apart.

Conversely, when a young wife first realizes that her husband is aging, she should understand that nature now impels him to compensate for physical by mental devotion and she may have even to face some form of the above choice whether it is better to be an old man's darling or a young man's slave. In him this is the nascent hour for becoming interested in her inmost wishes, aims, feelings, ideals, and to help her actualize them. In extreme cases he may come to devote himself to dancing attendance upon her wishes and even whims unless she herself has the good sense to restrain him from this fatuity, for by cleverly humoring and restraining him she can just now make him very plastic to her will. Thus her problem sometimes is to save him from an infatuation for her that might become ridiculous and that some wives are foolish enough to love to display. She must, however, learn to develop in and accept from him better succedanea for the more libidinous eros and to do this she must enter more sympathetically and intellectually into his life, as instinct now impels him to enter into hers. The impulse in the physiologically younger partner of every married pair to anticipate the age of the older one, if wisely met, may result in greater sanity and more true happiness for both. Who does not know fortunate cases where just this has occurred, rare though they may be and many as are the wreckages that have resulted from too great age disparity? If the wife tends to be in the mother image and the husband in the image of the father, a rich and rare blend of parent and mate love is sometimes seen. The feelings of the ideal bridegroom for the ideal bride are never without a strong ingredient of the affection he once cherished for his own mother, while one factor of her love for him was transferred from or first developed toward her father. At the same time each has a small ingredient of parental feeling toward the other, as if they were each child and each parent to the other. In all such unions the younger partner rejuvenates the older far more than the older ages the younger.

In all of us oldsters the problem of personal hygiene looms up with new dimensions. In our prime we gave little attention to health. The body responded to most of the demands we made upon it. If we were very tired, we slept the sounder. We paid no attention to minor ailments, which soon righted themselves. We ate or drank what, and as much as, appetite called for; exposed ourselves to wind and weather, heat and cold, wet and dry, with impunity. We could go without sleep a night or two if necessary and feel but little the worse for it; could abuse our eyes, nerves, heart, digestion, muscles, and more or less escape all evil consequences; could work at top speed and with an intensity that rung up all our reserve energies for days or weeks if need be, and could feel sure that our good constitutions would enable us to bear the strain and to more or less promptly recuperate. But now our credit at the bank of health begins to run low. We must husband our resources lest we overdraw them. Overdoing is a veritable bugaboo. There are certain symptoms we must never disregard on pain of days of lessened efficiency. We have had one or more signs of special weaknesses we must heed. There are some things that we must rigorously refrain from eating or doing. There is a weak organ, too, that must be humored. Appetite has perhaps been too keen and must be reined in. We must select the items of our dietary with discretion and self-restraint. A typical respondent says he can still indulge his love of hill-climbing, bicycling, swimming, and even skating, and exercises with diverse gymnastic apparatus that he has had set up in his garage, to say nothing of golf, which he holds to be best of all, and autoing, which has become with him a veritable craze. All these things at the age of seventy-five he still does occasionally but is becoming shy of doing so lest he be thought trying to seem young. He lately stole out alone at twilight to skate, when one urchin called to another, "Hey, Johnnie, doesn't that old man skate bully?" He said he felt like cuffing him for calling him "old" and hugging him for praise of his performance.

One correspondent says in substance that he did his best mental work evenings, continuing usually until at least one o'clock in the morning and then tumbling into bed, perhaps after a half an hour spent on a novel as a nightcap or brain sponge, and falling at once into profound sleep undisturbed by dreams and with hardly a change of posture till nature's demands were entirely satisfied. Now all his serious study can best be done by daylight and particularly in the early part of the day and he has a simple set of routine prescriptions for going to bed and to sleep. He occasionally awakes and even arises before morning, knows the sounds of all the night watches and is generally aware of the early dawn despite darkened windows, and is sometimes disturbed by troublesome dreams. He needs less sleep as measured by hours but is more dependent upon its soundness. Again, he sometimes feels moody, depressed, irritable, and wonders if anyone observes it. He has a new horror of nerves, of constipation, of age lapsing to dotage, anecdotage, and garrulity or taciturnity. If anything goes physically wrong, he recuperates more slowly and blesses his stars that his good heredity pulls him through, and nurses his weaknesses the more thereafter. He has a notion that by keeping at work all he is able to, he is conserving an energy that by letting up, if he is ill, will be drawn upon to restore him to condition; whereas if he were habitually idle this reserve would be thereby dissipated. With all the precautions and handicaps thus entailed he is still sometimes able to attain a high state of morale, to feel again the old youthful joy and exuberance of life, although it now has a new and unique quality. There are also certain new ambitions he dares not express. He even longs for new adventures before it is forever too late. He realizes that all his life he has been more or less repressed by "the fear of living" and would now entirely escape it. He is not content to grind over the old mental stores but would reach out into other fields and find new ones. He fears intellectual stagnation and routine as the senses begin to grow dull and that he is not well nourished mentally or suitably prepared for old age and the psychic marasmus to which it is so prone.

The old tend to grow stale and sterile of soul from two causes: lack of fresh mental pabulum and abatement of the power of creative ideation, and so their mentation lapses and they become fatuous about trifles and feel that just as they must live circumspectly lest their body suffer some sudden collapse so their psychic self may crumble into senility and the subtle processes of disintegration and dementia slowly supervene, a decline of which we are usually far less aware than of physical decay. All these considerations, however, may and together should constitute a splendid stimulus to activity. The very danger of decline or breakdown is a spur to develop the higher powers of man in this their time.

In such experiences we seem to have a condition of great interest and also of practical importance. Physical infirmity and accident which compel special attention to body-keeping often result in such added care to hygienic condition that we are actually better and more effective for the impairment. Just as an old man who takes special care not to fall or to take risks is often safer from injury than a stronger and less careful man, so in mental work consciousness of certain shortcomings may act as a spur to take more pains and so to do superior work. To this is added another stimulus. A senescent knows that his friends and enemies will be liable to ascribe any imperfections in his intellectual output to failing powers, and his horror of betraying this is an added incentive to do his very best. If his last product could be his best, he could die happier, and he cannot bear the thought of exhibiting signs or stages of senile debility. To be willing to accept the allowances that his hostile or even his amiable critics would be willing to make for his years is craven. His chief danger is lest the standards of self-censorship for his performances should unconsciously decline and that he should come to judge his own inferior work as superior. Of this the history of literature has countless examples, more perhaps than of the opposite tendency.

Unquestionably, too, there is a certain maturity of judgment about men, things, causes, and life generally that nothing in the world but years can bring, a real wisdom that only age can teach. But to observe and rely on this to compensate for thoroughgoing rigorism in demonstration or mastery of copious details is a fatality too often seen. Finally, we must realize that our own brain work must be done with less of the afflatus that often aided us in youth or in maturity. Once our best ideas came to us in heat after a warming up of our faculties, perhaps into an erethic or second-breath state. We found ourselves in the grip of a sort of inspiration that carried us on perhaps far into the

night or impelled us to exceptional activities for days
or even weeks and brought a reaction of lassitude in
its train. But now, not only is this generally less or
lacking but our mentation must be more stated, our
hours of intense application must be kept within bounds,
and there is the perennial danger of overdoing and its
penalties are surer and more severe. Thus with age
we must develop a new system or method that recognizes
and comports with our true mental age. We must have
safely passed the Scylla and Charybdis of affecting to
be younger than we are and of aping or adhering too
conservatively to the manners of thought and feeling
characteristic of earlier youth, on the one hand; or, on
the other, we must escape the opposite attitude that
often supervenes later in the very old of vaunting their
years and posing as prodigies of senescence. In a word,
the call to us is to construct a new self just as we had
to do at adolescence, a self that both adds to and sub-
tracts much from the old personality of our prime. We
must not only command a masterly retreat along the
old front but a no less masterly advance to a new and
stronger position and find compensation for what old
age leaves behind in what it brings that is new. What,
more precisely, is this latter?

Youth should anticipate the wisdom of age and age
should conserve the spontaneity of youth, for this latter
becomes not less but only more inward as we advance
in years. As the eye dims and the dominance of optical
impressions over attention declines, we see ideas clearer
and follow the associations of thought rather than those
of the external world with some of the same freedom
as that which comes to dreams when we close the eyes in
sleep. So, when audition becomes less sensitive, we turn
to the voices of inner oracles. If current events impress
and absorb us less, we can knit up the past, present, and
future into a higher unity. As the muscles grow weak

the will, of which they were the organ, grows strong to make the new adjustments necessary, while easy fatigue suggests renunciation and the acceptance of fate. Love that is less individualized may become not only broader but stronger. We worry because we feel we have not made the new adjustments necessary or unsealed all the new sources of wisdom and strength. Symptoms call upon us to develop hygienic sagacity and censoriousness may be only a negative expression of a higher idealism that longs for a better world. Schleiermacher [4] developed this thought, insisting that age was not only conserved but renewed youth, that no one should feel old till he feels perfect, that age brings us into contact with new sources of life and gives a new sense of the independence of the soul from the body, not thus presaging a higher post-mortem existence but being itself an entirely new life.

If I were charged with the task of compiling a secular bible for the aged, I would include two great and historic sections from Aristotle.[5] In the one he describes virtue as the golden mean between the extremes of excess and defect, as, for example, courage between timidity and foolhardiness; liberality between avarice and prodigality; modesty between bashfulness and impudence; courtesy between rudeness and flattery; vanity between solemnness and buffoonery, etc., in each of his twelve spheres of life. In the other passage he characterizes the magnanimous man as slow, dignified in speech and movement, forgetful of injuries, not seeking praise, open and not secretive because unafraid, attempting but few things but those things of gravity, neither shunning nor seeking danger, ready to die for a great cause, more disposed to bestow than to receive benefits or favors, inclined to be proud to the proud and kindly to the meek

---

[4] *Monologen.*

[5] *Ethics,* Book II, Chaps. 3 and 6 and Book IV, Chap. 3.

and humble, always animated by the effort to make his conduct in life as nearly ideal as possible—or, in a word, making honor his muse and striving always to be worthy of it. Now, most of these traits belong more to the ideal of old age than to that of any earlier period in life. The most advanced regimen and hygiene of to-day —personal, mental, moral, social, political, judicial, and even religious—have little better to suggest for old age, in which all the qualities here implied should culminate, bringing poise and philosophic calm.

This brings me to the main thesis of this book, which is that intelligent and well-conserved senectitude has very important social and anthropological functions in the modern world not hitherto utilized or even recognized. The chief of these is most comprehensively designated by the general term synthesis, something never so needed as in our very complex age of distracting specializations.

In the first place, it has been noted that withdrawal from biological phyletic functions is often marked by an Indian summer of increased clarity and efficiency in intellectual work. Not only does individuation now have its innings but the distractions from passion, the lust for wealth and power, and in general the struggle for place and fame, have abated and in their stead comes, normally, not only a philosophic calm but a desire to draw from accumulated experience and knowledge the ultimate, and especially the moral, lessons of life—in a word, to sum up in a broader view the net results of all we have learned of the *comédie humaine*. Taylor even considers the climacteric as not pathological but as "a conservation process of nature to provide for a higher and more stable phase of development, an economic lopping off of functions no longer needed, preparing the individual for a different form of activity." Shaler, too, noted "an enlargement of intellectual interests;"

405

and there is much in experience and literature to confirm this view. The dangers and excitements of life are passed. Normal men tend to become more judicial and benevolent and these traits suggest new possibilities for the race as vicariate for the loss of the power of physical procreation. Many think these phenomena are more marked in women but even men who seem to have crossed the deadline at fifty or even forty are sometimes later reanimated. Apperceptive data have increased facility for getting together, perhaps even into a new and larger view of the world and there may come a genuine psychic erethism or second-breath, half ecstatic, as the soul on the home stretch expatiates "o'er all the world of man a mighty maze, yet not without a plan."

There is, thus, a kind of harvest-home effort to gather the fruitage of the past and to penetrate further into the future. It is especially interesting to note that this is a stage of life in which most of the Freudian mechanisms and impulsions fail to act or strike out in new ways and very different ones take their place, which as yet lack any adequate psychology, much as this is needed. This is the wisdom of Solomon and the Psalmists, the vision of the mystics, and it exists only in those senescents who have found the rare power of developing and conserving the morale of their stage of life, which, as always, consists in keeping themselves at the top of their condition. The Binet-Simon devotees have furnished us with no inkling of how physiological and mental age are related in the old. Only when we know this shall we be able to evaluate the mentality of real sages wise in the school of life. This kind of sapience has a value quite apart from and beyond the methods of our most advanced pedagogy. St. John thinks that there is a certain rejuvenation due to a change from *a posteriori* to *a priori* habits of mind and that subjectivity and perhaps introversion now have their innings. However this be, ripe old age has been a slow, late, precarious, but precious acquisition of the race, perhaps not only its latest but also its highest product. Its modern representatives are pioneers and perhaps its task will prove to be largely didactic. It certainly should go along with the corresponding prolongation of youth and increasing docility in the rising generation if we are right in charging ourselves with the duty of building a new story to the structure of human life. Thus, while old age is not at all venerable *per se* we have a mandate to make it ever more so by newer orientation, especially in a land and age that puts a premium upon its splendid youth, who are now often called to precocious activities that sometimes bring grief and disaster because we have been oblivious of the precept, "Old men for counsel."

True old age is not, as we have seen, second childhood. It is no more retrospective than prospective. It looks out on the world anew and involves something like a rebirth of faculties, especially of curiosity and even of naïveté. Moreover, age is in quest of first principles just as, though far more earnestly and competently, ingenuous youth is. We have seen that Plato taught that the love and quest of general ideas was the true achievement of immortality because it brought participation in the deathlessness of these consummations of the noetic urge, for to him philosophy was anticipatory death because it involved a withdrawal from the specific and particular toward the vastness and generality of the absolute.

But to-day normal old age cannot be merely contemplative. True, our very neurons do seem to aggregate into new and more stable unities as if the elements of our personality were being bound more closely together, perhaps in order that we might survive some disruptive crisis or that our souls might not be torn apart by the wind if we chance to die when it blows.

But now we must conceive the synthetic trend as chiefly in the pragmatic service of mankind. Our message must not be a mere *morituri salutamus,* however cheerful, but must have a positive and practical meaning and our outlook tower should have a really directive significance.

One outstanding and central trait of good old age is disillusionment. It sees through the shams and vanities of life. Many of the most brilliant intellectual achievements of youthful geniuses in thought construction are precocious achievements of the insights that more properly belong to this later stage of life. Even Carlyle's *Sartor,* Hegel's *Phänomenologie,* Schopenhauer, Nietzsche, Emerson, and many more, to say nothing of Jesus and Buddha, show premature age. Young men who occupy themselves with the highest and most abstract philosophical problems are unconsciously affecting or striving to anticipate the most advanced mental age and many of them who discourse so sapiently on "experience" are really those who have had very little of it. The ancient Hindus knew this for, as Max Müller tells us, the wise grandfather rises above all the superstitions of his progeny, who still worship the old gods while he has come to revere only the great One and All and to see all faiths and rites as but painted shadows that fancy casts upon the unknown, while he awaits the blessed absorption into Nirvana.

Fewest of all are those who ripen to senescence in religion and realize that there is no external god but only physical and human nature and no immortality save that of our offspring, our work, or our influence. All who fall short of this are arrested in juvenile if not infantile stages of their development. So, in all matters pertaining to sex, marriage, and the family, most remain slaves of the mores of their age and do not recognize the pregnant sense in which love and freedom, the greatest words in all languages, should somehow be wedded, even though we do not yet know how. Only when the age of sex passes can we look dispassionately upon all these problems and glimpse the ways that easier divorce, backfires to lust and prostitution, some of which current hypocrisy still taboos the very mention of, can bring. So, too, in other social and in our economic conditions we are drifting perilously near to wrecking reefs. The very basis of our civilization is in the greatest danger for want of the very aloofness, impartiality and power of generalization that age can best supply. We oldsters do see these things in a truer perspective and the time has now come to set them forth, despite the penalty of being voted pessimistic and querulent.

With all these problems so wide open by and since the war crying out for solution, surely senescents who have retired and enjoy a superacademic freedom, with no responsibilities to Boards, institutions, or corporate interests; with no personal ambitions, no temptations of the flesh, and leisure for the highest things, have here an inspiring function which they must rise to. Age, with a competence sufficient for its needs, freed from anxieties about a future state, with none of the dangers young men feel lest they impair their future careers, should not devote itself to rest and rust (*Rast Ich, so rost Ich*) or to amusements, travel, or self-indulgence of personal taste, much as the old may feel they have deserved any and all of these, but should address itself to these new tasks, realizing that it owes a debt to the world which it now vitally wants it to pay. Great founders of great institutions have acknowledged this debt and striven to pay it in the service the rich can render. We intellectuals cannot pay it in their coin, but we owe it no less and must pay in the currency we can command.

Thus, old age is not passive and peace-loving but brings a new belligerency. Many of us longed for the physical ability to enter the war as soldiers and we did our "bit" in ways open to us with as much zest as our juniors. We not only want but need spiritual conflicts and feel reinforced aggressiveness against ignorance, superstition, errors, the sins of cupidity, and lust. What a list of evils we could make which we wanted to attack in our prime but lacked courage to grapple with! One of these is the current idea of old age itself. We have too commonly accepted the conventional allotment of three-score-and-ten as applicable now, but the man of the future will be ashamed and feel guilty if he cannot plan a decade or two more of activity and he will not permit himself to fall into a thanatopsis mood of mind or retire to his memories or to the chimney corner because an allotted hour has struck.

If we have lived aright, nature does give us a new lease of life when passion and the bodily powers begin to abate and the very danger of collapse, as we have seen, is in itself a spur. The human race is young but most are cut off prematurely. It is ours to complete the drama, to finish the window of Aladdin's tower, to add a new story to the life of man, for as yet we do not know what full maturity really is and the last culminating chapter of humanity's history is yet to be written.

Never, then, was the world in such crying need of Nestors and Merlins. What a priceless crop of experience in these postbellum days remains unharvested for want of precisely the objectivity, impartiality, breadth, and perspective that age alone can supply! These were the qualities that enabled the venerable Joffre to make his masterly two-weeks' retreat at the Marne. It was done against the will and wish of every one of his younger generals, who now admit that he saved Paris and the war and that he was, in a sense, a true superman. The world never so needed the wisdom, which learning cannot give, that sees the vanity and shallowness of narrow partisanship and jingoism, of creeds that conceal more than they reveal, of social shams that often veil corruption, the insanity of the money hunt that monopolizes most of the energy of our entire civilization, and realizes that with all our vaunted progress man still remains essentially juvenile—much as he was before history began.

What the world needs is a kind of higher criticism of life and all its institutions to show their latent beneath their patent value by true supermen who, like Zarathustra, are old, very old, with the sapience that long life alone can give. We need prophets with vision who can inspire and also castigate, to convict the world of sin, righteousness, and judgment. Thus, there is a new dispensation at the door which graybeards alone can usher in. Otherwise humanity will remain splendid but incomplete. Heir of all the ages, man has not yet come into his full heritage. A traveler, he sets out for a far and supreme goal but is cut off before he attains or even discerns it. The best part of his history is yet unwritten because it is unmade.[6]

Now that the pressure of outer reality and its duties remit, attention tends more to focus on self and intro-spontaneity and mentation may take on a slightly dreamy character in that it is less under the dominion of the objective environment, from which there is a new sense of freedom. The demand for rigorous proof of one's theorizations is somewhat less insistent and critics of them are felt to be lacking in insight. There is a slight shift from inductive to deductive thinking and as the senses begin to grow dim their verification of our speculations seems a trifle less imperative. Experience has furnished masses of data that yet remain unco-ordinated and as we feel the need of a deeper synthesis

---

*In the last few paragraphs I have, thanks to the courtesy of the editor of the *Atlantic Monthly*, freely used material from my anonymous article on "Old Age" in the January, 1921, number.

we grope our way to a bed-rock of first principles that will explain the riddle of life better and give it more unity and give us new personal satisfaction. Tendencies that have been repressed during our active life revive.

Perhaps we take up fads or occupations that have hitherto had only a secondary place in our lives or indulge ourselves by giving them now the first place as centers of interest. Now at last we can do things we have long wanted to do but for which we have had no time or strength. We can also now indulge our taste in reading in fields we have long desired to know better, can abandon ourselves to the enjoyment of music or the fine arts; or we travel, collect, or occupy ourselves with horticulture, agriculture or farm life. Again, there are more reveries and these most commonly gravitate to things about us or especially to the remote past. Thus we often revive and idealize old situations and incidents. We think of things we said and did and supplement them by imagining what we could, would, or should have said and done and fill lost opportunities fuller of "might-have-beens." Yet many as are the lost chances such retrospect brings to view, and imperfect as we realize our responses to circumstances and the environment have been, we are rarely oppressed by regret and still less often by remorse, so that the wish to relive our lives is never very strong. The flaws in our surroundings or our errors in judgment, even in moral conduct, are usually regarded with leniency and viewed with a certain detachment, however clearly they are seen and however impersonally they are judged. This is in part because we have to accept them as inevitable and are trying to make a virtue of so doing, but yet more perhaps because we are consoled by the fact that had our mistakes been very grave we should not have attained our advanced age in such good condition of body and mind. Thus we make our very age a kind of vindication of our course of life. We find yet more comfort in the fact that we discover so many points in which things might have been worse. We have escaped so many perils and survived so many trials that have overwhelmed many others that, on the whole, we deem ourselves among the fortunate of the earth.

I am inclined to think that the above, instead of being an optimistic should rather be regarded on the whole as a pessimistic view of old age. Fielding Hall tells us that in Burma, where it is purest, Buddhism teaches men to "die thinking on their good deeds." I cannot believe this is final but opine rather that old age has its positive duties to the present and to the future as well as its privileges and immunities. To be sure, if sex love is the mainspring of the most and best in the human psyche, it follows that when this goes there is little worth while left in us. Hence, the implications of the new analytic psychology are most tragic for senescence and man is doomed to spend the shriveled remnants of life in the contemplation of its only real stage, which is now gone or fast vanishing. I urge, on the contrary, that the facts of the soul-life of the aged teach us very clearly that if the *vita sexualis* has been anything like normal, we graduate from it into a larger love of man, nature, and being itself which can never be complete till the urge of sex has waned.

What are these facts? First, the very incident that the old tend to develop more sharply their own individuality as the powers of genesis decline points in this direction. Senescents in the post-climacteric acuminate their personality, sometimes to the point of idiosyncrasy and eccentricity. The *Ich-trieb* now has its innings. This selfishness of the old, repulsive and unsocial as are now its commonest manifestations, expresses a deep instinct that is really groping toward a new and higher type of personality, evolving a new synthesis of the

413

factors of life when the chord of sex shall have passed in music out of sight. It means man's reaffirmation of the self and of the will-to-live, although this points not, as the immortalists would argue, to a post-mortem rehabilitation of the ego but only expresses again the fact that man is as yet incomplete here and that even the old now die prematurely because they have not yet learned how to build the last story of the house of many mansions.

Again, as sex love declines friendship takes its place. Old lovers, and husbands and wives if happily mated, become friends and find new joys in these new relations. How we prize old friends and feel closer even to those of our contemporaries we have known but slightly! A fine old man of my acquaintance made a systematic effort by many letters to get into touch with all his old schoolmates who were living and to learn all he could of those who were dead. Another felt wronged whenever a friend of earlier days died and he had no word of it. Yet another wrote to a venerable colleague whom he knew but slightly, but whose career he had followed, exhorting him "not to die yet a while" because he would feel more lonely in the world with him out of it. There is a unique loyalty of veterans of war toward each other, although they are little together and do not always get on well with each other if they attempt intimacy. Moreover, there is a new type of interest in young people and in children, whom even grandmothers do not so much fondle and pet as indulge and serve in ways mothers do not always sympathize with. The "Borrowed Time" clubs of old men and young people's associations are both based chiefly upon the gregarious instinct which is strongest among adolescents, before woman has taken her place beside man, and among senescents when the charm of sex as such abates. Most of the scores of associations and fraternities of men of

mature years are for material advantage and the typical
clubman has failed to find, or else has lost, the normal
anchorage of the true home. The homosexual friendships of the old are not chummy and do not demand
close contact. These have been far too much neglected
and their cultivation, which is greatly needed, is possible
under modern conditions as never before. It is interesting to know that an old people's journal is projected.

Love in the aged also tends to broaden into the higher
and more sublimated form of interest in the subhuman
world, in animals, plants, trees, gardening, and country
life generally. The charm of a rural contrasted with
an urban environment increases. How often the old
take pleasure in planting or setting out trees they will
never see mature or bear fruit and in building homes
they know they can at best live in but for a short time.
Burbank knew and Burroughs felt this and Cato said
that all the aged should dwell in the country, as so many
of the old Romans did. The aged rarely have animal
pets but they do feel a new dread of destroying life.
They love scenery and commune with forests and mountains; revisit their rural boyhood homes and find deep
satisfaction in reënvisaging old landmarks.

They are, as we have seen, very susceptible to climate
and to weather changes, which they often become
sagacious in predicting, and sometimes keep note of
rain, snowfall, temperature, wind, the phases of the
moon, etc., and are not only accredited oracles in weather
wisdom but are appealed to as local weather bureaus
with amazing memory for exceptional climatic phenomena for years back. Thus it is that their sympathies
often widen until they become almost animistic for
things without life and may come almost to personify
ships, vehicles, and machines. What takes place within
the soul of an old man alone with nature our imperfect
psychology cannot tell; nor does he yet know. It is

415

something resumptive, preparatory for mingling with the elements, as he will ere long do. His consciousness is a poor witness of what transpires in the depths of his soul, for he only knows that the experience of such influences gives him a new poise and calm that is sweet if it is also sad. It is in such experiences that our nature points the way to the chief palliative of the ghastly death thought. In this direction lies the true way back to the all-mother of life, to the great womb of existence whence we come and to which we must all return.

By various devices nature tends to keep the number of males and females nearly equal. But when long periods of hardship, especially wars, reduce the relative number of males, this inequality is rectified by an increase in the number of males born; while in long periods of tranquillity females tend to outnumber males. This is well established by the statistics of natality. Whether nature would thus make good any such sharp reduction in the relative number of females is less demonstrable, because there is no such cause of sudden decimation of this sex. Women do not go to war with each other. This suggests the question whether nature also tends to regulate the proportion between the old and the young where this has been abnormally disturbed. We have already seen that in new communities opened up and settled by vigorous younger men the relative number of old men, though not of old women, soon increases because it is the most viable who respond to the call of adventure and pioneering and who thus, barring the effects of hardship, tend to live longer than the less enterprising who remain behind. Selection was less operative for women who went because their men did. So far as we may identify youth with progressiveness and age with conservatism, we may safely conclude that nature does exercise the same regulative function here as in making good sex disparity. At any rate, radical new departures always bring reactions. Now, young communities and countries have short, old ones long, memories. In the former, experience counts too little; in the latter, too much. The one tends to act perhaps too precipitately, the other to deliberate too long. In one, precedent and tradition have but little, in the other excessive, weight. The one tends to make the most and best of their present opportunity, while the other is chiefly concerned that no good thing of the past be jeopardized. Thus, the tide of progress, which is always marked by alternating waves of reform and stabilization, is regulated and the most fundamental moral basis of all party distinctions is age. In this sense there are always two, and only two, sides to every question; two, and only two, parties in every state, town, and family: the old and the young. Their harmonious action and reaction constitutes the most favorable condition for real progress. Age is far-sighted and synthetic, youth myopic and analytic; but public and private welfare need both, just as science needs both the microscope and the telescope.

All sciences, most of all those that deal with man, are liable to lack the perspective that only age can give to orient them to direct their researches toward problems of most value and hold them steadily to their true course. Even the ablest and most ingenuous of our young sociologists are most prone to lose sight of wider relations and come to focus in partial and extreme views, for extreme opinions are always easiest and in trying to cope with theories too vast for our powers even sane and vigorous minds show the same traits as feeble, neurotic, and infantile ones, which find even the problems of their limited personal lives too hard for them to solve.

In the field of psychology we have now perfected a methodology of introspection that seeks to be as exact as physics or chemistry in going back to elemental sensations as if they were elements from which all higher forms of mental activity were to be evolved by logic as rigorous as mathematics itself and that ignores evolution. We also have a behaviorism that focuses upon activities and physiological processes and would evict the term consciousness, which is the muse of introspection. The psychoanalysts, again, are most genetic and would evolve nearly all psychic phenomena from sex by mechanisms that are as sacred to them as were innate ideas to scholastics and philosophers before Locke, and their work is still taboo to most orthodox psychologists. Fourth, we have the testers who are intent upon applying psychology to the grading of intelligence and the standardization and calibration of abilities. All this work is valuable but how grievously we just now need the broader synthetic view that only age and experience can fully realize and really ought to supply. Age sees more clearly than youth that studies of the brain, of children, of instincts, animals, prehistoric man, the insane, defectives, the sexes, intellect, will, feelings, and even of the history of philosophy and religion are essential for a sound knowledge of man. For to the real anthropologist nothing human is alien. He alone sees that the real value of all such special work is what it contributes to enable us to make our lives fuller, better, and more worth living.

In religion, most of even our authorized leaders show symptoms of dementia præcox in clinging to juvenile attitudes that should have long since been sloughed off. They still antagonize Darwinism, the higher criticism, and the great philosophies of pantheism, which, rightly interpreted, constitute the religion of mature and normal senescent souls. In this oldest of all culture fields the world has suffered most grievous arrest. The fact that in this direction the old have generally so often been most reactionary, if not infantile, is one of the most grievous of all their shortcomings. Here they should lead, as in more primitive times they often did. The church has too little use for its aging teachers but prefers young clergymen. Happily, however, a few of them are now helping to build this higher story of the culture temple of the race and have bid adieu to the mad immortality quest born of the age of sexual potency and which should decline and die with it. In this, as in perhaps no other field, old age should thus be constructive and build mansions for itself and it will never attain the dignity nature suggests for it until it does so. This does not mean that its verdicts should be authoritative for other periods of life since, as with each of these, its findings are not absolute but true only for its own stage. But when senescence has found and accepted the faith that fits its nature and needs, this will at least serve to mitigate the fanaticism of young converts, rebuke ratiocination, which has so long impelled immature minds to make dogma out of religious literature, and check the intolerance of intellectual orthodoxy.

So in all departments of life the function of competent old age is to sum up, keep perspective, draw lessons, particularly moral lessons. Homer, tradition tells us, was an old man who synthesized many legends before unorganized, somewhat as Moses was said to have done in composing the Pentateuch. The dialogues of Plato that deal with the deepest problems are, by general consent, ascribed to his old age. Most of the prophets were old and even the Gospel, which represented the terminal phase of apostolic inspiration, is ascribed to the very aged John. The Confucian system is preëminently a product of the senium that had seen the vanities of the world; and especially of all cults of the transcendental. Herodotus, Thucydides, and Strabo were said to have been old. Wells' synoptical history not only meets the needs of the old but is something a wise old man might well have undertaken. The popular lectures of not a few leaders of science—DuBois-Reymond, Helmholtz, Huxley, Haeckel, and many others—are products of fertile minds unifying their life work, as befits scientists, before their powers fail, subjecting it to the supreme test by acceptance of the consensus of competent contemporaries and thus affirming the influential immortality of the authors.

The late James Bryce, at the age of 84, said words of supreme wisdom on national and international affairs at the Williamstown conference. Who is not heartened to know that Ranke wrote his famous *Weltgeschichte*—I think in five volumes—beginning at the age of 85; that Michelangelo was drawing the plans of St. Peters at 90; that Cornaro wrote his last version of *The Temperate Life* at 95; that W. S. Smith made his memorable trip around the world alone at the age of 80; that Durand edited a volume of his at 110. And it is satisfying to find not only scores but hundreds of such records, ancient and modern.

Again, if youth creates, age not only conserves but organizes. Both these functions are essential in human society and are related somewhat as are reproductive and connective tissue, as we saw in Chapter VI. Both youth and age seek truth and thrill when they feel a deep sentiment of inner conviction. But age lays more stress upon the pragmatic sanction of working well and can better understand even Loyola and Machiavelli. Thus it came that while men in their prime conceived the great religions, the old made them prevail. Thus, too, instituted and dogmatic religion owes its existence chiefly to men past the meridian of life. The old did not invent belief in supernatural powers or persons but needed and used it to sustain their position when physical inferiority would have otherwise compelled them to step aside and so they made themselves mediators between gods and men. They directed and presided over rites and cere-

420

monies and took possession of the keys of the next world, enforced orthodoxies for the sake of order, and established and equipped the young to aid them in this work. They were behind the scenes and held the secrets, realizing the utility to society and also to themselves of much for which they had lost the primitive ardor of belief. Thus the revivalist and the reformer have always found the old arraigned against them. Perhaps they resent "new bottles" even more then they do new wine.

In the domain of sex, so vitally bound up with religion, the Hebrew race first taught the world and most of this wisdom came from the old, against whom the rise of romantic love was one of the greatest revolts in the history of culture. In many primitive societies the old, as we have seen, initiate the young of the same and even of the opposite sex into its mysteries, and in modern mores, as for example, in France, the counsels of the old are still of influence in the matings of the young. It is they who insist on prudential considerations and warn against venery and the follies into which blind Eros may lead. They have seen and know each scene in the stormy drama to the fall of the curtain. Thus to-day, though less only in degree, the sharpest phase of the eternal warfare between the old and young is just where it was in the ancient tribes in which the old barred the young from the females. Youth seeks indulgence and resents the restraint and control for which the old stand.

This eternal war between the young and the old begins at birth and increases with every restraint and prohibition imposed on the former by the latter. The infant would subject its mother's life to its service and the psychoanalysts who urge that we begin life with a sense of omnipotence are quite as near right as those who, like Schleiermacher, found this stage of life characterized by a feeling of absolute dependence, of which he thought all religions are formulations. Both are always present and

421

in incessant conflict, now one and now the other predominating. The child revolts, yet must submit and obey its elders. It asserts its freedom by defiance, evasion, running away, by deceits, by fancies of escaping all control and doing all it wishes. It seeks to lead its own life and to live out completely its present state regardless of all the claims of the future and of all domination by adults, whose very existence much of his play ignores. The father especially is a tyrant and is often hated as well as loved. Younger children are always bullied by older. Every school grade seeks to dominate that below. The teacher is always imposing a wisdom that is not yet demanded by the child and that is accepted by it unwillingly, cramming the memory pouches with things that can be only imperfectly appreciated, picking open buds of interest and knowledge before their time, imposing standards that are too grown up, checking natural expressions of instinct and insisting on discipline, training, the often painful acquisition of skills and conformity to manifold conventions. There is always a sense in which the school is an offense to the nature of the child. Older minds prescribe what must be learned, and how, and when, and the scholiocentric still predominates over the paidocentric method of education.

The state also subjects youth and enforces rights of property and person to which the young have to be broken in. All kinds and degrees of apprenticeship and the age and meaning of attaining majority are prescribed. In many lands the parents control the marriage of their offspring as they do property and the older make and administer laws for the younger. After all these forms and degrees of servitude of the younger to the older it is no wonder that the former not only very often show symptoms of revolt all the way from the cradle to complete maturity but, along with gratitude and respect, also cherish, if more unconsciously, an enmity that they can neither entirely express nor control against all kinds of masters, perhaps especially when their power and authority begin to wane with age. The push of the advancing upon the retiring generation is not consciously to feed fat such ancient grudges by subjecting elders in their turn as they were once subjected and yet there is a deep and persistent sense, which even psychology has but little realized, in which every advance in history, every insurrection or rebellion, every protestant movement against the established order or custom, and every reform in religion, politics, or life generally is only an expression of the eternal revolt of youth against age, of which the extreme reaction of parricide is the symbol but which is the deep psychogenetic root of every degree of failure in care and respect. LeBon [1] sees and well presents the insurrectionary tendencies rife in the world to-day but does not realize the extent, nor does he find or seek the ultimate cause, of the present universal "revolt." Thus the aged everywhere still suffer from the imperfections with which they and even their remote forbears exercised the parental function.

On the other hand, it should not, of course, be forgotten that there is always the more obvious and countervailing tendency to respect parents as age brings the insight that in what they compelled and forbade they were wiser than we, and to feel grateful that they did not leave us to follow our own sweet wills. Just so far as we come to realize not only how they lived for their children and did so wisely and well we both love them more for all they did for us, and, if we are wise, we realize that their counsels may still be helpful and we draw the moral that there is always somewhere a wisdom superior to our own, an experience from which we may profit, and an authority somewhere to which we must always remain

---

[1] *The World in Revolt*, New York, 1921, 256 pp.

docile and toward which our proper attitude is that of a loyalty that is essentially filial. It is of this impulse that all kinds of ancestor worship are belated expressions, while at the same time it is compensatory for all ill wishes and treatment directed toward them while they lived. In a finished civilization the old will enjoy their full meed of reverence while they are yet alive and every sort of post-mortem canonization will be seen to be only the symbol of a *devoir present*.

Perhaps in the large Aristotelian sense of the word politics is, *par excellence,* the work of and for old age. Statecraft must look not at the transient fluctuations of current and popular opinion but must look beyond the present or the next election, must rise above the selfishness of party interest and look to the far future. It must think not in terms of the exigencies of the hour but of decades and generations and not of local or partisan but of national and humanistic interests. From the patriarchs down the old have been the wisest shepherds of the people and if young men have succeeded in diplomacy it is because they have been prodigies of precocity who have also devoted themselves to the intensive study of history, which is at best only a proxy for experience. To have read ever so exhaustively of a war of a century before, for example, can give the young student no such sense of its horrors, nor of the urgency of using every honorable means of averting it, as to have actually lived through it with a vivid personal memory of its incidents. Veterans of old wars would be cautious about entering new ones.

Thus it is well that the old are with us "lest we forget" and in exigencies we often turn to them if living and read and quote them with respect long after they are dead. Great statesmen are those who have not only identified themselves with the past, present, and future of the nations they serve but beyond this have felt themselves charged with the interests of mankind as a whole. We surely need all possible ripeness of knowledge and maturity of judgment in this field and if the span of experience personally demanded by leaders could have been a full century, many of the great disasters that have befallen the race might have been avoided.

The fact is that, as the Athenians seemed to the old Egyptian priest who had known of Atlantis, we are all children who have to play the rôle of real adults because the latter have not yet arrived, so they we have come to think ourselves really mature.

Again, if the young are the best advocates, the old are by nature the best judges. They can best weigh facts and ideas in the scale of justice. The moral faculties ripen more slowly. Thus the old can best supplement the technicalities of law by equity and give ethics its rights in their verdicts. They should be the keepers of the standards of right and wrong and mete out justice with the impartiality and aloofness that befit it. Even in private life we have a judicial function, which, though often ignored and even resented, is also often sought and respected if we have the tact to praise and do not become censorious. Our approval or disapproval, even if mild and unspoken, may count for more than is admitted or even realized by our family and friends.

Such philosophy as my life and studies have taught me begins and ends in the thesis that the supreme criterion of everything, including religion, science, art, property, business, education, hygiene, and every human institution and everything in our environment, is what it contributes to make life longer, fuller, and saner, so that each individual shall live out more completely all the essentials in the life of the race. If the best survive, it is not the good but the bad and unfit who die young. To have lived long but narrowly is just as bad. Both have really only half lived and it is just those who have failed

425

of realizing their full humanity in this life that most feel the need of another and imprecate the cosmos as having cheated them if it has not provided one. A rich old age is thus the supreme reward of virtue. Thus what is education but fitting us for a more advanced stage of life. It consists largely in giving to the young the products of older minds and thus advancing our mental age beyond our years. Childhood longs to die into youth and youth into maturity and so the latter in its turn should long to pass away into age. And how childish much in the adult world seems to those who have achieved the true sage-hood of age; and how unripe, full of folly, vanity, error, and passion! How little the world has realized its debt in the past to aging men and women in whom knowledge has ripened into wisdom and how much more age owes and will yet give to the world when human life becomes complete and realizes its higher possibilities!

Now, too, many of those who attain advanced years are battered, water-logged, leaky derelicts without cargo or crew, chart, rudder, sail, or engine, remaining afloat only because they have struck no fatal rocks or because the storms have not quite yet swamped them; or, to change the figure, because they have withered, not ripened, on the tree. How many of us really ought to be dead because we are useless to ourselves and to others. It is because there are so many such that the rôle assigned to the best of us is often so hard and so repugnant to our nature and to our needs. Hence it comes that we are not only handicapped but are sorely tempted to accept a sham old age that is false to all the best that is in us, instead of justifying and illustrating a better one.

Thus, in fine, all not later than the fourth decade or whenever they note that their youth has fled or that any of their powers have begun to abate, should not only boldly face the fact that they are aging but begin serious preparations for old age, so that this stage of life be not only happier but more efficient than it is and that it render to the world a service never so needed and never so possible to render as now. Men and women in all the earlier and often in the later postmeridional phases of life are cowards in facing for themselves and arrant tricksters in deceiving others about their physiological and psychological age. If all the psychic energy now directed to concealment, pretense, and the maintenance of illusions here were put to better uses, then health, prolongation of life, and efficiency in later decades, to say nothing of happiness, would be greatly increased. The dawn of adolescence, like that of senescence, has its peculiar possibilities and its very trying probationary years before the age of nubility; but youth always has the advantage, if it will only utilize it, of the counsels of those who have weathered its storm and stress. There is a vast amount of wreckage from which puberty often suffers. The old, however, have no older initiators into the last stage of life and must find or make their own way as best they can. But they should realize that all the fluctuations and circumnutation phenomena they experience in the middle decades of life are gropings toward new adjustments in the domain of hygiene and morale that are necessary when their income of vital energy does not quite balance its expenditure. All these phenomena are really only labor pains by which nature is trying to bring into the world a new and higher and more complete humanity. To repeat, our function is to finish a structure that still lacks an upper story and give it an outlook or conning tower from which man can see more clearly the far horizon and take his bearings now and then by the eternal stars.

The old who are really so, who are not merely spent projectiles, relics, vestiges, or ruins that time has chanced to spare, do sometimes attain vision and even prophetic power, and their last real words to the world they are leaving are not like the inane babblings of the dying, which friends so often cherish, but are often the best and most worth heeding by their juniors of all their counsels. Some have told us that if the long-awaited superman ever arrives, he will come by way of the prolongation of adolescence and others have said it would be by the fuller maturity of man in his prime. No doubt both these stages of life would be enriched and potentialized, but his first advent and his greatest improvement over man of to-day will be in the form of glorified old age. Nietzsche was right in making Zarathustra old and he himself was the overman whose message he brought to the world. He was intent on the future of man and not on his present, still less on his past. Thus the ideal old man will be chiefly concerned for what is yet to be. Whatever he knows of history, he is more concerned with the better history not yet written because it has not yet happened. If he thinks of his childhood and his forbears, he thinks still more of posterity. His chief desire is to see the young better born and better provided for so as to come to a fuller maturity.

In fine, it cannot be too strongly urged or too often repeated that at present we know little of old age and that little is so predominantly of its inferior specimens, its unfavorable traits and defects and limitations, that the old have been prone to repudiate their years. Some even in the seventies and eighties to whom I ventured to send my questionnaire resented it as imputing to them an age they denied all knowledge of, while others had come precociously to not only accept a padded life but to even crave services and sympathy and demand privileges and immunities to which they were not entitled, thus growing querulous because of a helplessness more affected than real. The fundamental passion of the normal old is to serve, to subordinate self, and, if in some ways they must be served, to help others in turn in such ways as they can. This instinct of expropriation of self is the voice of nature pointing to the effacement that awaits them. The fact that age is so often selfish should not blind us to the fact that in its true nature it is altruistic and thus in its later stages often finds its greatest trial in the progressive abatement of its power of actually benefiting others. Its greatest bitterness is that it must be so much ministered to, and one of my correspondents regretted that he could not die at sea or his corpse, when he was done with it, be left to nature so that his relatives might not have the fuss of a funeral and burial. Indeed, he seemed to have grown morbid about the trouble he was thus to make them. Even the new love of the country and of inanimate as well as animate nature into which they are soon to be resolved may be another outcrop of the deep but blind and groping immolation motive. It is love disengaging itself from persons and special objects and perfecting itself by attaining its goal, which is nothing less than the love of, and the resolution of self into, the cosmos from which we sprang. Hence there is a sense in which chemistry and physics, and even the Einstein doctrine of relativity, are studies of man's immortality.

Old age and death are eloquent of voices that call us to come home or back to nature, the all-mother, and to the earth from which we sprang and which is the terminal resting place of all who have gone before, with whose remains our dust will mingle. The more we know of the chemistry and physics of matter and energy, and even of the history, constitution, and contents of the earth's crust, the less dreadful do the grave and the processes that take place in it seem, and the less prone are we to become cowards, slackers, or malingerers in facing the Great Enemy. What we know of what is still often called brute matter shows it to be so much more dynamic and lawful than life and life is so much more fecund and complex than mind that there is now a new and most pregnant sense in which the way of even physical death is upward, not downward. Who, too, yet knows just how much of the charm of æsthetic contemplation of inanimate nature or even the urge that impels science to know ever more of it is due to what it does and will entomb. At any rate, as we realize far more clearly that none of the sons of men ever did or ever can come back, we can now find some compensation in the ever clearer understanding of the immortality of our somatic elements and see the meaning of the deep instinct that inclines the old to the country and to closer communion with nature as they withdraw from life.

The greatest influence of the old upon the young has, from time immemorial, been near the dawn of puberty, when almost every race initiates youth into manhood. This, too, is still the age of most conversions and church confirmations. Here education culminates and here, too, in a sense, it began and extended slowly upward toward the university and downward toward the kindergarten as civilization advanced. The age of nubility, which follows, is the period of the greatest break with the preceding generation for young couples generally set up for themselves and the increase of the interval between generations generally means a prolonged period of subjection and docility. When a third generation was added and grandparents became common in the families, conservative influences were increased, and if four living generations ever become common in the same family progress would probably be retarded and great-grandparents would think grandparents more or less radical or innovative, so that it is well that the former do not linger superfluous on the stage for this would make the tension between the past and the future too great. Thus the Great Silencer's work of oblivion is benign for the race.

SOME CONCLUSIONS

Such excessive contemporaneity of generations is not the goal of eugenics, for while it tends to prolong life it also increases the average span of years between generations and the longer-lived are also more fecund. Should it ever come that ancestors of half a dozen or a dozen generations live together, the advance of the world would probably be greatly retarded, perhaps to the point of stagnation. Therefore, for both their influence and for our love of them it is fortunate that they are well dead and live only in our memory, in the vitality they have bequeathed to us, and in the works that follow them. As it is, it is old minds and those that they have mainly influenced that have kept evolution, which is more charged with culture stimulus than any influence in the modern intellectual world, so largely out of our educational system. It is due to them that so large a part of Christendom has repudiated the higher criticism, another great achievement that has reanimated all scriptures and made them glow with a new light and has given insight and zest where before there was a confusion and indifference that kept religious consciousness so medieval and ultra-conservative. It is psychological age that makes statesmen suddenly confronted with new and vast world problems too large for them take refuge in the counsels of Washington, which were wise in their day but utterly inadequate for meeting the issues of our own time.

The World War was not primarily a young men's war, for most of them were sent by their elders and met their death that the influence of the latter might be augmented. Men may be made senile by their years without growing wise. Thus the world is without true leaders in this hour of its greatest need till we wonder whether a few score funerals of those now in power would not be our greatest boon. A psychological senility that neither learns nor forgets is always a menace and a check instead of being, as true old age should be, a guide in emergencies. Thus we have not grown old aright and are paralyzed by a wisdom that is obsolete or barnacled by prejudice. How often is it said of reforms great and good that they are earnestly needed and entirely practical but must wait for their accomplishment until certain venerable but obstructive personages of a generation that is passing are out of the way, because they are prone to think the old good and the new bad, and that every change, therefore, must be for the worse. Thus many live too long and undo the usefulness of their earlier years.

In fine, not only has the Western world now lost the exhilarating sense of progress that has for generations sustained and inspired it but civilization faces to-day dangers of decay such as have never confronted it since the incursion of the barbarians and of the Moslems into Europe. Other more disastrous wars are possible. Class hatred and the antagonisms of capital and labor, national and individual greed, race jealousies and animosities, the ferment of Bolshevism, the ascendency of the ideals of *kultur* over those of culture in our institutions for higher education in every land, industrial stagnation and unemployment, the crying lack of leaders and the dominance of mediocrity everywhere, the decay of faith and the desiccation of religion, the waning confidence in democracy: these are the prospects we must face if we are not to flee from reality and be cowards to life as it confronts us. If men still believed in an omnipotent all-wise god they would expect him to now intervene by a new, perhaps a third, dispensation such as Renan believed in. But the good old All-Father that saved a remnant and drowned the rest in the days of Noah and that sent His Son later to save the world when it seemed lost is dead and survives only as a memory, and we realize to-day that man must be his own savior or perish.

432

SOME CONCLUSIONS

There seem at present three and only three ways of escape, each of them radical, arduous, slow, and perhaps desperate, and which only those who have the supreme power of presentification or the genius that sees all problems in terms of the here and now can clearly discern. The first of these is (1) eugenics. We must learn to breed a better race of men. This is, indeed, a religion and already has its apostles and martyrs and a growing body of disciples who are propagandists of its new gospel. But the obstacles of ignorance and prejudice are appalling. The fact remains, however, as poor Nietzsche realized, that if man cannot surpass his present self he is lost.

(2) Others, like H. G. Wells to-day and like Comenius in his day, see our chief hope not so much in nature and preformation as in nurture and epigenesis and would reconstruct, vastly enlarge, and unify our entire educational system, reversing many a present consensus to the end of ultimately obliterating all national boundaries and racial prejudices and organizing a world state, "a parliament of man, a federation of the world."

(3) Others, like Metchnikoff and Bernard Shaw, look for salvation in the prolongation of human life that man may have the longer apprenticeship he now needs in order to wisely direct the ever more complex affairs of civilization. Compared with the task it now imposes, the wisest and ablest are only children and the disasters of our day are because young Phaethons have thought they could drive the chariot of the sun when in fact they were *"nicht dazu gewachsen."* If man could live and learn, not seventy but two or three times seventy years, and could begin to be at his best when he now declines and retires, he might know enough to guide the world in its true course. He must absorb more knowledge, and of a different kind, and assimilate it better in order to secrete the wisdom now needed. As the adolescent decade pre-

433

pares for maturity, so the senescent decades must prepare for old age and look forward to it with all the anticipation with which youth now looks forward to maturity. The limitations of old age must be made spurs to its greater efficiency just as so many in middle life have had to do with the chronic handicaps of poor health. Two prevalent traditions must be ruthlessly broken and destroyed. The first is that old people's hold on life is so precarious that medical care is less likely to be rewarded with success than at earlier stages of life. The fact is that normal and healthy age is not only immune to many diseases common to middle life but often has exceptional recuperative powers, while even under present conditions the percentage of deaths is not so very much increased at seventy. Physicians who specialize in gerontology could do very much here. The other vicious tradition is that retirement or marked abatement of activity should occur at a certain age. This ought to be always a personal matter and all who can really "carry on" should do so with all the powers they possess as long as they are fully able.

An "Indian summer" should be both expected and utilized to the uttermost for this is a precious bud of vast potentialities. In it we already glimpse the superhumanity yet to be. We can already guess something of the soteriological functions that now lie concealed and are yet to be revealed in it. It brings a new poise and a new perspective of values and hence a new orientation and new and deeper insights into essentials. The very fact that the old who have approximated ever so remotely this ideal have so far been exceptions and, in a sense, "sports" should at least open our eyes to the fact that the great all-mother can still show her original wish and intent.

The old are remarkably and uniquely suggestible in all matters that pertain to the suppression or augmentation of life. They give up and die prematurely as victims of a tradition that it is time for them to do so and they survive no less remarkably not only troubles and hardships but even surgical operations if they feel that they can do so. We need not be faith-curers but must be vitalists and believe in some kind of *élan vital* or creative evolution, as opposed to materialistic or mechanistic interpretations of life, to understand the true psychology of age. It is the nascent period of a new and unselfish involution of individuation which is impossible under the domination of egoism. The new self now striving to be born is freer from the dominion of sense and of the environment and has an autonomy and spontaneity that is reinforced and recharged with energy from the primal springs of life, and man may well look to this as one of the great sources of hope in his present distress.

With the sublimation of sex in the Indian summer of the senium, thus, comes normally a higher type of individuation than is possible before. It is freer from passion, sense, selfish interest, clearer and farther sighted, but sees the identity of the individual and the race with which it is becoming incorporate. This is the first step toward the final merging into mother nature. The isolation from the outer world that comes with dimming senses, the abatement of erotism, and the reduced vocational activities are compensated for by a new noetic or meditative urge that comes straight from the primal sources of all vital energy and gives a new and deeper sense of these and, if we are philosophical, brings a new sympathy with vitalistic theories like those of Lotze, Samuel Butler, Fechner, and Bergson, to say nothing of Schopenhauer, Nietzsche, Bernard Shaw, or the long line of evolutionists before Darwin, which goes back at least to Heraclitus. This final rally of powers just when the processes of bodily decay are accelerated, which in times past sometimes took the form of outbreaks of prophecy, admonition, or clairvoyance as to the meaning of present tendencies for the far future of the race and the further development of which is one of the great present hopes of a world in which the processes of degeneration are now being greatly accelerated, can be nothing else than the birth throes of a new and higher stage in the evolution of man. The task now rests upon us to intensify and prolong this stage and to assure it to an ever larger number. We already see that we here escape from many, and must learn to escape from more, of Metchnikoff's disharmonies in life. Sometime we shall both breed and educate for it, make it the ideal and goal for the young, and look for and heed its deliverances in the favored old. Having attained it, although death will seem all the darker by contrast with its regenerative light, man can meet it with less regret because he will not feel that he must be consoled by the sequel of another life. All forms of belief in the latter are, in fact, only surrogates expressive of a deeper faith and these symbols of it have served the precious purpose of keeping alive in his breast the sense that his life here was an unfinished fragmentary thing. The true Indian summer of life, when its possibilities are developed, is all that they mean, for in it all man's belated powers will ripen and the final harvest of his life be garnered.

As to death, normal old age loves it no better than do the young. Metchnikoff, who postulated an instinct for death as the reversal of the love for life and which he thought should supervene at the end, looked for it in himself when he faced imminent and certain death at nearly three-score-and-ten; but in vain. The late Secretary Lane, facing it, was praised for saying, "I accept," but the psychologist doubts whether anyone ever did or could welcome death understanding it to be extinction. The suicide may murder his instinctive will to live; the martyr may die in the hope of a better world beyond; the disappointed lover or the coward to life may turn to it as the lesser of two evils. A man may surrender his life as a sacrifice to a cause he deems greater than self but it is nevertheless a supreme sacrifice. A soldier accepts the fatal thrust of the bayonet and a criminal mounts the scaffold or sits in the death chair because he cannot help it. For how can life accept its own negation? It can never hope to know more of it than the sun can know of shadows, which are where it is not. Thus the old are no wiser and no more willing to die than the young, if indeed they are as much so, because it means more to the latter who have more to lose by it. All that philosophy or religion can do is to direct our minds from its full and stark envisagement.

Growing old hygienically is like walking over a bridge that becomes ever narrower so that there is progressively less range between the *licet* and the *non licet,* excess and defect. The bridge slowly tapers to a log, then a tight-rope, and finally to a thread. But we must go on till it breaks or we lose balance. Some keep a level head and go farther than others but all will go down sooner or later.

Several of my respondents say that they never on any account admit to themselves that they are old and a few advise us to avoid by every possible means all thought of death, using every method of diversion from it. One thinks that to dwell upon this theme is positively dangerous because the thought tends to bring the reality. I believe, on the contrary, that such an attitude is not only cowardly but that it involves self-deception because the *memento mori* is in fact always present, if unconsciously, in the old and to face the Great Enemy squarely really brings easement and safeguards us from a thanatophobia that may have far more dangerous outcrops. To have once deliberately oriented ourselves to death before our powers fail gives us a new poise what-

437

ever attitude toward it such contemplation leads us to.

My own conclusion that death is the end of body and soul alike, while it gives me a profound sense of satisfaction as having reached and accepted the final goal of all present culture tendencies which all serious souls feel impelled toward but which many of them still fight down also brings me, I frankly confess, a new joy in and love of life which is greatly intensified by contrast with the blankness beyond. As a dark background brings out a fading picture, so whatever remains of life is vastly more precious and more delectable day by day and hour by hour than it could possibly be if at the door of the tomb we only said *au revoir*. The very minutes seem longer because the departure into eternity is so near. Although death treats our psyche just as it does our soma, this is not so bad on our present views of the universe and insight lifts us above the need of consolation and even gives a sense of victory though Death do his worst, which those who expect another personal life never attain. And so I am grateful to senescence that has brought me at last into the larger light of a new day which the young can never see and should never be even asked to see. Thus if any of them should ever read my book thus far I would dismiss them here and in the following chapter address myself to the aged alone. That Jesus faced, and consciously, this absolute death at the close of his career seems to me now to have been made clear by modern critical and psychological investigation. But it was a sound pedagogic instinct that led the evangelists to veil this extreme experience of their Master.[8]

---

[8] See my *Jesus, the Christ, in the Light of Psychology*, Chapters VII and XI.

CHAPTER IX

THE PSYCHOLOGY OF DEATH

The attitude of infancy and youth toward death as recapitulating that of the race—Suicide—The death-wish—Necrophilism—The Black Death—Depopulation by the next war—The evolutionary nisus and death as its queller—Death symbolism as pervasive as that of sex—Flirtations of youthful minds with the thought of death—Schopenhauer's view of death—The separation of ghosts from the living among primitive races—The thanatology of the Egyptians—The journey of the soul—Ancient cults of death and resurrection in the religions about the eastern Mediterranean, based on the death of vegetation in the fall and its revival in the spring, as a background of Pauline Christianity—The fading belief in immortality and Protestantism which now at funerals speaks only of peace and rest—Osler's five hundred death beds—Influential, plasmal, and personal immortality and their reciprocal relations—Moral efficacy of the doctrine of future rewards and punishments—Belief in a future life for the individual being transformed into a belief in the future of the race on earth and the advent of the superman—Does man want personal immortality—Finot's immortality of the decomposing body and its resolution into its elements—The Durkheim school and the Mana doctrine—Schleiermacher—The Schiller-James view of the brain and consciousness as repressive of the larger life of the great Autos—The views of Plato and Kant—Have God and nature cheated and lied to us if the wish to survive is false—Noetic and mystic immortality by partaking of the deathlessness of general ideas—Views of Howison, Royce, and others—Is there a true euthanasia or thanatophilia—Diminution of the desire for personal immortality with culture and age—Thanatopsis.

FROM infancy to old age the conceptions of death undergo characteristic changes in the individual not unlike those through which the race has passed. The death fear or thanatophobia is, thus, a striking case of recapitulation. The infant, like the animal, neither knows nor dreads death. The death-feigning instinct in animals is only cataplexy and the horror of blood that some herbivora feel is not related to death. From Scott's 226 cases [1] and my own 299 returns to questionnaires [2] it

---

[1] *Am. J. Psychology*, vol. 8, p. 67 *et seq.*
[2] "A Study of Fears," *Am. J. Psy.*, vol. 8, pp. 147–249; see also Street, "A Genetic Study of Immortality," *Ped. Sem.*, vol. 6, p. 167 *et seq.*

appears that the first impression of death often comes from a sensation of coldness in touching the corpse of a relative and the reaction is a nervous start at the contrast with the warmth that the contact of cuddling and hugging was wont to bring. The child's exquisite temperature sense feels a chill where it formerly felt heat. Then comes the immobility of face and body where it used to find prompt movements of response. There is no answering kiss, pat, or smile. In this respect sleep seems strange but its brother, death, only a little more so. Often the half-opened eyes are noticed with awe. The silence and tearfulness of friends are also impressive to the infant, who often weeps reflexly or sympathetically. Children of from two to five are very prone to fixate certain accessories of death, often remembering the corpse but nothing else of a dead member of the family. But funerals and burials are far more often and more vividly remembered. Such scenes are sometimes the earliest recollections of adults. Scrappy memory pictures of these happenings may be preserved when their meaning and their mood have entirely vanished and but for the testimony of others they would remain unable to tell what it was all about.

Little children often focus on some minute detail (thanatic fetishism) and ever after remember, for example, the bright pretty handles or the silver nails of the coffin, the plate, the cloth binding, their own or others' articles of apparel, the shroud, flowers, and wreaths on or near the coffin or thrown into the grave, countless stray phrases of the preacher, the music, the incidents of the ride to the graveyard, the fear lest the bottom of the coffin should drop out or the straps with which it is lowered into the ground should slip or break, a stone in the first handful or shovelful of earth thrown upon the coffin, etc. The hearse is almost always prominent in such memories and children often want to ride

440

in one. This, of course, conforms to the well-known laws of erotic fetishism by which the single item in a constellation of them that alone can find room in the narrow field of consciousness is over-determined and exaggerated in importance because the affectivity that belongs to items that are repressed and cannot get into consciousness is transferred to those that can do so.

Children often play they are dead, even when alone. They stretch out in bed, fold their hands, and hold their breath as long as they can to see how it feels to be dead. A few in fancy feel ill, imagine doctor and nurse, go through the last agony, imagine others standing about weeping and praising them, or perhaps picture themselves as the bystanders and see the imaginary death of a friend and try to weep. Real grief is hard for them and late to understand and they often think tears a pretense. They sometimes pick out pretty coffins for themselves or their chums and imagine becoming burial frocks. The odor of varnish from a coffin sometimes has an incredible persistence and power to call up feelings and emotions. Many children fear the corpse will wake and sit up—"he is not dead but sleepeth," etc. Many are the records of how by calling, touching, pounding, or otherwise doing either forbidden or commendable things children strive to provoke or coax their dead relatives to awake.

Death has many degrees to children. The buried body is deadest. It is more so in the coffin than before being placed there. A very sick person who may die begins to be invested with the same awe. Lying in bed by day, the doctor, the silent nurse, the smell of medicines, often suggest that death has begun. Toward very old people children feel something of the same awe because they must soon die. According to some of our data some young children are incipient necrophiles, persistently trying to stroke, handle, or even kiss and hug the corpse. Scott's curves indicate that up to and at the age of five death is more likely to be interesting if not attractive, while at about nine its real horror first begins to be felt. Some, at a very tender age, acquire associations that persist for years, perhaps through life, and which are liable to be evoked by specific instances. This is, for example, the case with the sight and smell of tuberoses, a black box or boat, a crepe veil or bow on a door, hat, or garment, tolling of bells or even the ringing of them, etc. Certain phrases in Scripture and in some morbid cases all allusions to death are liable to cause hysterical outbreaks. Some thanatophobes in whom these infantile fetishistic fears persist cannot go past an undertaker's show window but go far around to avoid it. One such young man felt a sudden and strong aversion toward a young lady to whom he was attached as soon as he learned that she was employed in an undertaker's establishment. These aversions often spring up suddenly, perhaps in the form of a convulsive sob, tears, or inexplicable depression, although they are usually of infantile origin. Children's funerals and interments of pets are now represented by a small literature.

For young children the dead are simply absent and curious questions are asked as to where they have gone, when they will return, why the child cannot go with them. The infantile mind often makes strange mixtures of its own naïve constructions with adult insight. The distinction between psyche and soma, of which death is the chief teacher, is hard for the realistic minds of children. Told that Papa or Mama rest or sleep in the ground, they ask why they are there, where it is so cold and dark, why they do not wake, what they eat, who feeds them, impulsions in the race that primitive burial customs often elaborately answered by preparing bodies for reanimation, leaving food and utensils with the corpse, etc. When told of heaven above, children have strange, crass fancies, such as that the body is shot up to

442

heaven, the grave dug open by angels, the body passed down through the earth and then around up, etc. It generally gets out of the grave and goes to its abode by night.

As ideas of the soul begin to be grasped it is conceived as a tenuous replica of the body hovering about somewhere, sometimes seen though rarely felt. It may even be talked to or fancied as present, though unseen. Children's dreams of the dead are often vivid and rarely dreadful. In general the child thinks little or nothing but good of the dead and the processes of idealization, aided by adults, often almost reach the pitch of canonization so that later the memory of a dead parent may become a power in the entire subsequent life of sentiment as if all the instincts of ancestor worship were focalized on the individual parent. Indeed, we find some adults who maintain quiet sacred hours for thought of or ideal communion with their departed dear ones and such yearnings, of course, make a favorable soil for the ghost cult of spiritism. This component of our very complex attitude toward dead friends is also the stratum that crops out in the holy communion sacrament of the ghost dances of our American Indians, in which the souls of all the great dead of their tribe are supposed to come back and commune with their living descendants. Just in proportion as the dead are loved does death work its charm of sublimation and idealization, and just as a child of either sex has loved the parent of the other will he or she idealize a chosen mate snatched away by death. Thus, too, one factor in the belief in immortality is love that must conserve its object though deceased, this factor being quite distinct from the transcendental selfishness that would conserve our own ego. Young children often seem rather to rejoice in than to fear death. The excitement of all its ceremonies is new and impressive. Some even express a wish, after a funeral is over, that someone else would die. In their funeral games they quarrel as to who shall assume the central rôle of the corpse, which they feign well. One abnormal four-year-old tried to kill a younger mate and I find records of a number of pathological children who have actually done so, largely in order to enjoy the excitement of death, funeral, and burial. A sweet young girl was found dancing on the fresh grave of her younger sister, chanting, "I am so glad she is dead and I am alive," suggesting not the ancient days of famine when every death left more food for the survivors so much as jealousy at the diversion of parental attention and care to the younger child.

Neurotic children often play with unusual abandon, as if to compensate for the depression, when they have just left a room where brothers or sisters have breathed their last. A small boy who lost his father said, "Now I will milk, cut wood, bring up coal," etc., attempting thus to assume the father's rôle, perhaps even putting on some of his attire; while girls whose mothers die become more tender to their fathers or the other children, feeling themselves to be in some degree the surrogate of the mother. Just as children of tender age far more often fear the death of others than they do their own, so they vastly more often wish the death of those they hate than they feel any suicidal impulse. Children's propensity to play with death-shudders in their talk and thought was well illustrated in the case of two girls of perhaps seven whom I overheard while they were watching a man on a very high roof. One said, "Oh, I wish he would fall right down backwards and kill himself." "And they pick him up all bloody," giggled the other. "His bones all broke," said the first. "And put him in a black box in the grave," said the second. "And all his children cry," said number one. "And starve to death," added the other. They were getting more excited and spoke lower as they passed out of my hearing. The horror and also the fascination of rooms in which people have died often shows a conflict that is psychologically the same.

If death is thus distorted by misconceptions in infancy it looms up as a great and baffling mystery to fledgling *youth.* So little is it really understood by them that it is hard to utilize the fear of it even for motivating hygienic regimen. To tell a boy or girl in the teens that it has been proven that by conforming to certain established laws of health life may be prolonged on an average of fifteen years seems to them a far cry and it has little power as an incentive because they are so absorbed in living out all the possibilities of the present. There are certain perils, too, in using the death fear as a euthenic motive for the young. Yet during adolescence the death problem often becomes a veritable muse inspiring endless dreads, reveries, perhaps obsessions and complexes of the most manifold kind, especially in neurotics, in whom infantile impulses and adult insights are strangely mingled, producing weird perversions in later life. All these mazes we can never thread without a knowledge of the impression death has made upon the impressionable soul of man at every stage of life and perhaps most of all in the adolescent period, when youth first comes into close contact with the death thought.

When the young are achieving adulthood at the most rapid rate they are often overwhelmed with a sense of insufficiency, inferiority, or incompleteness against which they have to react as best they can. Tolstoi gave us a good illustration of this from his own boyhood. His tutor flogged him and he reacted as the only way in which he could "get even" by not merely the thought of suicide but the vivid imagination, well set in scene, of himself as dead and his father dragging the horrified tutor before his beautiful corpse and accusing him of having murdered his son, while the friends around

445

bemoaned him as so brilliant and so tragically slain. It seems strange that at that period of life when both vitality and viability are greatest and the will to live seems to have its maximal momentum the death thought is so prone to be obsessive. But death is very hard to conceive and interpretations of what it really means differ with every age, race, individual, and perhaps almost every moment of life. It is so negative, privative, and human nature, like physical nature, abhors a vacuum so much that the soul balks not only at the idea of annihilation but at every thought of the arrest of life. Recent studies of children's suicides show that although they begin at the early dawn of school age they are augmented by all repressions of their natural interests and instincts. Only at puberty or after, when the life of the race begins to dominate that of the individual, do children begin to comprehend what death really means; and even then, as the 58 suicides of German school children per year from 1883 to 1905 show, many, if not most, are sudden and impulsive and probably the majority, at least those of pubescent girls, are largely for the sake of the effect their death will have upon those nearest them. What child has not seriously considered suicide, at least in reverie? Several partial censuses have been unable to find one.[3]

As to the death wish, this may be often felt and even expressed impulsively on some special provocation and then the realization of it may bring not only horror but

---

[3] L. Proal, *L'éducation et le suicide des enfants*, Paris, 1907, p. 204; G. Budde, *Schülerselbstmorde*, Hanover, 1908, p. 59; E. Neter, *Der Selbstmord im kindlichen und jugendlichen Alter*, 1910, p. 28; L. Gurlitt, *Schülerselbstmorde*, n. d., p. 59; Baer, *Der Selbstmord im Kindesalter*, Liepzig, 1901, p. 85; Eickhoff, "Die Zunahme der Schülerselbstmorde an den höheren Schulen," *Zts. f. d. evangel. Religionsunter. an höheren Lehranstalten*, 1909, vol. 4; Eulenberg, "Schülerselbstmorde" in *Der Saemann*, 1909, vol. 5, p. 30; Gebhard, "Über die Schülerselbstmorde," *Monatss. f. höhere Schulen*, 1909, vols. 3 and 4, p. 24; Wehnert, *Schülerselbstmorde*, Hamburg, 1908, p. 81.

in neuropathic children may set up a prolonged and morbid corrective process to strangle it. We have many cases in which overtenderness to parents or relatives, which had become so insistent as to be troublesome, was motivated by the impulse to atone for a vivid death wish that took form in a moment of anger. In general we have only a life wish for our friends and reserve the death wish for enemies. Even in the most highly evolved emotional lives this is perhaps only a question of predominance, for psychoanalysts tell us that never was there a death, even of a lover, that did not bring some small modicum of joy to the survivor, swallowed up and overwhelmed as this component might be in grief. Were this not so, comforters and consolers would have no resources. We strive to think that our dear ones are happier, comforting ourselves with memories, and ascribe to the dead superior powers of transcendental enjoyment; while, conversely, no savage ever killed the bitterest foe of his tribe without elements of pity or perhaps phrases to atone for the soul of the victim or to his friends by saying propitiatory words or performing placatory rites. Even hell and devils never kill the soul and there are spots and spells of remission of torment so that surcease and nepenthe are not unknown, even in the inferno.

The death thought in some of our data seems to be spontaneous, that is, it may break out obsessively, not only on the slightest occasion but without any ascertainable cause. Some young people have spells of crying with wild abandon at the thought that they must die, which sometimes seems to sound out to them as if from the welkin. It is worst nights. It seems so unspeakably dreadful that they cannot steady their voice. The thought in the infant prayer, "If I should die before I wake," etc., made one child more or less neurotic for years with horror of hell and judgment and she was wont

447

to fancy herself found dead in the morning and used to pose for it to look her best. This, too, plays its rôle in revival hysteria. Some who have been very near death by drowning or other accident magnify this experience in memory until it may come to haunt them. Indeed, it seems characteristic of adolescence that although it may occur at later stages of life, in some quiet hour, perhaps when alone on the shore or in the forest or in a wakeful moment at night, the thought, "I must die," seems to spring and fasten upon the soul like a beast of prey. It flashes out with great and absorbing vividness. Occasionally a voice seems to pronounce the sentence. In a few cases it is so intense that a child fancies itself in the act of dying and springs up in terror. Probably all morbid fears of death are regressive or reversionary and have childish features. One clergyman was so haunted by it that he could not conduct funerals and only after years was he able to find self-control in the conviction that he might live on till Christ's second coming.[4]

---

[4] Mersey "La Tanatophilie dans la famille des Hapsbourg," *Rev. d. Psychiatr.* Nr. 12, 1912, p. 493, describes the strange case of love of death in the daughter of Ferdinand and Isabella and also Charles V. The former, after the death of her husband, Philip the Beautiful, whom she loved with a consuming jealousy, had his body embalmed and only with great difficulty could she leave the coffin where it lay. Sometimes she had it open for a time to kiss the bare corpse and did so with the greatest passion. This state had periods of remission and exacerbation. The history of Charles, too, can be paralleled in many modern instances, while dreams show us still more clearly how necrophilic man can be.

Witry says that from his own practice he believes thanatophobiacs are almost always from the professional or upper middle classes, those from the lower classes meeting death with more stoicism than those of the upper. Catholics, he says, have little fear of death. Thanatophobes are usually neuropaths of degenerate heredity. One of his cases, a girl of 18, was suddenly seized by a violent fear that she was to die within an hour. She was put to sleep by suggestion and woke up normal. A woman teacher of 49 had three acute attacks, cured by suggestion. A middle-aged physician, after being drunk, had acute fear of death and Hell, which yielded to medical treatment. Old priests, we are told, are especially subject to it if neuropathic or *"scrupuleux."* Some feel it acutely when, after fighting a long reluctance to do so, they have compelled themselves to make a will.

THE PSYCHOLOGY OF DEATH

In my teens in the country I often, and with a willingness that was hard for myself or my parents to understand, took my turn in watching with the sick and dying neighbors or "setting up" with corpses. On two occasions, once entirely alone, I performed as best I could the office of "laying out" the body of an old neighbor who died in the middle of the night. Other young people of my acquaintance were generally very ready to perform such offices although they involved great nervous tension, and in general a companion watcher was sought or provided. Another personal experience illustrates the persistence of juvenile attitudes toward death in mature life. As a boy in the country I had to pass, in going to and coming from the village, a lonely country church yard, by which I used to run and in which many of my relatives for generations were buried. Only a few years ago I yielded, during a sojourn at the village inn,

---

Ferrari, "La pour de la morte," *Rev. Scient.*, 1896, vol. 5, p. 59, describes several cases of tolerably healthy people who have had sudden premonitions of death, with acute fear, and who have shortly thereafter died, some of them from no ascertainable cause. Hence he raises the question whether an obsession of death can be so strong as to cause it.

Fiessinger gives a case, which he thinks directly due to the symptoms of *angina pectoris,* and discusses whether patients should be told their disease and its gravity, in view of this possible phobia.

Ferrero, "La crainte de la morte," *Rev. Scient.*, 1895, vol. 3, p. 361, thinks the natural man has little fear or thought of death and its representations in art and religion are not painful, on account of the sustaining influences of our organic sensations. Still, the thought of death does have much influence upon our ideas, and to some extent our sentiments. The mathematical chances of death plays a small rôle in affecting the choice of professions. It is only the prospect of impending death that shocks. Chronic invalids have little fear but only hope for life, for example, consumptives, while to some, for example, Indian widows, lovers, it is attractive. Hence he thinks it normally indifferent and sometimes agreeable but becomes an object of fear only by association.

Levy, "Die agoraphobie," *Wien. allg. medizin. Zeitung,* 1911, nr. 10, gives a case of an agoraphobia that was rooted in a very distinct dread of death by a special disease. A Dubois psychotherapeutic conversation, which proved the fallacy of its grounds and to which the patient attended, although with great effort, did not quiet but only increased excitement. Excitement and exhaustion were the chief symptoms and the case yielded only to isolation and rest.

to the whim of revisiting this graveyard by moonlight one midnight. I forced myself to climb over the high black entrance gate, for all was surrounded by a wall of dark-colored stone and by a row of pine trees. I walked deliberately through the graveyard and back, striking a match on my grandfather's tomb to light a cigar as a culmination of a kind of bravado that left nothing that an observer could detect as indicating anything but perfect poise and control. I did not even quite shudder when, as I stood amidst the grave stones, a dark cloud obscured the moon, and after walking back and forth there for a time I leisurely clambered out and went back. But the strange thing about it all was a nervous tension, the flitting fears and fancies that had to be kept under and that constantly impelled me to turn and run. On returning I found myself in a state of high nervous excitement and realized that almost any sudden unexpected shock would have caused me, as the sudden obscurity of the moon nearly did, to yield to precipitate flight.

Thus, we see in the young buds of about all of the many and diverse attitudes the race has assumed toward death. Most of them are polymorphic and perverse, some merely organic residua of long phyletic influences. Thus, as in sex, the components of the death attitudes are early present but are not organized into unity until puberty, when the racial experiences in both fields come to be more or less unified. It would seem that death has no business with young people or they with it and that it is as absurd for them to occupy themselves with it at this age as it would be for them to worry about posterity before the dawn of adolescence. Since the life and growth of the psyche and soma are now at their flood-tide, it would seem that every intimation of death would be not only foreign to the very nature of young people but would be arrestive of the course of nature and should be veiled in reticence, like sex, before its time, with only provisional answers to the genuine questions about it. Indeed, the above data seem to show that the genetic impulse itself seems to shield the child by diverting it from the central fact of death to countless irrelevancies, trivialities, and accessories. Just as the instinct of the race has blindly striven to avoid sex precocity, if not to delay puberty, and more consciously and purposively to enforce a period of repression between the age of pubescence and that of nubility, so myth, primitive religion, and especially Christianity, have provided ways of mitigating, even for adults but more especially for the young, the nameless horror of direct envisagement of the fact that all must die and cease to be, body and soul, or, like the Nirvana cult, to make this conviction more tolerable.

Indeed, it is probably a normal instinct of compensation that often leads young people to visit morgues and perhaps dissecting rooms, to develop a certain immunity from such obsessive tendencies as the above.[5] Great earthquakes, disastrous floods, and, above all, war and pestilence compel us to face the death thought at close quarters for a season and there are always those who revel in describing it in its most gruesome details, although there is a tacit consensus of the press to sup-

---

[5] A striking illustration of this comes to me, as I write, in a popular song with lugubrious music that many of my young friends persist in singing and humming as if haunted by it.

SOME SWEET DAY

Did you ever think as the hearse rolled by
That some day or other you must die?

In an old churchyard, in a tiny lot,
Your bones will wither and then they'll rot.

The worms'll crawl up, the worms'll crawl in,
They'll crawl all over your mouth and chin.

They'll bring their friends, and their friends' friends, too;
You'll look like hell when they're through with you.

451

press the most horrible of them. Soldiers have to be hardened to inflict it in its most direct and personal way, as, for example, by the bayonet, as well as to keep cool when they are first under fire and to carry on and not turn and flee in panic when their comrades are torn to pieces about them. Such experiences, while they often mature the unripe and give a new poise to character, also tend to make human life seem cheaper, so that it is not strange that wars are followed by crime waves and especially by marked increase in assaults. For disguise it as we may, war is at root licensed murder and its heroes are they who have killed the most of those who have been declared enemies. Indeed, it is self-evident that the normal man who can deliberately stake his life in a fight in which he knows that he must either kill or be killed does so because he realizes that there is something that he values more than he does his life, and to have had one such experience marks an epoch of the utmost moral import. Perhaps it is not too much to say that only those who have made this supreme sacrifice in spirit are finished and complete men.

When death holds high carnival and whole populations are depleted, long periods of readjustment follow and human nature breaks out in strange ways. Defoe's very realistic though fictive story of the Great Plague showed this. J. W. Thompson [6] says that the Black Death, A.D. 1348–1349, swept away at least one-third of the population of Europe and brought in its train economic chaos, social unrest, profiteering, lack of production, phrenetic gayety, dissipation, wanton spending, recklessness, greed, debauchery, avarice, hysteria, and decay of morals. The nerves of the people were shattered. Goods were without owners but everything movable was immediately appropriated by survivors. Prices first shrank very low

---

[6] *Am. J. Sociology*, March, 1921.

and then rose to preposterous heights. The Plague was like an invasion and there were great migrations for years. There was administrative inefficiency for the trained class was cut down. The machinery of government almost stopped and there were thousands of ignorant and incompetent men in important public places. The church was no better off and it had to press unfit raw recruits into its service. Flagellants exhibited a mixture of religion and sex rivaling the psychology of the crusades. Thought went off on all kinds of tangents. There were charlatans, mind-readers, sorcerers, witch doctors, soap-box preachers, and the Pied Piper very likely really did lead the excited children with his mad antics and wierd music to wander off with him until, as in the children's crusade, they were lost. Thompson points out that although there are many points of difference, there are more very significant analogues between the after-effects of this plague and those of the World War. A Danish historian estimates that in the latter ten million soldiers died in battle or of wounds, three million were permanently disabled, and probably some thirty million more people would have been alive to-day but for it. Such a decimation of Europe has certainly brought social, economic, and psychological changes that it would take us long to evaluate.

Meanwhile, we cannot entirely escape the looming prospect of a far more disastrous war that may yet come. W. Irwin [7] has cleverly hit off some of the possibilities of the awful holocaust that death would probably celebrate if such a conflict ever came to pass. Instead of liquid flame we have now Lewisite gas, which is invisible, sinks, and would search out every dugout and cellar, while it also attacks the skin and almost always kills, having a spread fifty-five times greater than that of any other

---

[7] *The Next War*, New York, 1921.

poison gas. He quotes an expert as saying that a dozen Lewisite air-bombs of the greatest size and under favorable atmospheric conditions would practically eliminate the population of Berlin and we even have hints of a gas beyond this. Gas will very likely be the chief weapon of the future war. Moreover, the bombing airplane has a range, of course, far beyond any gun. Bombs grew in size during the war from that of a grapefruit to eight feet in length, with half a ton of explosives and gas-generating chemicals, costing some $3,000 each and the planes carrying these will be directed by wireless, so that the airplane is thus the supergun. Hitherto warfare has been directed against soldiers, but in the future it will be against whole peoples and this generation may see a great metropolis suddenly made into a necropolis. Formal declaration of war, too, will become as obsolete as a Fauntleroy courtesy. Killing will be not by hand but by machinery; not in retail but by wholesale. War will be not between individual nations or small groups of them but will embrace the entire world, even the East, so that there will be no neutrals. Tanks will be used as super-dreadnoughts and poison gases will perhaps paralyze the soil for years, as indeed they have done to some extent in eastern France. Thus if war in the future becomes one hundred per cent efficient in the use of the resources at present at its command and those that it is only the part of common sense to anticipate, the depopulation caused will be incalculable and the world may experience again all the phenomena that Europe did after the Black Death, and perhaps more.

There is an evolution larger than Darwinism and far older than science in which all who think have everywhere and always believed. The common phenomena of growth suggest it to every mind. It is almost of the nature of thought to seek origins and to trace things to their simple beginnings. Indeed, the most perfect knowledge of anything is the description of the processes of its development. Special creation myths, cosmogonies, and religious theories of the world and man, philosophies and histories, are all products of the same deep instinct to know the cosmos as a whole and also its parts genetically. And it is a deep and dominant noetic instinct that has given us the far more highly evolved evolutionism that now prevails in every department of human knowledge. Thus, even those who oppose its recent applications to man are only halting at the last step in a path that all have traveled far and long.

The will-to-live, the struggle for survival, the *élan vital*, libido, etc., are only new names given to the impelling forces of the growth-urge in its higher stages; but these have become types and symbols, if a bit anthropomorphic, of all the more basal and earlier processes by which the homogeneous tends to differentiate itself. Thus we may conceive the universe as being from the first in labor to produce life. Everything that lives hungers to do so more intensely and as for man " 'tis life of which our nerves are scant, more life and fuller—that we want." Macrobiotism was the term used to designate the lust to maximize our lives, to make them vivid and long, and to exhaust all the possibilities of human experience; but, more especially, to enlarge the pleasure field and narrow that of pain, which is arrestive. We want to enjoy everything of which man's estate is capable and we want it here and now. In youth, particularly, we long for wealth, knowledge, power, strength, fame, health, and beauty because these make us glow and tingle with life. The things to which we ascribe worth and value are those that enhance the joy of living. All of them are only forms of the affirmation of the will-to-live or fulfillments of the wish to be well, happy, and of consequence to ourselves and others. Progress, reform, enlightenment, enterprise, efficiency, are terms used as we climb the heights of the excelsior mount of promise. "More life and fuller"—we want nothing else here or hereafter.

But death, ghastly, inevitable death, is our goal. It is the great and universal negation of life and coregent with it of the world. All that lives must die. How the death-thought sometimes springs like a beast of prey from its ambush upon youth when life is most intense and how it blights, sears, stings, and wounds but nevertheless charms and fascinates! Here is the first of all dualisms, the greatest of all contrasts, and the most universal of all conflicts. Death is dissolution, defeat, retreat, abnegation, the processes of which begin with life itself and even the old who still "carry on" know that they must soon become carrion and that no funeral pomp or tomb can do more than camouflage putridity in order to divert us from the horrid thought to escape which the very concept of the soul itself was entified and immortalized, just as all the devices of modesty and all the precepts of sexual morality were evolved to divert us from the envisagement of bare sex organs and acts. Death is not only the king of terrors but to the genetic psychologist every fear is at bottom the fear of death, for all the scores of phobias that prey upon man are of things and of experiences that abate life. Death is thus a matter of infinite degrees from the loss of a penny or a sore tooth to that of a friend or to our own extinction. Freudians rightly ascribe many ailments of mind and body to abnormalities and disharmonies of sex love, which presides over the life of the race. But this now needs to be supplemented by quite another and probably no less important psychoanalysis that will show, when it is explored, that the fear of death or of life-abatement for the individual is no whit less pervasive and dominant than are love and hunger, which are so often said to rule the world. Only one psychologist has, although but very partially, recognized this and his findings are résuméd as follows.

W. Stekel says that not only has death played a great rôle in poetry, folklore, myth, religion, and art, but it is a more or less disguised theme of many dreams, especially those of neurotics.[8] He urges that not only the death fear but the death wish, masked in very diverse symbolic forms, is extremely common in the dreams of psychopaths. He ascribes a thanatic meaning to very many factors that analytic Freudians have usually interpreted as having only a sexual significance and holds that the same mechanisms apply to both. He would have all psychoanalysts look for the death thought, which he believes hardly less common and quite as disguised and illusive as sex, not only in dreams but in the illusions of the insane. To our bestial unconscious self, which in these experiences escapes the censor, the ego is supreme and finds its ultimate goal only in the destruction of others; and if it does not kill those in our way, it pictures their death or finds some way for their removal. This, indeed, is involved in the realization of very many of our secret hopes. A woman loves a man whom she cannot see and so she dreams that her child dies, for she knows that he would attend the funeral and there see and also pity her. A man has more or less unconsciously ceased to love his wife but suppresses the realization of the fact from his waking consciousness and so dreams of her as talking with his grandfather, long since dead. Another man in a like state of mind dreamed that his wife suddenly and mysteriously vanished.

The most common death symbols are going away, a journey, wandering; or there may be still more remote focalization of the death wish upon sandals, feet, footsteps, a path, going home, passing through a narrow

---

[8] *Die Sprache des Traumes*, 1911, pp. 214–284.

street or door, growing small; or even vehicles of any sort or anything suggestive of transportation may signify death. Instead of a skeleton or skull the dream may conceive death under the form of a rider, huntsman upon a white or black horse, a deaf mute—suggestive of the silence of the grave—or blindness, symbolic of its darkness; a doctor, perhaps Doctor White or Doctor Black, a tailor cutting a thread, a messenger, raven, black cat or dog, thirteen, a clergyman, priest, weeping willow, a woodman felling a tree, a mower or reaper, a small house or room, fire or flood.

Death in our unconscious is a wondrous masquerader and it very often appears as sleep. The grave is a bed; the churchyard, a dormitory; catacombs, berths. Water symbolism, too, is very common, for example, the crossing of a dark river to the other shore, a boat, a narrow strait, a stormy or a deep dark sea across which we pass to an island or a new continent, the abode of the dead; and we speak of going out with the ebb of the tide, shipwreck, stranding, etc. Death may also appear as a fire that consumes or purifies. Processions and even crowds may suggest burial or funerals; and so sometimes do festivals or even weddings. A chest or trunk may mean a coffin, and graduation or even promotion in school may stand for "passing out." Sometimes the basis of the primitive impulse to kill, which made man a wolf to his fellow-man, may crop out in dreams or insanity without either camouflage or repression and the sleeper tries poison, pistol, dagger, knife, etc. Perhaps man still has in his unconscious, deep down at the bottom of his soul, the sin of father-murder, as some now tell us, and reaction to this brings remorse and later a sense of atonement from the original sin and guilt for which man has for ages sought remission and fancied resurrection. At any rate, many psychoneurotic souls seek to compensate for instinctive death wishes by excessive tenderness to friends and relatives, whose removal, they realize with horror, they have sometimes caught themselves desiring. Nietzsche says that we should never pity the old who are about to die; but under the law of bipolarity the worship and even the tyranny of the dead hand, or mortmain, has sometimes developed to such a degree that the dead have been or should be made to die again to free us from their control.

If these views are at all correct, our larger, older unconscious soul is still full of reverberations of suffering, inflicting, and observing death. Man became man when he knew that he must die, and to defer or escape death has been the basal motivation of all of his culture. That he might not starve he accumulated property, the primitive form of which, as Leternau has shown, was food. To escape death by the rigors of climate he devised clothing and shelter. To avoid it by wild beasts and human enemies he devised weapons and organized the hunt and warfare. To keep himself alive when attacked by disease, the medicine man and later the healing art were evolved. Now he insures not only against death but against the partial death involved in the loss of limbs, accident, and illness; he safeguards his person and his goods by codes and law courts; and regulates diet, regimen, mores, and social hygiene with a view to more and fuller life. All these institutions are impelled by the instinct of self-preservation, reinforced as it now is in man by the knowledge of his mortality. Man may thus be redefined as the death-shunner. He does not and cannot begin to realize how much he fears death and dreads it now and always has. The reason for this is that while the knowledge that he must die is so certain and ineluctable, the opposite impulse to forget, repress, and deny this fact also has behind it the momentum of ages. The rank, raw death-thought that our late dear ones are, and that we shall soon become, masses of rotting putridity, most offensive of all things to sense and sources of loathsome and mortal contagion, is so rarely allowed to escape its inveterate censorship that we are all liable to become neurotic toward it if it does so.

One envisagement of an erstwhile dear one who had become this most loathsome of all objects drove Buddha to renounce his throne, wealth, and family, and to become a mendicant and a seeker for, if not an antidote at least a palliative for the awful death-thought. The great religion he founded is essentially a religion of pity for man because he is doomed to die. Its founder aspired to be the world's great consoler, accepting frankly the stark and gruesome thought of death with all its horrifying implications.

Schopenhauer, who had a very morbid fear of death till near the close of his life, when it seemed to quite abate, developed views about it that have had immense influence throughout the world, especially in Germany. He believed his views to be modern expressions of ancient Hindu philosophy and also that all systems of philosophy are primarily either comforts for or antidotes to death.[9] The power behind creative evolution he calls the will-to-live, which is blind and unreasonable. "It is not the knowing part of our ego that fears death, but the *fuga mortis* proceeds entirely and alone from the blind will with which everything is filled." Only the will as it exhibits itself in the body is destroyed by death. We should no more dread the time when we shall not be than we regret the time before birth when we were not. The infinite time before us is no more dreadful than the infinite time that preceded us. As of sleep, we may say: Where we are, death is not; and where death is, we are not. "If one knocked on the graves and asked the dead whether they wished to rise again, they would all shake

_____

[9] *The World as Will and Idea,* vol. iii, p. 249 *et seq.*

their heads." We were enticed into life by the hope of more favorable conditions of existence and death is disappointment and return to the womb of nature, who is all the while entirely indifferent to both our birth and death. Only small minds fear it. It is to the species what sleep is to the individual. All that exists is worthy only of being destroyed.

We come into life buoyant and happy but before leaving it have to pay for all the joy by pain enough to compensate. True, the intellect, which is an individual acquisition, is sloughed off by death, while the will is given its freedom again. "The will of man, in itself individual, separates itself in death from the intellect," so that new generations get new intellects. This is the truth that underlies the doctrine of metempsychosis or palingenesis and is the faith of half the world. Here, too, roots the philosophy of eternal recurrence. The present generation in its inner metaphysical nature, that is, in its will, is identical with every generation that has preceded, but we do not recognize either our previous form of existence or the friends we once knew in a former state because the intellect, with its memory and perceptions, is only phenomenal and individual. Christianity gave itself a needlessly hard task in representing the soul as created *de novo* and in failing to recognize that pre- and post-existence support each other. "Death is the great reprimand which the will-to-live, or more especially the egoism which is essential to this, receives through the course of nature, and it may be conceived as a punishment for our existence. It is the painful loosening of the knot which the act of generation has tied with sexual pleasure, the violent destruction coming from without of the fundamental error of our nature, the great disillusion. We are at bottom something that ought not to be; therefore we cease to be." The loss of our individuality is thus only apparent or phenomenal. "Death is the great opportunity to be no longer I." "During life the will of man is without freedom. Death looses his bonds and gives him his true freedom which lies in his *esse,* not in his *operari.*" Individuality is one-sided and "does not constitute the inner kernel of our being" but is rather to be conceived as an aberration of it. Thus death is a *"restitutio ad integrum."* The wise man wishes to die really and not merely apparently and so desires no continuation of his personality. "The existence which we know we will all give up; what we get instead of it is, in our eyes, nothing because our existence with reference to that is nothing" (Nirvana).

It is an illusion to place the ego in consciousness because in fact "my personal phenomenal existence is just as infinitely small a part of my true nature as I am of the world." "What is the loss of this individuality to me who bear in me the possibility of innumerable individualities?" Individuality is thus "a special error, a false step, something that had better not be, nay something which it is the real end of life to bring us back from." Death is, thus, the awakening from the dream of life, which is made up of trivialities and contradictions, time being only one of the principles of individuation and having no absolute existence but being merely a form of knowledge of it. Will is the true thing itself. It is human nature that is perdurable. It is true that we know only even our will as phenomenon and not what it really and absolutely is in itself. Knowledge is entirely distinct from will but the latter is always and everywhere primal. The inveterate blunder of philosophers is to place the eternal element in the intellect while in fact it lies solely in the universal will and struggle to live, which is indestructible. We cannot know it because of the essential limitations of consciousness *per se,* but in the true being of things free from these forms the latter distinction between the individual and the race disappears and the two are identical. The continuation of the species is really the image of the indestructibility of the individual.

We are lured into life by the hope of pleasure and retained in it by fear of death; but both are equally illusions. It is strange that the only thing in us that really fears death, namely, the will, is precisely that which is never affected by it. "Thus, although the individual consciousness does not survive death, yet that survives it which alone struggles against it, namely, the will." Neither the intellect nor anything in it is indestructible for knowledge is only secondary and derived from the objectivizations of the will. "The intellect is dropped when it has served its purpose. Death and birth are the constant renewal of the consciousness of the will, in itself without end and without beginning, which alone is, as it were, the substance of existence." When in death the will is separated from the intellect, it feels lost because it has so long depended on it, and hence we fear. Life is only a heavy dream into which the will-to-live has fallen. To the dying we may say, "Thou ceasest to be something which thou hadst done better never to become." Thus generations of individuals are constantly reappearing, each fitted out with new intellects. But every new form of life is only an assumption in another form of the same will. Thus for Schopenhauer death is emancipation of the will from its slavery to consciousness, a breaking down of the wall it has erected between individuals, a regression to the ultimate momentum that underlies evolution, so that new individuals made of the same will, but disencumbered of the limitations life and mind impose, are ever starting again. The race is immortal and even back of that nature herself is still more so. The rhythm of life and death does change the nature or the form of the eternal currents of existence.

But, leaving Schopenhauer, we must go back to the

very beginnings of humanity to realize all that the death-thought has done in the world and to understand how man has always wrestled with it, tried to fight it down, and devised so many ways and means of escaping from it. Probably there was never a stage of human life so low that corpses were not separated from the living and put away by themselves, so that necrophilism hardly seems to be an atavistic psychic rudiment. Man disposes of corpses by fire, water, or inhumation, towers of silence, tombs, cemeteries and other homes set apart for them, while animals do nothing of this kind. He alone cannot endure the spectacle of the fate that nature provides and so shroud, coffin, flowers, monuments, shrubs, trees, serve to divert attention from what is going on in the sepulchre below.

But the great diversion, coeval with the beginning of corpse disposal, was the conception of a soul separable from the body and surviving it, and this is as old as animism. Other factors, of course, contributed to the primitive belief in souls but when and wherever it arose it became the chief distractor from and the great negator of the death-thought. Now, as the body is not all, death is not complete and some part of us, however tenuous, lives on. Let the carcass rot. We can now focus our attention upon a spirit that outlives the flesh and this invention is the chief panacea mankind has found against the most gruesome of all its ills. In the very crudest and crassest form of belief in a separable soul lie the promise and potency of all the quellers of death-thoughts that have arisen from it; and so, when in the course of time it came that the air was becoming as full of ghosts as the earth was of corpses, they too had to be partitioned off from the living and given their own abode beyond some river, sea, mountain or other barrier, or beneath or above the earth. Whatever betide, the souls of the departed must be driven and kept away by apotropic rites or by sacrifices, the motto of which was *do ut abais*. Thus the living had to herd the souls of the dead as they had their bodies in order that they themselves might be free and sane. This was a great achievement, which spiritists and psychic researchers tend to undo, for ghosts must be laid just as bodies must be buried and the decomposing souls that appear in seances are only less offensive to common sense than the mouldering bodies are to sense.

Thus the fear of death has always called attention more strongly than anything else to the soul and to psychology. Something leaves the human body at death and has some power of independent existence; but just as the body must be put away so ghosts must be laid or driven off. In primitive culture the souls of the dead tend to linger near the body. Sometimes widows are plunged into water to drown off the souls of their dead husbands before they can marry again. Some tribes turn out *en masse* at stated times to frighten away the spirits, as they do to get rid of vermin and rats or to clean house. Ghosts may be burned in effigy. A window or hole in the roof must be opened for the soul of the dead to escape and afterwards closed. The body is carried several times around the house so that the soul cannot find its way back. Those unjustly treated or not buried may return for vengeance. Some think tombstones were primitively to hold down the souls of the dead, just as the Tiber was turned and Attila buried in its bed and it was then made to flow back again so as to keep him in the land of spirits. In Gurney's *Phantasms of the Living* ghosts have their chief power at or near the moment of death. It is one of the great functions of the medicine man to dispose of the spirits of the dead and many rites were devised to relegate them to some place appointed. The living have their own domain and their own rights, which the dead must respect. Only the witch makes havoc with this order by bringing back the souls of the departed. Thus many kinds of barriers grew up between the living and the dead—distance, oblivion, a stream, a belt of fire, a deep chasm, a high divide, etc., so that the ghost world became hard to get to or from. Thus, in general, man does not wish to go to the realm of ghosts or to have them trespass upon his preserves. The New Zealanders conceived such preserves for their dead over the precipice of Reinga; the Fiji Islanders in their deep and fiery cañons; the Sandwich Islanders in the subterranean abodes of Akea; the Kamchatkans in an underground Elysium; the Indians in a Happy Hunting Ground; the Greenlanders deep under the sea; the old Teutons in Walhalla, the temple of the slain with its columns of spears and roof of shields; and the Greeks and Romans in the realm of Pluto. There are many roads and many ushers to conduct souls to their own home—sunbeams, the Milky Way, paths through caverns, or over the rainbow bridge Bifröst; while in Greece Charon and in Egypt Anubis carried souls across or through the interval or partition. In all these ways man has sought to conceive of the souls of the dead as effectively shepherded in folds of their own.

Other studies show that there is a sense in which every incident of a funeral tends to lay ghosts. If we simply hear at a distance of the death of our friends, we are far more liable to receive visits from their revenient spirits or dream of them as alive than if we have actually seen them buried, because all the incidents of this ceremony bring home, even to our unconscious selves, the fact that they are really dead and gone from us, soul and body. Thus the tears, Scripture reading, badges of mourning, and even the expense tend to reef in our sense of our dead friend's personality and to make it powerless to project ghostly phantasms, because such ceremonials are cathartic and preventative of all such hallucinations.

466

Thus, at this stage of the story of the immortality cult we have two worlds well apart and the *Jenseits,* or the realm of death, can perhaps be reached from the *Diesseits* of the body only by a long and dangerous journey that the psyche must take after leaving the soma to moulder. Why has man always stood in such awe of the ghosts of even his friends? The answer is not simple. It is partly because he wanted to be free from their constraint. They included his parents, from whose control even youth, at a certain stage, wants to be well rid. Even his dearest ones might cherish some secret grudge that could now be indulged in with impunity. As spirits they have certain unknown new powers for mischief, whereas if they were enemies they could use these powers for revenge. Toward the dead we generally have a bad conscience. They can often read our secret motives while we cannot read theirs. Thus man propitiated the pallid shades of Orcus by offerings and sacrifices to abate their malevolence and secure their good-will. However remotely he banished them, he has never been able to realize the fact that they were utterly dead forever, soul as well as body. All his will to rid himself of them has always stopped short of entire fulfillment.

On the contrary, some of the great dead he has not only immortalized but deified. Others may still come back at midnight in a dream or vision at some weird haunted spot or in dire emergencies; or if conjured by constraining spells of sufficient potency; perhaps if they have not been rightly buried; or to deliver some pregnant message; or, again, to pronounce a curse or benediction. It is generally hard for them to get to us and also, having done so, to make their presence felt and they are perhaps so exhausted by this effort that they can tell us nothing; while it is given to but few mortals to visit their abode and come back unscathed and to fewer yet it is given to bring back others with them.

SENESCENCE

One of the most momentous steps in culture was taken by the ancient Egyptians, whose religion, more than that of any other race, might, in view of our recent knowledge of it, be called the cult of the dead *par excellence*. The new step here taken consisted, in a word, in making the postmortem status of the soul dependent upon virtue in this life, thus enlisting the mighty power of the next world in behalf of morals. Their famous book of the dead presupposes "a religious belief in the actual revivification of the body," because of which hoped-for event the Egyptians took the greatest possible care to preserve and afterwards to hide the bodies of the dead. This famous book treats of the soul's journey through Amenti, of the gods and other residents there, with formulæ that will deliver the migrant thither from foes. It contains prayers and hymns to the great gods intended to recommend him to all of them; texts that must be inscribed on both the amulets and bandages of the mummies; plan and arrangement of the mourning chamber; the confession before the assessors; the scene where the heart is weighed in the hall of Osiris; and a representation of the Elysian fields, etc.

At death, relatives and mourners emerged from their houses to the streets, placed mud upon their heads, fasted, and priests pronounced an oration describing the good works of the great dead. There were sometimes accusations and formal judgments by the forty elders as to whether or not the burial should be in due form to convey the soul to the gods. If the verdict was favorable, the gods were entreated to admit him into the place reserved for the good; if not, he was deprived of burial and must lie in his own house. If there were debts, the body was given to creditors as a pledge until the sacred duty of redeeming it was performed. The details of embalmment during the seventy-two days of mourning were given in great profusion for each part of the body.

Each bandage had its text and the tomb must be made a proper dwelling place for the ka, or soul, which will stay there as long as the body does. Each process, pledget, and wrapping, had its name and there was an elaborate trade in bitumen, which is the meaning of the word mummy.

The people felt great satisfaction in preserving and seeing the simulated features of their ancestors, whom they came to regard in some sense as contemporaneous. The welfare of the soul in the nether world depended upon the completeness of all the funeral processes. At the height of this central cult of Egypt, bulls, antelopes, cats, crocodiles, ibis, hawk, frog, toad, scorpion, snake, fish, hippopotamus, cow, lion, sphinx, were sacred to the gods and were mummified, while the scarab was loaded down with symbolic meanings and became central in all funeral rites. These ceremonials did not decline until the third or fourth century of our era and only when Christianity taught that the body would be given back in a changed and incorruptible form, did it cease to be necessary to preserve it with drugs. This necrophilism was all for the sake of the soul and both expressed and strengthened belief in it. The cult of no race has been so saturated with thanatism.

In all we know of the folk-soul there is no more striking illustration of geneticism than the slow but sure establishment in recent years, by comparing ancient myths and rites with the findings of excavations, of the fact that in the great countries about the eastern Mediterranean, especially Thrace, Asia Minor, and Egypt, the highest religious consciousness of these races was expressed in elaborate cults of death and resurrection, to have participated in which is said to have made the celebrants over and initiated them into a new and higher life. All was so secret and oath-bound that it found little representation, save the most incidental allusions in

469

history and literature, so that it was reserved for modern research to uncover, reconstruct, and understand its tremendous power.

Osiris, Persephone, Attis, the lover of the all-mother Cybele, Demeter and Dionysius in the Eleusinian mysteries, Astar in her restoration of Phanæus and many others, some with very high and full and some with very scanty and fragmentary developments of the myth and cult, died and perhaps went to Hades and came back bringing, now one, now many with them. Typical of these ceremonies were the funereal sadness, death dirge, wailings, active symbolic manifestations of grief and despair, as if to attain the very acme of psychalgia. The great, good, beautiful, divine hero is not only dead but has perhaps gone over into the nether-world to defy death and the power of evil in their stronghold and to conquer and bind them. There is, then, a phase of painful, anxious, silent suspense. Will he succeed and return or will he fail and never reappear? Then, when the tension is at the very breaking-point, comes the thumic ebb, rebound, or reversal. Someone whispers or cries aloud, "He has won and comes back," and then all is changed. Lights flare out in the darkness. Instead of tears and sobs there is joy unrestrained, congratulations, embraces, and soon frantic ecstasy, leaping, shouting, wine, song, revelry, bells, fireworks, and sometimes in degenerate days, drunkenness and gluttony with the sacramental elements and, in token of the triumphs of the higher love, perhaps carnal debauch and revelry and always ecstasy and inebriation with euphoria. Thus from three to six centuries B.C. men strove to attain an immunity bath that should safeguard them from all excessive pain and pleasure of life by participation in a pageantry or dramatization of the eternal struggle between the greatest evil, death, and the dread of it and the greatest joy of the most intense living, thus ensuring

470

their souls against being led captive by the pleasures or pains of life, neither of which could be so extreme as these, by keeping wide open the way from the extremest depression to the maximum of exaltation.

Now all this rests in every case where it can be traced upon the retreat of the sun and the death of the world, symbolized by winter and the return of spring, reinforced, of course, by the alternations of day and night. These deities or their prototypes were originally gods of vegetation and their resurrections are vernal. The everlasting bars that broke were snow and ice. The king of glory that came in when the gates were lifted was spring, the conqueror, or dawn; and in these secular changes of the year are found the first preformations of the soul and the momentum that still subconsciously reinforces belief in a life after death and supplies always an anodyne and often an antidote for the death-fear.

It was on this basis that Christianity, especially as interpreted by Paul, arose.[10] The culminating event in its story took place in the few days between the burial of Jesus and the Pentecostal outburst. Never in history, if it be history, and never in the subject story of Mansoul, if this be the stage on which it was all accomplished, has there been such an *au rebours* from the nadir of depression of the disciples, because the type-man of their race, who had grown to their minds to be a fully diplomated God-man, was completely dead—and that in shame and ignominy—and his corpse sealed up to moulder and rot in a rock. Then came first the timid and then the plenary conviction that He had conquered death and even hell, risen from the dead, walked and conversed with friends in an attenuated body and had visibly ascended to Heaven and God. Once fully convinced that this was all veritably true, witnessed and attested by every sense

---

[10] See my *Jesus, the Christ, in the Light of Psychology*, Chap. XI, "Death and Resurrection of Jesus."

and proof, the great incubus of ages was thrown off and Death, the supreme terror, was abolished. This brought an ecstasy or intoxication of joy called the gift of the Holy Spirit, which possessed the lives of believers. The ecstatic disciples shouted in weird unknown tongues until onlookers thought them "full of new wine" (Acts 2:13, 15), gazed all day into Heaven, henceforth the home of souls, and had to be exhorted to cease their raving jubilations and go to work. In this exhilarating new joy and freedom they, and later their successors, met the nine persecutions, during which martyrdom became a passion and tender youths and maidens could hardly be restrained from throwing themselves to the wild beasts in the arena as the supreme crown and testimony to their faith.

So, too, Christian asceticism followed from the same motive. This life was mean and it mattered little how squalid it was, for it was only a provisional, probationary moment compared to the eternal joy and happiness where all real worths and values were confidently awaited and compared to which those of earth were only dross. "There is no death. What seems so is transition" to an infinitely higher state than this. Never did the other world so absorb the power of this. Visions, trances, homilies, poems, poetry and theology fitted the other world out with every good and the chief offices of the church were to keep the keys of the transcendental world and to wield its tremendous sanctions in a way to dominate life and determine good and evil. Thus never was the greatest *Verdrängung* (repression) that ever oppressed the human race so completely removed. The most essential claim of Christianity is to have obviated the fear of death and made the king of terrors into a good friend, if not into a boon companion, by this the most masterly of all psychotherapies. If it be only a pragmatic postulate or hypothesis or *Als Ob* (As If) in

Vaihinger's sense, it has worked well on the whole. Despite the ever present dangers of transcendental selfishness that prompts only to save one's own soul, it is nevertheless the supreme demonstration of the *"Allmacht"* (omnipotence) of the folksoul to minister to its own gravest diseases and banish its greatest enemy, the death fear.

Thus Jesus is most widely known as the Man of the Cross and the crucifix and even the fragments of the Cross are revered throughout the Christian world. In no other religion has the death of the founder had such prominence or efficacy. All the events of Holy Week have been wrought out in great detail by tradition and art. Its story is the world's great masterpiece of pathos. The ecstasy of the passover represents the culmination of the conquest of the death-fear by Mansoul. The gift of the Holy Spirit was simply the conviction that death itself was dead. For centuries preaching consisted of nothing else than telling this story, which was the gospel of the gladdest of all glad tidings. If Christ is not arisen, our faith is vain. To doubt this has always been the most culpable of all heresies save that of atheism itself.

Thus night, day; sleep, waking; autumn, spring— cadence the soul to life and death. To these were added the higher symbolisms of sin and holiness, illness and health, old age and rejuvenation, crushing despair and triumphant hope, pessimism and optimism, with the latter and not the former, as had often been the case before, final and triumphant. Every known race of man initiates the young at puberty by a ritualized pain and pleasure treatment that anticipates all this. Youth was isolated, made to fast, scarified, tattooed, made to endure extreme hardship, fatigue, sometimes partial burial; and then followed remission, dance, feasting, perhaps orgies, only after which did the young become full members of the tribe. Thus it is the inveterate consensus of man through all his history that on the threshold of mature life each individual should be oriented to its sovereign master's pain and pleasure by extreme experience with each in turn, as if thereby to develop the power of elasticity, resilience, and reaction, and to impress upon it throughout all its profoundest depths the conviction that there is no defeat that should not be followed by victory, no darkness so black as that which just precedes day, no virtue like that which has just overcome evil, no passivity that will not tend to react toward progressiveness. Indeed, this is a kind of modulus that Christianity has impressed upon the entire occidental world and it is this that has given it its courage, *élan,* and enterprise. This is the chief imprint it has left upon the human soul, even for those who have forgotten or denied all its tenets. Thus there is a deep psychological sense in which all those who have not passed rigorously through the experience that Christianity symbolizes by the phrase "dying and rising with Jesus" are not initiated into life and remain immature.

It is they who are more liable to be arrested in the trough of the wave and to become discouraged or even melancholic and when they meet the ills and hardships of life to flee from reality and seek some refuge from its stern demands, because life in them has not conquered death. They have not learned the great law of taking their pleasure and pain in the things they ought and in a measure proportionate to each. Indeed, modern psychotherapy is, for the most part, a new application of this old mode of rescue for such souls in distress. Maeder [11] has well and wisely found all its processes typified in Dante's descent into hell at the nethermost center of the earth where Satan himself was; and his emergence a slow ascent up the purgatorial mount to the infinite joys of paradise, first under the guidance of a human sage

---

[11] *Guérison et Evolution dans la Vie de l'Âme.*

and then led by Beatrice, a type of the supreme self-directing oracle within. Dante, as everyone knows, called his poem a comedy because it had a happy ending, but every modern novel and drama is constructed according to the same formula that Christianity made current.

And who would read a story or see a play in which at the end the hero or heroine did not achieve all they desired? And, again, why do we love to experience all the desperate miseries to which our favorites in story and on the stage are subjected before the happy dénouement begins to show but that we are dead sure that in the end both the villain and the virtuous will get their deserts. Indeed, at least one German "pithiatric" psychiatrist prescribes a drastic experience of the story of the Cross as a therapeutic method in certain cases. All this, of course, has no reference to the question whether the story is all fact or all fancy. The psychologist only studies its effects and its inner mechanisms, which, save for those who have grown scrupulous under the influence of modern controversy, are no more relevant than is the historicity of Hamlet, Lear, or Portia to the audience in a theater. In the patristic and in the Middle Ages, and even now, children and neurotics have suffered almost to the point of stigmatization at any realistic description or at the Ober-Ammergau dramatization of the items of the crucifixion and feel with all the vicariousness that sympathy can yield the thorns, bitter cup, nails, spear, etc., as we have elsewhere shown in detail.[12]

But despite all the realistic pedagogy of the church the conviction of another life is very rapidly fading from the modern consciousness and even within the church itself is becoming an ineffective shadow of a shade. Dr. George A. Gordon of the Old South Church, Boston, preaching to the Congregational State Association in

---

[12] See my *Jesus, the Christ, in the Light of Psychology*, Vol. II, Ch. II.

1902, said: "We ministers of the Lord Jesus Christ know as no other persons in the community what a paralysis has come over intelligent and thinking people in regard to the reality of the other life. So many doubt it; so few have any strong confidence in regard to it." This opinion, of course, was posited not only on the confidences of the pastor's study but also on the confidences of the sick room and the death chamber. The tendency has steadily increased and in funeral services we hear little of future rewards and punishments and only of rest and peace. The old evidence from death-beds is fallacious.

Sir William Osler [13] says:

I have careful records of about five hundred death-beds, studied particularly with reference to the modes of death and the sensations of the dying. The latter alone concerns us here. Ninety suffered bodily pain or distress of one sort or another, eleven showed mental apprehension, two positive terror, one expressed spiritual exaltation, one bitter remorse. The great majority gave no sign one way or the other; like their birth, their death was a sleep and a forgetting. The Preacher was right: in this matter man hath no preeminence over the beast—"as the one dieth so dieth the other." [14]

---

[13] *Science and Immortality,* Boston, 1904, 54 pp.

[14] G. Lionel Taylor (*The Stages of Human Life,* N. Y., Dutton, 1921. 363 p.) says that there are four stages in the process of what he believes to be normal dying: first there is an appealing, anxious, puzzled look at the approach of a great crisis, as if wondering what the person will meet in the great darkness that is supervening, all not without an element of fear; then there supervenes a peace and poise, in which stage leavetakings are often made; third, when the last breath is drawn there is a strong impression on the bystanders that there has been a real departure, that something very actual has left, so that the body is no longer the friend. Then for perhaps an hour there is on the face of the dead a look of unnatural beauty and tranquillity which slowly fades and corruption begins.

Some in contemplating their own demise think chiefly of the isolation it involves. The most sympathetic friend can only go to the brink of the dark river which we must all cross absolutely alone. Suicide lovers sometimes vainly attempt companionship. Those about to die who are conscious of their impending departure may bid sad farewells to their friends. Aging and sickly people conscious of an impending end but with their faculties intact realize the inevitableness of dying alone no matter how

This belief persists, thus, only as a dead article of faith which men no longer live by. It is a desiccated herbarium specimen and not a living plant. If common observation did not sufficiently show this, it has appeared very significantly and statistically in many recent studies.[15] These showed that it diminishes progressively as we go up the educational grades from high school through the university and that, in general, the more cultivated man becomes, the less he believes in any form of personal survival. If we had a similar investigation of the old as compared with the young, my own partial studies incline me to believe that this conviction of personal persistence beyond the grave in general loses its force in senescence, as indeed it becomes vital only at adolescence. If it be thus a creed that first blossoms with the advent and tends to decay at the close of sexual life, we have a new key for understanding both its function and its limitations. True, it often persists, if only feebly, as with the momentum of a spent force, in those who have not fully realized the senium, although they all do not wish to be conserved as old as they really are but to be rejuvenated as they once were.

---

many friends are about but are silent about it with an instinctive reluctance to betray any of the perturbations which weaklings, patheticists, and hystericals seek refuge in.

To others the thought of their own death centers in the idea of their body. They see themselves in thought pale, rigid, insentient, and follow the fate of their corpse in every detail at least up to interment or cremation, and some cannot resist a rather strong imaginative experience as to how their living sentient body would feel the rigidity, the cold, the treatment to which it is subjected, the gazing of friends, a custom which some interdict.

A third group focus on the cessation of activities which begins in the dimming of the senses and the weakening of motor or other powers, and here, too, we find two attitudes: that of compulsive but regretful renunciation, and the other of longing as for rest. In this sense death begins with the first abatement of powers, and as we have time slowly to adjust to progressive enfeeblement we do so more and more readily.

[15] See especially J. H. Leuba, *The Belief in God and Immortality*, 1916, 340 pp.

SENESCENCE

In what follows we believe it will appear that upon analysis by mechanisms akin to metonymy or synecdoche the vigor with which we have clung to a belief in personal is really motivated by a deeper belief in racial immortality and that in this latter, when the strophe of life is succeeded by its antistrophe, the deeper faith tends to come out and true sages realize what the soul meant by what the tenuous and falsetto faculty called faith blindly groped its way toward.

The psychic factors that have so overdetermined the hope-wish of personal immortality are as follows.

I. First is the desire to be remembered and esteemed by survivors. The soul abhors oblivion somewhat as it does extinction. We wish our friends not only to think of us but to think well of us. How satisfying this is both to those who die and to those who live is seen in Confucianism, where ancestor worship vicariates for belief in personal immortality. It would almost seem that some of the good and great would think more of the certainty of being canonized in due time or perpetuated in the form of bronze or marble, or enrolled in some temple of fame, than of personal immortality. At any rate, this mundane, would in some degree compensate for the loss of celestial perpetuation. Those who die in more or less full consciousness are prone in their last moments to dwell upon their friends far more than they do upon their own future state, as if the enshrinement they chiefly sought were in the hearts and minds of those they leave behind. Conversely, those who die alone, friendless, or with the execration of survivors, cling the more to the rehabilitation that death itself always tends to bring. On the basis of questionnaire data it would seem that some about to die shudder more at the thought that others would think they were totally extinct at death than from inwardly facing this conviction for themselves. We want others to think we are enjoying the best the universe can provide for its favorites, because in that case they will think more highly of us since we have obtained the diploma of the cosmos, that we have stood the test and have graduated *summa cum laude* from the terrestrial cu riculum. Perhaps if we were early Christians we should begin to "put on airs" and affect the manners of a higher life here to impress our own valuation of ourselves upon others. An ancient sage would rather that others thought him bad and hated him than to be forgotten. Thus, in fine, if all knew that they and all their good deeds would never fade from grateful memory of their descendants, the conviction of a conscious personal existence beyond the grave would lose one of its preforming determinants and reinforcements. Therefore, those concerned to keep alive the fate and hope of another life should foster any agency that keeps the memory of the dead green. There really ought to be those who sum up effectively the good lessons and meaning of every life when it closes, as a kind of mundane judgment day so that no good influence be lost and no warning fail to have its due effect—a court of the dead to pass impartially upon each life as it sets out to sea. We censor books and are beginning to test eugenic marriages, etc.; and so, if all knew that upon their death an impartial tribunal would pass upon their lives in the interests of the common weal, even if their verdict came late or was given only to those most interested to know, ethical culture would mark a great advance and the fear of death, instead of consoling itself with belief in a future life, would be set to work in the interests of normal lives here.

II. The second mundane surrogate for transcendental immortality is doing things that will affect those who survive or will perpetuate our will and works to those who know little or nothing of us or of our name. Many last wills and testaments benefit those who knew nothing of the donor. Many such have reared buildings, started movements, built organizations, written books, invented, created works of art, transformed the face of nature with an instinct of workmanship in which all thought of self was merged. All our lives are thus greatly influenced by those who are unknown. The egoistic element tends to merge in a disinterested desire to make part of the world in some way better for our having lived. Sometimes, indeed, anonymity is actively striven for and the individuality of benefactors is hidden. The phobia here is that we may have lived for naught. Here the idea of God as an All-Discerner who sees virtue and vice, and rewards or punishes in secret, coöperates. Such hidden service to the race, with no thought of any compensation here or hereafter, has a unique charm all its own. Scientific discoveries and beneficent inventions have sometimes thus been given freely to all without any personal benefit and without a personal label. True love sometimes lavishes every gift, opportunity, and joy upon its object, with no stipulation of love or gratitude or even recognition in its turn. Indeed, the possession of wealth compels more or less attention to this field of the immortality of influence. Unlike the pauper, the millionaire must forecast if he would try to shape the future; and even if great givers attach their names to their bequests, they know that to most who profit by them their name will soon mean nothing. Jubal invented music and wandered afar and when he came back he found a great festival in honor of his art and of his name, but could not identify himself and was cast out as an impostor. "Jubal's fame and art filled all the sky, while Jubal lonely laid him down to die," supremely happy in the thought that he had done the race a great service. To love and serve man is far higher than to love and serve God, for we can do nothing for Him save in this way and He needs and expects no help from us save this.

Men come and go but institutions and influence go on forever and those who start them share their mundane deathlessness long after they are forgotten. The cup of cold water illustrates the way of the gentleman or lady born and bred, best attested by the desire that others be happy and not that they themselves shine, be aggrandized, or have pleasure. This is the most ideal conduct and appeals most strongly of all things to the two great and ultimate standards of conduct, namely, honor and an approving conscience. And as we achieve this we belong to the order of the immortals and have triumphed over death. Desjardins, the founder of the order of the new life, said in substance, "We are never so impelled to snap our fingers in the face of death, to despise all its pomp and horror, and to defy him to do his worst to body and soul, as when we have just performed some such act of pure but passionate duty or kindness." Then only can we truly feel that "no evil can befall a good man living or dead" and that the cosmos is moral to the core.

III. The third killer of the death-fear is children and posterity. To die childless, knowing that our heredity that began with the amœba and came down to us in an unbroken line dies, sharpens the sting of death; while, on the other hand, to have many well born and well reared children to rise up and call us blessed is one of the best antidotes to its baleful psychic virus. As every one knows, every creature, man included, lives about as long after the maximum power to propagate as his offspring requires to become mature, so that the prolongation of the period of immaturity means the prolongation of old age. Our foremost duty is to transmit the sacred torch of life undimmed, to give the maximal momentum and right direction to the nature and nurture of offspring and to bring rising generations to their full maturity—that is the highest criterion of an ever rising nation, including civilization itself. The true parent lives not only in and

for the children but is the ancestor of their souls as well
as of their bodies and even his belief in a future life is a
good or bad thing according as it affects this. We feel
this life incomplete, unfinished, and in need of a supplement because its possibilities are as yet unrealized. But
we feel all this so much the less if we have children, while
the dread of the inevitable hour becomes that of a kind of
second or dual death for the childless because not only
they but their line die in them. Yet, on the other hand,
they have less ties and so less to lose, even though they
may feel that they have, in a sense, lived in vain. What
parent was ever so world-weary, so strong a believer in
postmortem joy, that he would not rather live on here
and see his children's children thrive than go on hence to
any conceivable future state? Those who leave offspring have had less time to develop morbid fears of
Lethe's waters and if they expect to enter a great peace
beyond, they often find their chief joy in contemplating
the fruits of their loins on earth. We have seen how the
death thought begins with the life of sex and when the
latter, if it has been normal and happy, comes to an end,
death has already begun and we are advancing deeper
into the shades of the dark valley, so that there is already
less to lose. Thus the death of the aged is less tragic and
less inconsolable; and, what is far more important, normal and cultured souls think and care progressively less
about another life.

IV. As for the good old doctrine of personal immortality, we cannot yet escape the great law that the next
life is compensatory. If men are wretched here, the
future becomes a refuge and grows not only actual but
attractive; while, conversely, if this life is rich and
abounding, the next tends to fade. No Christian age
was ever so heedless of the latter as our own. For most
intelligent, prosperous women, and especially men, it has
lapsed to little more than a mere convention or trope or

fetish of an effete orthodoxy, and hell is at most only a nightmare of the past, a childish phantom. Our actual *modus vivendi* is as if another life did not exist and death were the end. No priestcraft can longer make men content with misery here in the hope of compensation hereafter. All make the most and best of this life as if it were all they were sure of and the motto of most believers is, "One life at a time and this one now." Only in a kind of secondary falsetto Sunday consciousness do their thoughts turn to the future and does a flickering hope that death is not the end appear. Extinction is black by contrast in proportion as life is bright, happy, and absorbing, so that the death dread is in some respects growing as our life becomes richer, while it is at the same time being more and more banished from consciousness. The chief attractiveness it now has is that it brings rest and peace, for our tropes of it are more and more borrowed from sleep. Thus if the idea of the negation of life was never so dreadful, there was never such diversion from its closer envisagement. Thus, too, although suppressed, it was never so potent a factor in governing conduct, in improving hygiene, and providing for our offspring. Although we take a chance at saving our souls by church membership it is more and more bad form to discuss such matters. The real treasure of the soul is laid up elsewhere than in heaven and the growing phobia of death has now psychotherapies that are more and more effective. Its power is far greater than we know and there are endless uses to which it can yet be put in helping on the world's work. Just as every pain that depresses the vital spirits a few points on the scale of euphoria, though they still remain far above zero, inclines to death, so when life is at its optimum or flood-tide man is wonderfully immune and recuperative in body and soul and the higher up the euphoric scale we live, the more difficult it is to fear or even think of death.

Thus every legitimate fear of death is in a sense a life-preserver and -prolonger. Our business is to live and not to die, to keep at the very top of our condition and as far as possible from death, which is the *summum malum*.

As to the relation of these four immortalities, nominal, influential, plasmal, and orthodox, to each other, geneticism and the revelations of the dynamism of the folk-soul have shed much new light. This may be summarized in the statement that each of them is correlated with all the others. Even he who is chiefly intent on perpetuating his name is gratifying the deep instinct of transcending the limits of his own personal life and to know that he is remembered is not without consoling power even in the loss of property or if the conviction arises that death means extinction; while, conversely, the prospect of death in utter obscurity and of being completely forgotten tends to reinforce any or all of the other immortalities. Were we to rehabilitate hell in a modern sense, one of its horrors would be a sentence of summary oblivion even to our friends: "Let his name be forever taboo from mention or even from memory." Of course, we shall all sooner or later fall under this sentence despite all our pathetic efforts to leave durable names behind.

As to anonymous influence, we are all sure of it to a degree, for the world we are born into is made by those who preceded us and we help to shape the future. In the social field we have endless illustrations of a service that involves more or less emulation. The case in point is a woman I knew who, having lived a most disinterested and self-sacrificing life, when told that God would reward her in the next world replied that she had never had either conviction or interest about another life but had been too busy doing good to think about it. If another life was in the order of things, all would be well, but if annihilation were in store, that, too, would be just as welcome, for she had found her pay in the satisfaction that each day's work brought. She had no children and wanted no outer recognition but was content that her good deeds registered in others' lives would follow her and nothing else really mattered in her scheme of life. The point is that in any other ages or environments the same instinct to enlarge life might have found expression in either of the other forms. Some even commit colossal crimes from a perverted form of *Geltung's* propensity. Because they cannot be potent for good they make themselves so for evil. Anonymity is often a passion and finds outcrops not only in religion and philosophy but also in science. Indeed, very much of our civilization is composed of innumerable influences originated by those whose names no history or *Acta Sanctorum* have preserved and are products of this deep basal trend in the human soul.

As to plasmal immortality, who knows how much of all the good done in the world, if traced to its genetic roots, comes straight from the original momentum of the instinct to make the world better for posterity? To be sure, many of them are now broken erratic trends, forgetful of their source, which is really a nest-building instinct so irradiated and sublimated as to have lost orientation toward both its origin and goal. The first constructions in the world were nidifications. The first animal societies were stirpicultural. The primal examples of self-sacrifice were for the young. Everything for the world is good that squares with the functions of parenthood broadly conceived, and all is bad that contravenes it. Psychotherapy is slowly leading us to the astonishingly new insight that aberrations of the life-transmitting, young-rearing propensities constitute very many if not most of our mental abnormalities and that the rectification of these functions has marvelous therapeutic efficiency. The race is immortal, at least back to the first protozoan and indeed infinitely beyond. And so, in the future, our race and it only is immortal to the cosmic end. If we are tips of the twigs of a vast buried tree, these twigs may become themselves roots of a yet greater one and even a true superman may yet be born in the line of any of us. Thus, perhaps all the other immortalities have their dynamogeny in the instincts of parenthood.

As to the venerable belief in personal immortality, it was of course selfishness transcendentalized so as to subordinate every other goal in life to that of insuring our own happiness in a postmortem world. And we have to-day only contempt for the squalid ascetic who made his life miserable with the prime end of saving his own soul. But this crude doctrine now stands forth in a very new light, for psychology shows it to have been an ugly cyst or cast that enclosed and sheltered through hard dark ages a precious and beauteous thing now just emerging. Its content, as now revealed by analysis, is really man's ineluctable conviction that his own life was insignificant compared with its larger meanings. Its real lesson is the subordination of the individual to the greater whole toward which it gave him a correct *Einstellung*. The close attachment of this doctrine to the ego was incorrect, for the self is only a trope or metaphor of the race, but even this was necessary at an earlier stage of race pedagogy. The transcendentality ascribed to a self freed from the body was inevitable because that was the only symbol by which the greater life of the race could be described or comprehended. This belief stored up and conserved the psychic promise and potency that is now again flowing over by transfer to the other outcrops of the immortality instinct. It did not say what it meant but was a pragmatic masterpiece, like so many great creations of the folksoul. From the soul of the race it went straight home to that of the individual and if it overstressed individuation for a time, that, too, was

486

at first needful. Had man not so long or so inevitably believed in the great work of saving souls for the next world, he would now be less effective in saving them from the evils of this world. Had he not so cherished the conviction of a future heaven, he would have lost much of the very energy of his soul, which now strives to transform this world into a paradise and to populate it well. Thus we have here a great field in which the laws of the transposition of psychic trends into their kinetic equivalents, with very many different forms but with persistence of identical content, are abundantly shown. Man's instinct has always been right and only his more superficial conscious interpretations of it wrong.

Excess or defect of either of at least the first three immortalities hypertrophies or dwarfs the others. The doctrine of conscious personal survival was not only developed in unconscious conformity to this principle but has an even more important pedagogic rôle for the young than we had hitherto supposed. It is a pragmatic, artistic, and in no sense a scientific fact. It utterly fails before the criteria of reason but it has worked far better results than it could have done had these requirements been alone regarded. It should not only be inculcated in the young but has immense therapeutic value and to doubt this is only another side illustration of the fact that cultivated adults have, the world over and particularly in our country, unprecedentedly lost touch with youth. Wherever the instincts of parenthood have not degenerated, it must be clear that belief in future personal rewards and punishments is a wholesome regulative of the lives of the young at a stage when feeling and impulse are at their strongest and before reason is mature.

V. But there is a fifth form of immortality concept somewhat more apart and uncorrelated with the others because newer and which comes from the lure of the infinitesimal elements which science now finds at the basis of the universe. What Dalton called atoms are now known to be planetary systems of unimaginably minute corpuscles, one thousandth the mass of an atom of hydrogen and, if they are solely electrical, "their size must be one millionth of the linear dimensions of an atom," or relatively as a period on the printed page is to a large theater. Their groupings constitute the chemical elements, so that matter is dynamic to a degree we cannot conceive; and if so-called inorganic matter were proven to contain germs of man and mind, this would add but little to the new marvel of it. Matter is so active and subtle that the modern conceptions of it that have come from the study of radium make us feel that in a sense it is more spiritual than we have ever conceived spirit itself to be. In this new world, which may be homogeneous with mind, there is nothing like death anywhere to be found, and there is an unbroken gradation from the corporative unity of electrons in an atom up to the aggregations of man in society—and some think further still. On this view death is not only non-existent but inconceivable. True, more complex aggregations are reduced to simpler, more transient to more permanent ones by it, but matter is not only not dead but more intensely active than mind, so that the student of the ultimate constitution of matter and the persistence of energy is in a sense studying immortality, for this is the basis from which all orders of animal nature arose and into which they will all be resolved.

Thus we are told that the new physics and chemistry are really investigating death and regeneration. Our brains have little sense of the marvelous and lawful processes that underlie all their activities. While we have deemed evolution upward, there is another sense in which it is a fall or a series of departures from a more durable and elemental state, so that the gain is not all

one way and catabolism has its own attractions. If our
lives affect these more permanent electrons, this is survival and our ego is only part of a larger continuum and
is without end or beginning, although inconceivably
changed. The disintegration of our elements is the
harvest-home back to the cosmos from which we arose
and may involve increase, not decrease, to the sum total
of good. This unselfing or "fusing with all we flow
from" is the direction in which love, whether of man,
woman, animals, or nature itself, as well as subordination of self to others and the world, inclines us. Thus
the conscious soul of man is swept by tides of which our
poor psychology as yet knows but little. Should such a
conception of the world become general, it could still
use many of our religious phrases, litanies, and symbols,
but they would be inundated with fresh meanings.

Jean Finot's book [16] is marvelously learned, his view
is unique, and his style fascinating. It rapidly passed
through fourteen editions and was translated into many
languages. He has almost nothing to say of the soul, so
that his volume might be entitled The Immortality of the
Body, or Death, the Great Illusion. He is bitter against
theologians for having made death such an all-dominat-
ing fear fetish in the world. Tolstoi feared death all his
life and writes, "Nothing is worse than death, and when
we consider that it is the inevitable end of all which lives,
we must also recognize that nothing is worse than life."
We are told that the dread of it poisoned the life of
Daudet and that Zola trembled before the thought,
"which obsessed him and caused him nightmares and
insomnia." Renan says, "We may sacrifice all to truth
and good, which are the ends of life, and when we have
done say, 'Following the call of this interior siren we

---

[16] *The Philosophy of Long Life,* Tr. from the French by Harry Roberts,
1903, 305 pp.

have reached the turn where the rewards should lie. Oh, dreadful consoler, there is none!' The philosophy which promised us the secret of death stammers excuses." Finot says, "A study of the evolution of death in the literature of the past and to-day would become almost a history of literature itself." "The meditations of the fathers of the church and the monks of the Middle Ages would shine particularly in this concert of vociferations against death ('If the slightest wound made on one finger can cause so great a pain, what a horrible torture must be death, which is the corruption or dissolution of the entire body'). We can look fixedly neither at the sun nor at death." Mme. de Sévigné says, "I am swallowed up in the thoughts of death and find it so terrible that I hate life more because it leads there." It is no great consolation to say with Renan, "We shall live by the trace which each of us leaves upon the bosom of the infinite." "All that lives is simply preparing for death." Belief in the perdurability of the soul is an alterative or placation, a mirage. Only Confucianism and Taoism, if they had remained faithful to the teachings of their creators, would close to their initiates all possibilities of an after life; but they did not remain faithful. Even Luther at the beginning of his campaign against Rome classed the dogma of immortality of the soul as amongst "the monstrous fables which are part of the Roman dung heap," although he later became reconciled to it.

The very fear of death has killed many. "Sick persons who gather from their doctor a presentiment of their term usually die before reaching it." The Western world should take heart from the millions of Buddhists who view the prospect of death with enchantment. For subjective idealists like Berkeley, who tell us that we can really know nothing of the external world, death only deprives us of our conceptions and we may really take consolation in the fact that our individuality is composed of a whole hierarchy of more or less independent centers, each of them made up of more complex units, until our ideas of immortality merge with those of the conservation of energy.

Finot's own views begin with his conception of "life in the coffin." "The underground existence of our body is far more animated than that which is led above the earth." "The fathers of some few human beings upon the earth, we become the fathers of myriads of beings within its depths," and man perhaps gives more pleasure to his grave companions than he ever enjoyed. He specifies nine species of insects, mostly strikingly colored flies and coleoptera, which in regular order, one after another, live upon and copulate, lay their eggs and rear their maggots in corpses that are paradises to them, and he praises the work of Francisco Redi who gave us "the admirable science of the entymology of graves," which now takes the place of the old ideas of Tartarus and the Elysian fields. The foods brought to the tomb and frankly meant for the dead, who were often conceived as hungry, were really consumed by the "worms" that devour us. He tells us of a young woman caught singing at a grave who, seeing that she was observed, remarked, "My mother liked the Casta Diva." The Greeks certainly did not believe that those beneath the earth were quite quit of existence and perhaps the first religion was that of the grave or tomb, which was a factor in the birth of patriotism. The tomb is democratic because all bodies suffer exactly the same fate if exposed alike to the elements. We may really be interested in "our offspring" in the grave, for they, at least to biologists, have more interest than do the poetic conceptions that we become flowers, trees, or drifting clouds. We may thus "facilitate the body's immortal diffusion into immortal nature."

Indeed, each of the thirty trillion cells of our body has its own partial elemental life and, while we live, these

partake in the general life of the common wealth. Each
has to eliminate waste, ingest food, and their energy is
such that "we should need a force of several hundred
thousand horsepower to kill simultaneously" and in-
stantly all these cells. Even molecules have infinitely
little lives, each after its own fashion. The chemist's
view of even putrefaction, which appeals so repulsively
to one of our senses, makes it interesting. Thus the elements of our body carry on after what we call death, for
life dwells in each cell and even molecule. The very first
germ was immortal. True, we cannot analyze the consciousness of a cell, if it has one. Back of all this there
is the life of inanimate nature. Again, many of the
organs and elements of our body continue to live and
grow, if sufficiently nourished, after the death of the
body as a whole, though a part does not have the power,
as in some animals, of regenerating the whole. The
heart has been revived after thirty hours of death. Bits
of skin have been removed and preserved and grafted
on to other bodies six months after detachment and this
process might go on indefinitely, the same skin being
transferred for generations to new bodies. True, organs,
like cells, lose their subordination at what we call death.[17]

At this point Finot introduces a very long argument
against cremation because it interferes with all these
processes. He seems to have a rancor against it that is
somewhat like that of the Western believer in personal
immortality against Oriental pantheism, which holds
that the soul melts into the universe like a drop into the
ocean. He finds great comfort in the scientific phenomena, which he résumés as "the life of so-called inanimate
matter," which, we are coming to realize, is by no means
dead. Indeed, molecules lead an intensely active life,
changing their place, perhaps vibrating, traveling, group-

---

[17] See Chapter VI.

ing themselves in very many different ways, so that metals have a kind of physiology and even therapy of their own. Perhaps, indeed, crystallized matter represents the most perfect and stable arrangement to which the particles of the body are susceptible. Thermodynamics shows us that motion and heat are related in metals as in our bodies. Metals suffer fatigue and recuperate from rest, as Bosé has shown. Perhaps even the soul of life is here and we are just beginning to know the powers of ferments, which seem on the borderline between the organic and inorganic. Both are subject to evolution.

Again, there is no sharp line between animal and vegetable life. Protoplasms are as different or must be so as individuals. Both have variability. Both the cabbage and the rat, as standard biological experiments show, breathe. Plants are affected by narcotics. Sick vegetables respond to some of the same medicaments that animals do, while some actually have a sensorium. Philosophers like Descartes have tried to break down all the identities between man and animals and give the former a unique place in the universe. Fechner, who believed plants besouled, and even Haeckel knew better, although Wundt insisted to the last that "all psychic activity is conscious." The unconscious, which comparative psychology must admit, opens the door downward toward the very dawn of life, so that perhaps even unicellular organisms have elemental souls. Very many of the earlier philosophers, when human thought was fresh and untrammeled by tradition, insisted on the unity of life and mind. For a long period animals were thought to be moral beings and courts were held in which they were tried. Indeed, we may conclude that "a living being is always living" and back of this life merges by imperceptible gradations into the larger life of the cosmos.

SENESCENCE

All religion, says Finot, is based on a belief in a soul independent of the body and while so many Western philosophers have insisted on a perdurable and even immaterial personality, there has always been a background of thought repressed by current opinion to the contrary view, till we have developed a kind of "sentiment of the end." In point of fact, those near death have first a feeling of beatitude, then complete insensibility to the outer world and to pain, and lastly great rapidity of thought, so that dying is a kind of beatitude. Finot thinks modern biology by its experiments, not on spontaneous generation but on the control of fertilization, has gone some way toward realizing the goal of the alchemists, which was to create homunculi; and he wonders whether man may not sometime be thus able to control the very sources of life.

Alchemy, which for centuries was the mystic philosophy of the wise but has seemed to modern minds only a mass of felted symbols that could never be resolved except in the new light shed upon it by the studies of A. E. Hitchcock, Silberer, and others, represents in one of its aspects a unique trend of the quest for immortality. The lower alchemist strove to reduce the baser metals back to a common element, menstruum, or materia prima, for which there were fifty mythological expressions, and then and there to transmute them into the purest and the most precious of all metals, gold. The later higher alchemy left all this behind and strove to bring not only life but the homunculus itself out of various rotting putridities or out of decomposition backward and downward to evolve something endowed with exceptional vitality. Near this devolutive pole lie the deep sources of creative energy, the antæus touch of which brings regeneration. So regression to the "within" causes the soul to arise from the body and the spirit from the soul. It is like the transmutation of experience into heredity

494

or individuality reinforcing itself by contact with the mighty spirit of the race. The personal is united with the world's will or with that of God and is transmuted into it. Symbols are always a product of "apperceptive insufficiency" but the higher anagogic meaning of many of them in the hermetic field is that askesis, sacrifice, the death of egoism, and renunciation lead to the great treasure, the new light, self-impregnation with Pneuma, a new birth, joy, the *summum bonum,* etc. To some alchemists this goal was like that of the Yogi cult, depersonalization if not annihilation, while to others it was more like a distillation of a quintessential supersoul from its sarcous base, as mercury and even lead are transmuted into gold. Palingenesis is the purpose not only of experimentation but of the prayer and meditation that must precede it. In the sex symbolisms the subject fuses with the object as the male and female principle unite in conjugation. Old age is regression or retreat toward the fountain heads of life and the new life may be formed within the old body before its collapse, so that there is no break of either conscious or physical continuity. Where and when there is most death, there is also most life, for the two are true reciprocals.

But the alchemists did not make gold nor evolve an homunculus nor achieve even spontaneous generation according to our criteria. Diligently as they sought for them, they never found the philosopher's stone, the fountain of youth, or the *elixir vitæ*. Active as were their immortal longings and intricate as were their products, they were all abortive. They groped toward chemistry and metallurgy and these came in due time, although they were no more products of it than the modern building trades are of freemasonry. But their quest for a transmortal life neither achieved nor was followed by any after results that seem to us to be of value.

Modern astronomy tells us that the stellar universe

is at least 250,000 light years in diameter, so that if one of the remoter stars went out we should not know it for that number of years. The extensions outside the range of even our Euclidean axioms which we now know were only provisional and where time is only a fourth dimension of space (Einstein); suns a million times larger than ours; thousands of millions of celestial bodies in all stages of evolution and devolution, yet all composed of nearly the same chemical elements as our tiny planet and all following the same laws of gravity, light, heat, the conservation of energy through all its transformations so that none of it is ever or anywhere lost, with illustrations of every stage of planetary development and dissolution, some of them probably evolving life and creatures far higher than man:—it is out of this universe that our world and we came and back into it we shall both be resolved sooner or later. As we advance in life we turn our backs to all this but when the retreat begins we face the stupendous whole of it again and death is freedom from the progressive limitations involved in individuation and a return home to the One and All. It is restoration, resumption, emancipation, diffusion, reversion, and all worlds and systems as well as men are thus destined to die of old age, perhaps by collision or other accident, since time is as boundless as space and the history of our solar system is but a single tick of the cosmic clock-work which we know is always running down even though it may have the power of eternally winding itself up again. If "our hearts like muffled drums are beating funeral marches to the grave," so is also the heart of the universe. As we "join the majority" when we die, so do suns that become extinct and those we see with the strongest telescope may be but a handful compared to those that within its range have suffered "entropy." Thus the true death thought is the transcender of all horizons and its muse points us straight to infinity as our goal. Along with this there is a deep conviction that there is no void or vacuum but that even though the existence of universal ether is now doubted by certain experts the cosmos is somehow a plenum full to repletion of being as it is of energy and teeming with the possibilities of even life far richer and more abundant than we can conceive. Thus we see again that personality is arrest, exclusion from all this, which ceases at death when we reënter the great current that sweeps onward all that is. Thus the solar system, earth, man, and finally our own ego involve descent as from a *summum* genus to an *infima* species This progressive individuation is at every step arrest which death removes and reverses, so that the energies which during all our lives have held up and hampered us by so many disharmonies and conflicts are gone forever.

VI. Next come the noetic theories of immortality. Gnostics, illuminati, mystics, logicians of the categories, and all who seek salvation and perdurability by the noetic way assume that as the soul leaves individual things and persons and passes to species, to genera, and on to the abstract and unconditioned, certainty increases until it tends to become cataleptic in the old Stoic sense. The ultimate goal is pure absolute being, knowledge of which brings ecstasy, love of, and identification with it. Self is merged and lost in the infinite. Negatively this seems not merely death but annihilation. It should be regarded positively as the great affirmation and realization of true existence and the proper and only true finish and completion of human life, the last stage of psychogenesis. It is involution, the at last fully developed counterpart and complement of evolution. To this the genetic life impulse with which each of us starts will take us if its trajectory suffers no arrest and does not swerve from its proper course. This ontological immortality is Oriental, eleatic, and frankly pantheistic. It is a product not

497

only of old thinkers but of old races and civilizations. It goes with retirement from and not with useful advent into the world. Those who begin this involution by, for example, knowing that they know, knowing that they know they know, etc., find that at the mathematical point when they reach the center of the involucre, the universe bursts in upon them. By tracing self-consciousness to its deepest root all that is conscious is lost in an unconscious that is utterly without bounds or orientation.

The religious instinct has always been vastly wiser than it knew but it always needs reconstruction, often radical in form. Thus, if at death the psyche is disintegrated as much as the body is and the disintegration goes down into molecules or any of the basal forms of energy, death is not absolute. The difference is like that between the mountains and the sea level when compared with that from the surface of the earth to its center. Hering and Simon tell us that what we have called heredity is really memory. The world beyond is like an ocean to an ant accustomed to its own ant-hill but floating out to sea on a straw. The subconscious is greater than the conscious and we do not dread this in sleep and so biology is greater than psychology, just as folklore is broader than psychology or philosophy. We want to feel ultimately forces and powers that are not our own, to be inundated with a larger strength, to fall back into everlasting arms. Thus, back of Christianity is an older, larger, meta-Christian, meta-human religion found in the love of nature, and old men ought to grow progressively interested first in animals, then in plants, then in the inanimate world, with a view to the ending of life in a pantheistic absorption.

This view has had another great reinforcement of late from studies that originated with Durkheim and Lévy-Brühl, from which it appears that back of primitive animism there are always found traces of some kind of mana cult, which is not unlike that of Om in India. Man is anthropic or upward-gazing. We address the sky not as "our father in heaven" but as a vastated navel-gazing orientation toward the source of all things. Schleiermacher, who conceived religion as absolute dependence and in his earlier writings made it pantheistic at root, sought to console a young widow who said that her whole soul went out to her dead husband and she could not possibly feel that he would be resolved back into the great One-and-All by saying that this should bring her no grief for it meant merging into the highest life of the infinite whole and no longer setting up for self—"If he is now living in God and you love him eternally in God as you loved and knew God in him, can you think of anything sublimer or anything more glorious? Is not this the highest end of love?"etc. Mailander held that pantheistic divinity died in giving birth to the world and that all its processes are self-destructive, pointing ultimately to a Nirvana; that everything is traveling the road to death, the desire for which is really the universal motive, so that we are unconsciously seeking this kind of absorptive death in all we do or say. Man's business is to know the great whole and thus he will enjoy the prospect of annihilation and attain the full and glorious will to die. We must be resolved back into primal energy, which is nothing only in the sense that it is too great to be defined.

Meyer-Denfey urges that no part of the soul can be lost any more than can any element of the body and that the fuller our life has been the more of these modifications of cosmic matter and energy does it effect. Pantheism has resources for meeting the death fear which the Western world knows little of. It should also be noted that to the psychologist consolations drawn from the persistency of the elements of our body in the above sense are related to world-soul theories merely by ambivalent variance. Psychogenetically there is little difference between concepts of absolute mind back of all conscious and sentient beings and those of preëxisting energy, stress, nebulæ, or any other mother-lye of the universe. The Schiller-James view is that matter limits the expression of the absolute mind back of all. Our brain is a thin place in the veil through which the great life of soul breaks into the world but always in restricted forms. The philosopher, Schelling, thought mind and nature at root identical but Schiller is more dualistic and regards the body as a "mechanism for inhibiting consciousness." "With our brains we are able to forget."

Still, the mind is in rapport, however dim, in contact, if not indeed continuous with a larger consciousness of unknown and perhaps universal scope that is disclosed to us in our subliminal self. On this view the brain does not secrete thought but obstructs it like a bad conductor, so that when the thought currents of the great Autos make the nerves glow, the phosphorescence or incandescence caused by the resistance of the brain is what appears to our fragmentary subliminal mind as consciousness. Ideation is thus a transmissive function of the brain and when it perishes, personality, which means limitation, is dissolved into the larger life of the whole. Mind stuff, like force and matter, may preëxist in minute and disseminated fragments, which our bodies mass and our brains combine into what we call souls. And on this view these fragmentary psychic elements, whether they be combined in a human or even animal ego or not, must also be immortal for all the reasons we are. Perhaps the highest combinations may be grouped into yet higher beings, which would be resolved back again into us on their way to more elemental states.

If our soul is the mouthpiece of an absolute soul, as the word *persona* is often interpreted to imply, inadequate though it be it is still to those lower mausolized souls somewhat as the more definite and absolute soul is to us; and as their voices are absorbed in us so we are in infinite being. We are bundles, vincula, or parentheses of more ultimate elements that preceded and will survive us, but we are somehow helping these immortal components on to their own goal, so that the real value of life is theirs and not ours. But if subliminal functions are most immortal, the dissolution of our consciousness might be desiderated, for organization obscures the ultimate reals and the massing of lower monads involves a larger sum of arrest, so that perhaps our lives really hinder rather than help on the cosmic process of evolution or redemption. As in chemistry the more complex combinations are unstable and tend to disintegrate, so the higher psychic compounds we cause and that make our minds persist a while will be resolved into lower and simpler ones that outlast them. Thus, at best the problem and conduct of our earthly life would be akin to that of a careful breeder who would leave permanent variations in the vegetable and animal species to be cultivated that would persist long after he himself is forgotten. If this soul of the world is conscious, as we are, death is lapsing down the evolutionary scale. But this ideolatry of consciousness is passing. And if the unconscious is higher and the basal cosmic energies are greater, more perfect, and more important than our psyche and soma, then we have lost our sense of direction and devolution is really upward.

VII. As to the philosophic attempts to prove the doctrine of personal immortality, no genetic psychologist can to-day despise even the most proletarian form of belief in a principle that survives death. Although the time is past when the old theological arguments for immortality are convincing, save to those whose religious development has been arrested, they will always deserve respect not only because they have done so much to sustain great souls in the past but because, as we now interpret them, they mean a larger and more complete life for man here in the future. Disregarding these, we must, however, briefly pass in review the chief views that the philosophic minds have evolved that the soul lives on.

We begin with Plato, who finds not one but many proofs of it. In the *Phaedrus* he finds it in the spontaneity and power of self-motion of the soul. In the *Timaeus* he finds it in the fact that the soul is the *chef d'œuvre* of the world, so wondrous and beautiful that the gods would and could not really let it die. Elsewhere he finds proof of its immortality in the soul's struggle for knowledge, the impulse to progress to ever more general ideas, which, as we have seen, he thought akin to death. Again, he deemed it immortal because he thought no sin or evil could kill it. Once more, as all that live must die, so the correlate must hold that all the dead live or, as Cebes puts it, the latter is a necessary postulate to the idea of life. The soul, too, is simple and undecomposable and so can never be destroyed. His doctrine of reminiscence was that we remember previous incarnations, preëxistence being long thought to be as necessary and as demonstrable as postexistence. Plato found Greek life and mind confused and sought by cross-examination and induction in the psychic field to attain a few fixed ideas that the soul could anchor to in the sophistic flux, minds be drawn together, and Greece thus saved from disintegration as the old theological views crumbled. The products of all this Socratic midwifery were basal concepts, the eternal patterns of which by participation in things made them real. These Aristotle and many later writers elaborated and defined as a table of categories and in nature they were interpreted as *summa genera* or fixed species or types. It was the persistence of belief in these that both Darwin and Locke attacked. The species and entities of the scholastics, which underlay even the doctrine of the Eucharist, and not only nativism and apriorism but all forms of philosophic realism, as well as absolutism, metaphysics, ontology, rational transcendentalism, the passion for deducing conclusions from presuppositionless data elsewhere derived, and even the Stoic and Kantian conscience—all rest upon the assumption of definite and abiding norms in nature or mind that are simple and undecomposable by psychic analysis and from which all thinking starts and in which it ends. Thus the doctrine of ideas has been the key not only to philosophic orthodoxy but to much of the thought and most of the great controversies of the world. Not only theologians but Descartes, Spinoza, Fichte, Hegel, and also no less but in a different manner, mystics, illuminati, rationalists, scientists in their quest for constants and laws of nature, and even the codifiers of Roman law, were all inspired by belief in attaining ultimate principles, and all these were looking toward immortality.

Now, all noetic theories of immortality agree in holding that it is attained when the intellect intuits or grasps one or more of these ultimate truths and thus partakes of or participates in their perdurability. They are so high and abstract that Plato considered philosophy not only as the withdrawal from sense and the world toward the solitariness of the infinite but as the active practice of death. Hegel thought them the inner constitution of the mind of God, and to know God is eternal life. The great bliss and peace of what Aristotle described and praised as the theoretic life have thus often been interpreted as a foretaste of heaven. Thus the love and struggle for knowledge have been said to be motivated by the desire for an incorporeal existence.

Wordsworth's "truths that wake to perish never," "high instincts before which our mortal nature trembles like a guilty thing surprised," is based upon the doctrine

of reminiscence. When the soul has attained the unconditioned, and even when it experiences a love that is felt
to be stronger than death, or a pure autonomous ought-
ness, or conceives the idea of God as the greatest and
best being, which Descartes said it could not do if such
a being did not exist; when it envisages a beauty that is
transcending and seems to take the mind above time and
space into pure being and whenever we reach generalizations of such a high degree that they include soul and
body, life and death, and all things else, man has been
told in countless ways that he was becoming immortal,
that in such experiences the soul was outsoaring mortality, as if the subject were parasiting on to its object,
absorbed in ecstasy of contemplation, till the subject and
object fused in a unique way. The soul that harbors
such great thoughts and has passed through such experiences thereby acquires a quality of permanence, whether
it acts by *apperçus* or by severe logical ratiocination.

All such arguments, however, from their very nature
are fallacious. Knowledge is not participation in this
sense. A being of low may know one of a far higher
order, but the chasm between subject and object remains
unbridged. To know beauty and power is not to attain
them. The further epistemological assumption that the
world of ideas is itself a projection, just as subjective
idealism asserted the world of sense to be, would also be
necessary. But even this colossal postulate would not
suffice for a world that is all eject and ends as well as
begins with man. On this hypothesis the mind creates
its own saving principle and was saved by its products.
Indeed, such a method begs the whole question, which
becomes again one of fact. Does or does not such a
power exist in our psychic nature? The only possible
support for such a hypothesis is the degree of coherence
of its own parts with each other and with experience.
All such arguments, however, are really pantheistic and

leave little room for personality but are rather destructive of it. Nothing individual can persist in the absolute for in it all distinctions are merged.

Connected with this view is that which assumes that because we have the idea of or the wish for immortality and because this is so generally implanted in human nature, the latter is a lie if it is not a fact. Of this class of proofs the most common are those that urge it because of its practical utility for morality. In the other-worldness of early Christian centuries, where eschatology was more developed than cosmology, fear of hell and hope of heaven performed the greatest service for virtue and its progress was advanced by these artificial and extraneous supports. The danger is lest they have undue weight and be relied on long after their function should have been progressively replaced by the conception of virtue as its own reward. Luther thought that the chief motive of morality would be gone if there were no future life. Andrews Naughton said there could be no religion without it. Theodore Parker said: "If I perish in death I know no law but passion." Chalmers urged that without it God would be stripped of wisdom, authority, and honor. Walt Whitman exclaimed: "If rats and maggots end us, then alarum! for we are betrayed." Human nature has been called a lie and God a liar if there is no future life and those who do not desire it have been called in reality already dead. It is a potent motive to escape eternal pain and secure eternal bliss for our own ego hereafter. "If," says one, "our souls do not hold the latchstring of a new world's wicket, then goodbye, put out the lights, ring down the curtain. We have had our turn and it is all so nauseating that even suicide is a welcome spectacle." One need only glance over a few of the five thousand titles of Alger's very incomplete and quite out-of-date bibliography upon the subject to be able to draw up a long list of desperate things that would happen in the world and that individual writers would do, or of imprecations on God's character and the nature of the universe, if it were proven false or if none of the strands in the complex net of theories and demonstrations that have been flung to the other shore should hold. All virtues, piety, honor, integrity, and civilization itself would perish, men become brutes, God a malign fiend gloating over the unbridled lust and supreme selfishness that would slowly sweep man from the earth, etc.

The most vivid portraitures of heaven and hell have been made. Isaac Taylor deemed the sun heaven although a later contemporary thought it hell, adding that its dark spots were the souls of the damned. The great comets in the last century were called hell making its rounds to gather its victims. The old Saxon catechist pronounced the setting sun red because it looked on hell. Thus the flood of evil now held in restraint would deluge the earth and chaos break loose if, when pay day came, men found a future life of rewards and punishments bankrupt.

All this assumes that it is proven because it has aided virtue and because a belief so general must be true. But even the good Bishop Butler argued that men must be prepared to find themselves misled—"Light deceives, why not life?" From childhood to the grave, from savagery to the present, man's history has been one of disillusion and disenchantment. His mind has been far more fertile of error than of truth. Few of his wants have been satisfied and no wise man would feel secure in arguing from desire to attainment. The impetuous diathesis of the West may have grown neurotic as it became free, rich, and powerful, but it is all unavailing. Despite all that pragmatism can say, truth is very different from utility. In view of all this we might, with Bishop Courtney, refute all proofs of post-mortem existence, insisting that all men die, body and soul, and are extinguished but at some appointed time their spirits are resurrected by the power of God. The other alternative is more familiar. "If our ship never reaches port and if there be no haven, it becomes us to keep all taut and bright, sails set, and to maintain discipline." All we want even of a future life is opportunity for virtue.

A special form of this argument from ideas to reality was developed by Kant. Reason always seeks the unconditioned by its very nature and nothing but the *summum bonum* will satisfy it. This includes two things, perfection and happiness, the two great desires of the ages. The ancients thought each implied the other. The old Hebrews believed that righteousness brought happiness in this world. The Stoics held that the highest joy was implicit in the practice of virtue from its very nature, while the Epicureans taught, conversely, that the highest happiness involved virtue. This does not suffice. The unity between the two must not be analytic but synthetic and causal. That is, each must bring out the other. In the world of experience this is not true and yet they belong together and so must find each other in a higher intelligible world.

Thus the very idea of immortality is the greatest perfection joined to the greatest happiness. They must be united completely. Whereas in the phenomenal world their development and union are only partial, there must be an infinite progression to bring them completely together because a being destined for perfection cannot be arrested. If this were the case there would be no perfect virtue and we are immortal because the latter must be attainable. Thus, heaven and hell must rise and fall together. True, the sense of justice by which we judge life, the drama, literature, and novels demands that the good always get their reward and the bad their punishment. This instinct is very deep and underlies law and society but we have no warrant for believing that the universe is built upon this principle. There is abundant evidence to the contrary. Neither intellectual intuition nor conscience are constitutive principles. Moreover, only the Western world demands personal immortality, so that the conviction that no evil can befall a good man is only a sentiment or postulate. Who knows but what it is only the *hubris* or fatal pride of man, which the gods would destroy, that has impelled him to believe that his wishes, ideas, or even his ego itself are too good to be allowed to perish.

Pluralistic views of immortality may be very roughly grouped together. Howison,[18] for example, makes pluralism absolute by advocating an eternal or metaphysical world of many minds, all self-active, the items and orders of experience of which constitute real existence, even time and space. About everything is logically implicit in their self-developing consciousness, and the recognition of each by the other constitutes the moral order. This makes an eternal republic or city of God, who is "the fulfilled type of their mind and the living bond of their union." They control the natural world, are sources of law, and are free, for their essence is mutual relation. In the world of spirits God is not solitary and there is room for the freedom of all. The joint movement that we call evolution is transient and can never enter the real world. Creation is not an event with a date but a metaphor. The key of everything is conscience and teleology. This view differs from Leibnitz's monadology only in denying grades and castes in these fulgurations of God. It makes objects in nature the manifestations of mental activity and therefore just as real as they. So the eternal reality of the individual is the supreme fact.

Royce, too, does not teach a psychology without a soul.

---

[18] *The Limits of Evolution and Other Essays,* New York, 1901.

Individualities are basal and teleological. They are aspects of the absolute life and therefore have a meaning. But in this present life, much as we strive to know and love individuals, there are no true individuals which our present minds can know or express. As we strive, therefore, to find real others, we realize that all we know of them is but a system of hints of an individuality not now revealed to us which cannot be represented by a consciousness that is made up of our own limited experience. Therefore the real individualities we loyally seek to express get from the absolute viewpoint their final expression in a life that is conscious, the only life that idealism recognizes and that in its meaning, but not in time and space, is continuous with the fragmentary, flickering existence wherein we now see so dimly our relations to God and to eternal truth.[19]

This argument, so dear to and so ably advocated by its author, is obviously suggested by the Kantian postulate. Is it true in fact, however, that the closest companionship, friendship, and even love do not take us to the real individuality of the objects of these impulsions? Though man has always been gregarious and social, it would seem that this instinct is abortive if Royce is correct and also that the reality of such an individuality as he postulates would not be conscious but rather transconscious or frankly unconscious.

Miss Calkins in her various writings, although not consciously intent upon proving immortality, belongs to this group. The constant sense of self, which she postulates in the teeth of the modern studies of multiple personality, harks back to Descartes and she seems to be a good illustration of Royce's persistent quest for a self that from its very nature cannot be known, a quest that in her has its chief strength, if analytically considered, in

---

[19] *The Conception of Immortality.* Also *The World and the Individual.*

the personal satisfaction coming from the subconscious reinforcement by reading and thinking in maturity of a juvenile stage of development, which originated in a theological and here deploys in a metaphysical stage.

C. T. Stockwell [20] assumes that there is something related to the germ plasm from which the individual sprang as it is to the rest of the body, and Shaler [21] concludes: "We may therefore say that the most complicated part of life is not that which goes out with the body's death but that which is cradled in the infinitesimal molecule that is known to us as the germ of another life evolution." Edwin Arnold [22] is platonic in assuming that life is so beautiful that "we may rightly feel betrayed if dysentery and maggots end everything." So our fears may be as ridiculous as those of Don Quixote hanging from a window by the wrist over what he thought was an abyss but, when the thong was cut, falling only four inches. Such an authentic and transfiguring Yes might be pronounced if we could recombine the chemical elements of a man analyzed in the South Kensington museum into a vigorous youth. An anonymous author asks why should the soul, the noblest and last goal of evolution, perish and the cosmos throw away its crown. It is the entelechy of all evolution. In general the best survive and only the worst become extinct. The great *biologos* has wrought from the beginning to give itself an organ to think through and mirror itself in, and this momentum of self-preservation is too great to be entirely arrested at death. So individuality must have absolute worth and be eternized because it is the key to and the paragon of existence. It must be an *ens realissimum* because it has cost so much. Democracy, too, hyper-

---

[20] *The Evolution of Immortality.*
[21] *The Study of Life and Death.*
[22] *Death and Afterward.*

trophies individuality. The Orient knew *one* was eternal; the Middle Ages knew a *few* were; and only lately did man begin to think *all* were so. Our motto, thus, must be *Impavi progrediamur* shouted with bravura. Self-conscious life is the highest of all possible categories, the model of all other units by which they are understood, and not merely a symbol of ultimate reality but the thing itself.

S. D. McConnell revives the somewhat patristic idea that man is by nature mortal but is also immortable and can attain another life by piety and knowledge, as of old the Eucharist developed the potentiality of another life or as the infant is a man, only dynamically. Man may become indestructible by a higher process of biogenesis. John Fiske, too, says, "At some period in the evolution of humanity this divine spark may have acquired sufficient concentration and steadiness to survive the wreck of material form and endure forever." To be deified by righteousness would be a fit climax. This life is a period of probation and gestation in a new sense. Thus, too, hell is obsolete and the bad die, so that the great choice is now between continuation and extinction. Some crude prelusions of this were found among the Taoists, who held that "the grosser elements of man's nature may be refined away and immortality attained even in this world." This could be done by an elixir of life, the desire to discover which a century or two before and even after Christ became in many places a veritable craze. So-called pills of immortality taken in connection with certain rites and regimen, like alchemy, which could make gold out of baser metals, would purge away mortal elements and transfiguration and sublimation might result, even for animals. But where do we draw the line between the mortal and immortal, for this may be as far above as the Taoists thought it was below us?

All arguments of this kind are provincial. Man may

be a mere microbe on our little dirt ball, which the high gods could hardly see if the lentiform Milky Way were the object-glass of a celestial microscope. What reason have we to think that the cosmos accepts us at our own valuation? The great sphinx has for ages suckled children at its breast only to destroy them with its claws and when men die it recks and cares not. As Fechner says, the plant world might say it was supreme and that insects, animals, and men lived to manure its seeds. Vegetation preceded, nourishes, and might at any time send out bacteria and miasma to rid the world of all animal life. Man is perhaps mean compared to the denizens of other worlds and even his type, so precious compared to individuals, may be worthless or serving other ends. Despite his decadent but titanic pride and monumental nescience of self he is really pathetic. So tempting to the vengeance of the gods is his pride that to be disappointed about another life serves him right. The great saurians were once the highest creatures and seemed the pets of nature and the goal of all, but although their period was far longer than man's they have passed. So, perhaps the superman will sometime quarry and explore, trace by trace, the evidences of a human biped representing our own stage of existence, and man as he is to-day be classified in a tongue as yet unborn. Are we really nearer any ultimate goal than was the amphioxus? We may be only a link to the higher man and that link may sometime be missing.

What right have we to assume anything so sacrosanct and fetchingly irresistible in the human type that the great Goodheart will never seek to evolve anything better but accept us as a stereotype of finality. Such suppositions are naïve and man as a race ought to rejoice if he can serve even infinitesimally in a greater purpose. In fact, in many quarters it is now bad form to even discuss the question of personal immortality because the world is becoming—in the phrase of Osler—Laodicean, indifferent, or even antagonistic to such views and leaves passionate affirmations of a future life, so in fashion in the days of Tennyson and Browning, to mystics, clerical rhapsodists, pectoralists, or to those steeped in cardiac emotions.

There are many reasons challenging the generality or strength of the desire for another life. From a questionnaire of the Psychic Research Society it was found that very many did not feel it of urgent importance, did not wish to know for certain about it, and many did not desire it, although a few, like Huxley, "would prefer hell, if the conditions were not too rigorous," to annihilation. Perhaps we are still haunted by submerged reminiscences of the immortality of our primeval unicellular ancestors, which, as we have seen, divide forever and never die. Man is certainly at present a very defective creature, a bundle of anachronisms with organs new and old. Even the aged die with a minority, and very often a majority of their organs and faculties charged with potencies of a longer life. Man may be not a paragon but a fluke or sport of the anthropoid apes and his death is commonly a gruesome execution by microbes, accidents, or hereditary handicaps. His sex nature may be abnormal. Unlike the beasts, he seems to have lost his hygienic or dietetic instinct or conscience. He knows more than he can practice. His consciousness is often abnormal and not remedial as it should be. It is very fallible, always partial, and by no means the oracle he has deemed it to be. It may be nothing but a thing of shreds and patches, extemporized, accidental, transient, made up of fragmentary outcrops of unconscious forces that, deep below the threshold, rule his life. To truly know himself he must go down stratum by stratum, study every outcrop of older formations, every denudation caused by disease, every psychic fossil of tics, obsessions, whims, every anatomical clue, every hint from comparative psychology, disease, crime, rudimentary organs of body or soul; and in his efforts to maximize himself must realize that if all the studies of his nature that have been made were to be depurated of the lust for a future life it would leave a vast void, for the passion for immortality has left its mark on all his cultural history.

But the fear of death and the forms of mitigating this fear are chiefly because man still dies young. If we had experienced and explored senescence fully we should find that the lust of life is supplanted later by an equally strong counterwill to die. We should have no immortality mania for we should be satisfied with life here without demanding a sequel to it. Our present dreams of all forms of post-mortem existence would become a nightmare. True macrobiotism means not only more years but completeness of experience, absence of repression and limitation. Had we lived out the whole of our lives and drained all the draughts of bitter and sweet that nature has ever brewed for us, we should feel sated. The fact is, man is now cut off in his prime with many of his possibilities unrealized. Hence he is a pathetic creature doomed to a kind of Herodian slaughter and because he has dimly felt this he has always cried out to the gods and to nature to have mercy. He has imagined answers to the heartrending appeal he shouted into the void: if a man dies shall he live again? and on the warrant of fancied answers has supplemented this by another life, which, when psycho-analyzed in all its processes, means only that he has a sense that the human race is unfinished and that the best is yet to come. And so it is. Man's future on this earth is the real, only, and gloriously sufficient fulfillment of this hope. It will be found only in the prolonged and enriched life of posterity here. The man of virtue will realize all desires and live himself completely out so that nothing essentially human will be foreign to his own personal experience.

Thus the wish for and belief in immortality is at bottom the very best of all possible augurs and pledges that man as he exists to-day is only the beginning of what he is to be and do. He is only the pigmoid or embryo of his true and fully entelechized self. Thus when he is completed and has finished all that is now only begun in him, heavens, hells, gods, and discarnate ghosts will all fade like dream fabrics or shadows before the rising sun. All doctrines of another life are thus but symbols and tropes in mythic form of the true superman as he will be when he arrives. The great hope so many have lived and died by will be fulfilled, every jot and tittle of it, not in our own lives but in the perfect man whose heralds we really are without knowing it. Deathbed visions will come true more gloriously than the dying thought. They hunger for more life but the perfect man will die of satiety passing over into aversion and the story will be completed not in a later number but in this.

Is there any true thanatophilia, the opposite of thanatophobia? Does the most complete and harmonious life bring not only the quest for death but an active striving toward Nirvana? Will man ever come to observe the approach of death in himself and in others just as we love to study and observe growth? The records of centenarians do not show it; nor do the superannuated now generally feel it. Even Nothnagel, who observed himself clinically almost up to the moment of his death, did not find it. True euthanasia is not mere resignation or the exhaustion of the momentum to live or satiety with life. We know nothing of truly natural death. But we do know that psychogenetically the old lust for personal immortality has made man now more anxious to prolong and enlarge this mundane life. We can no longer postpone our ideas of happiness. The great and good things man once expected beyond he now strives to attain here. He wants more, not less in this life because he expected so much of the other. Thus the belief in immortality is one of the psychic roots of modern hygiene although the question whether it can all go over into orthobiosis and humaniculture still remains open. If all were cut off in their prime, like Jesus, for example, another life would be even more desired and believed in, for the longer and better we live the less we care about it. Thus the answer to the problem of euthanasia strictly considered must remain in abeyance, at least until humanity is more complete. Biological studies and new therapies may develop, give more importance to, and help us to a far better knowledge of, the gerontic stage of life. At any rate, I hope and believe that the data I have gathered and presented in this volume may contribute its mite to make the status of the old more interesting to themselves and to increase the sense that they still owe important duties to a world never more in need of the very best that is in them.

THANATOPSIS

By WILLIAM CULLEN BRYANT

When thoughts
Of the last bitter hour come like a blight
Over thy spirit, and sad images
Of the stern agony, and shroud, and pall,
And breathless darkness, and the narrow house,
Make thee to shudder, and grow sick at heart;—
Go forth, under the open sky, and list
To Nature's teachings, while from all around—
Earth and her waters, and the depths of air—
Comes a still voice—Yet a few days, and thee
The all-beholding sun shall see no more
In all his course; nor yet in the cold ground,
Where thy pale form was laid, with many tears,
Nor in the embrace of ocean, shall exist
Thy image. Earth, that nourished thee, shall claim

THE PSYCHOLOGY OF DEATH

Thy growth, to be resolved to earth again,
And, lost each human trace, surrendering up
Thine individual being, shalt thou go
To mix forever with the elements,
To be a brother to the insensible rock
And to the sluggish clod, which the rude swain
Turns with his share, and treads upon. The oak
Shall send his roots abroad, and pierce thy mould.

Yet not to thine eternal resting-place
Shalt thou retire alone, nor couldst thou wish
Couch more magnificent. Thou shalt lie down
With patriarchs of the infant world—with kings,
The powerful of the earth—the wise, the good,
Fair forms, and hoary seers of ages past,
All in one mighty sepulchre. The hills
Rock-ribbed and ancient as the sun,—the vales
Stretching in pensive quietness between;
The venerable woods—rivers that move
In majesty, and the complaining brooks
That make the meadows green; and, poured round all,
Old Ocean's gray and melancholy waste,—
Are but the solemn decorations all
Of the great tomb of man. The golden sun,
The planets, all the infinite host of heaven,
Are shining on the sad abodes of death,
Through the still lapse of ages. All that tread
The globe are but a handful to the tribes
That slumber in its bosom.—Take the wings
Of morning, pierce the Barcan wilderness,
Or lose thyself in the continuous woods
Where rolls the Oregon, and hears no sound,
Save his own dashings—yet the dead are there;
And millions in those solitudes, since first
The flight of years began, have laid them down
In their last sleep—the dead reign there alone.
So shalt thou rest, and what if thou withdraw
In silence from the living and no friend
Take note of thy departure? All that breathe
Will share thy destiny. The gay will laugh
When thou art gone, the solemn brood of care
Plod on, and each one as before will chase

SENESCENCE

His favorite phantom; yet all these shall leave
Their mirth and their employments, and shall come
And make their bed with thee. As the long train
Of ages glide away, the sons of men,
The youth in life's green spring, and he who goes
In the full strength of years, matron and maid,
The speechless babe, and the gray-headed man—
Shall one by one be gathered to thy side,
By those, who in their turn shall follow them.

So live, that when thy summons comes to join
The innumerable caravan, which moves
To that mysterious realm, where each shall take
His chamber in the silent halls of death,
Thou go not, like the quarry-slave at night,
Scourged to his dungeon, but, sustained and soothed
By an unfaltering trust, approach thy grave,
Like one who wraps the drapery of his couch
About him, and lies down to pleasant dreams.

CROSSING THE BAR

By Alfred Tennyson

Sunset and evening star,
   And one clear call for me!
And may there be no moaning of the bar,
   When I put out to sea.

But such a tide as moving seems asleep,
   Too full for sound and foam,
When that which drew from out the boundless deep,
   Turns again home.

Twilight and evening bell,
   And after that the dark!
And may there be no sadness of farewell,
   When I embark.

For tho' from out our bourne of Time and Place
   The flood may bear me far,
I hope to see my Pilot face to face
   When I have crost the bar.

INDEX

Taylor, J. M., 231
Teachers, old and young, 385
Tedium vitae, 383
Temperament, changes of, in the old, 219 *et seq.*
Temperature and longevity, 283
Temptations of the old, 330 *et seq.*
Tessier, 232 *et seq.*
Testes transferred, 297
Thanatophilia, 515
Thanatopsis, 516
Thomas, W. I., 44
Thompson, W. G., 228
Three generations in a family, 430
Thyroid gland, 308
Tissue growing in plasma, 288 *et seq.*
Treatment of age, 195 *et seq.*
Trollope, Anthony, 130
Trollope, Frances, 108

Utecht, Byron C., 110

Vita sexualis, close of, 394 *et seq.*
Von Kleist, H., 16
Von Mueller, F., 24
Von Scheffel, J. V., 19
Voronoff, Serge, 306 *et seq.*
  results and criticisms of, 313

Walpurgis night, 74
Wandering Jew, 54
War, a greater, 453
  between old and young, 85, 421
  the great, effects of, on old and young, 135

Warthin, A. S., 212
Weather changes, interest in, by the old, 415
Weismann's views and their limitations, 248 *et seq.*
Wells, H. G., 30
White, Margaret E., 101
Whitman, Walt (poems), 148, 505
Whitney, Mrs. A. D. T., 108
Will-to-live, the, 455
Wilson, U. V., 126
Wisdom of the old, 406
Wish to live life over again, 342 *et seq.*
Wissler, C., 40
Witches as old, 72
Women as old as they look, 387
  older than men, 389
Wordsworth and immortality, 503
Work planned by some old people, 361 *et seq.*
World War, effects of, on relations of old and young, 431

Young best advocates; old the best judges, 425
  enfranchised by the war, 136
  men in philosophy, 424
  wives of old men, 398
Young, T. E., and the patriarchs, 50
Youth, and death, 445
  rivalry with age, 417
  of old age, 11
  traits of, viii

Zarathustra, 428

Family in America

AN ARNO PRESS / NEW YORK TIMES COLLECTION

Abbott, John S. C. **The Mother at Home:** Or, The Principles of Maternal Duty. 1834.

Abrams, Ray H., editor. **The American Family in World War II.** 1943.

Addams, Jane. **A New Conscience and an Ancient Evil.** 1912.

The Aged and the Depression: Two Reports, 1931–1937. 1972.

Alcott, William A. **The Young Husband.** 1839.

Alcott, William A. **The Young Wife.** 1837.

American Sociological Society. **The Family.** 1909.

Anderson, John E. **The Young Child in the Home.** 1936.

Baldwin, Bird T., Eva Abigail Fillmore and Lora Hadley. **Farm Children.** 1930.

Beebe, Gilbert Wheeler. **Contraception and Fertility in the Southern Appalachians.** 1942.

Birth Control and Morality in Nineteenth Century America: Two Discussions, 1859–1878. 1972.

Brandt, Lilian. **Five Hundred and Seventy-Four Deserters and Their Families.** 1905. Baldwin, William H. **Family Desertion and Non-Support Laws.** 1904.

Breckinridge, Sophonisba P. **The Family and the State:** Select Documents. 1934.

Calverton, V. F. **The Bankruptcy of Marriage.** 1928.

Carlier, Auguste. **Marriage in the United States.** 1867.

Child, [Lydia]. **The Mother's Book.** 1831.

Child Care in Rural America: Collected Pamphlets, 1917–1921. 1972.

Child Rearing Literature of Twentieth Century America, 1914–1963. 1972.

The Colonial American Family: Collected Essays, 1788–1803. 1972.

Commander, Lydia Kingsmill. **The American Idea.** 1907.

Davis, Katharine Bement. **Factors in the Sex Life of Twenty-Two Hundred Women.** 1929.

Dennis, Wayne. **The Hopi Child.** 1940.

Epstein, Abraham. **Facing Old Age.** 1922. New Introduction by Wilbur J. Cohen.

The Family and Social Service in the 1920s: Two Documents, 1921–1928. 1972.

Hagood, Margaret Jarman. **Mothers of the South.** 1939.

Hall, G. Stanley. **Senescence:** The Last Half of Life. 1922.

Hall, G. Stanley. **Youth:** Its Education, Regimen, and Hygiene. 1904.

Hathway, Marion. **The Migratory Worker and Family Life.** 1934.

Homan, Walter Joseph. **Children & Quakerism.** 1939.

Key, Ellen. **The Century of the Child.** 1909.

Kirchwey, Freda. **Our Changing Morality:** A Symposium. 1930.

Kopp, Marie E. **Birth Control in Practice.** 1934.

Lawton, George. **New Goals for Old Age.** 1943.

Lichtenberger, J. P. **Divorce:** A Social Interpretation. 1931.

Lindsey, Ben B. and Wainwright Evans. **The Companionate Marriage.** 1927. New Introduction by Charles Larsen.

Lou, Herbert H. **Juvenile Courts in the United States.** 1927.

Monroe, Day. **Chicago Families.** 1932.

Mowrer, Ernest R. **Family Disorganization.** 1927.

Reed, Ruth. **The Illegitimate Family in New York City.** 1934.

Robinson, Caroline Hadley. **Seventy Birth Control Clinics.** 1930.

Watson, John B. **Psychological Care of Infant and Child.** 1928.

White House Conference on Child Health and Protection. **The Home and the Child.** 1931.

White House Conference on Child Health and Protection. **The Adolescent in the Family.** 1934.

Young, Donald, editor. **The Modern American Family.** 1932.